Advanced Applied Interventional Cardiology

Guest Editors

SAMIN K. SHARMA, MD, FSCAI, FACC

ANNAPOORNA S. KINI, MD, MRCP, FACC

CARDIOLOGY CLINICS

www.cardiology.theclinics.com

Consulting Editor
MICHAEL H. CRAWFORD, MD

February 2010 • Volume 28 • Number 1

SAUNDERS an imprint of ELSEVIER, Inc.

W.B. SAUNDERS COMPANY
A Division of Elsevier Inc.

1600 John F. Kennedy Blvd. • Suite 1800 • Philadelphia, PA 19103-2899

http://www.theclinics.com

CARDIOLOGY CLINICS Volume 28, Number 1
February 2010 ISSN 0733-8651, ISBN-13: 978-1-4377-1800-3

Editor: Barbara Cohen-Kligerman

Cardiology Clinics (ISSN 0733-8651) is published quarterly by Elsevier Inc., 360 Park Avenue South, New York, NY 10010-1710. Months of issue are February, May, August, and November. Business and Editorial Offices: 1600 John F. Kennedy Blvd., Ste. 1800, Philadelphia, PA 19103-2899. Customer Service Office: 3251 Riverport Lane, Maryland Heights, MO 63043. Periodicals postage paid at New York, NY and additional mailing offices. Subscription prices are $264.00 per year for US individuals, $416.00 per year for US institutions, $132.00 per year for US students and residents, $322.00 per year for Canadian individuals, $517.00 per year for Canadian institutions, $374.00 per year for international individuals, $517.00 per year for international institutions and $187.00 per year for Canadian and international students/residents. To receive student/resident rate, orders must be accompanied by name of affiliated institution, data of term, and the *signature* of program/residency coordinator on institution letterhead. Orders will be billed at individual rate until proof of status is received. Foreign air speed delivery is included in all *Clinics* subscription prices. All prices are subject to change without notice. **POSTMASTER:** Send address changes to *Cardiology Clinics*, Elsevier Health Sciences Division, Subscription Customer Service, 3251 Riverport Lane, Maryland Heights, MO 63043. **Customer Service: 1-800-654-2452 (U.S. and Canada); 314-447-8871 (outside U.S. and Canada). Fax: 314-447-8029. E-mail: journalscustomerservice-usa@elsevier.com (for print support); journalsonlinesupport-usa@elsevier.com (for online support).**

Reprints. For copies of 100 or more, of articles in this publication, please contact the Commercial Reprints Department, Elsevier Inc., 360 Park Avenue South, New York, NY 10010-1710. Tel.: 212-633-3812; Fax: 212-462-1935; E-mail: reprints@elsevier.com.

Cardiology Clinics is also published in Spanish by McGraw-Hill Interamericana Editores S. A., P.O. Box 5-237, 06500, Mexico D. F., Mexico; in Portuguese by Reichmann and Alfonso Editores Rio de Janeiro, Brazil; and in Greek by Dimitrios P. Lagos, 8 Pondon Street, GR115-28 Ilissia, Greece.

Cardiology Clinics is covered in *MEDLINE/PubMed (Index Medicus), Excerpta Medica, The Cumulative Index to Nursing and Allied Health Literature* (CINAHL).

Printed and bound in the United Kingdom
Transferred to Digital Print 2011

Contributors

CONSULTING EDITOR

MICHAEL H. CRAWFORD, MD
Professor of Medicine, University of California, San Francisco; Lucie Stern Chair in Cardiology, and Chief of Clinical Cardiology, University of California, San Francisco Medical Center, San Francisco, California

GUEST EDITORS

SAMIN K. SHARMA, MD, FSCAI, FACC
Director, Cardiac Catheterization Laboratory, and Intervention Mount Sinai Hospital, New York, New York

ANNAPOORNA S. KINI, MD, MRCP, FACC
Associate Director, Cardiac Catheterization Laboratory, Mount Sinai Hospital, New York, New York

AUTHORS

CARLOS E. ALFONSO, MD
Instructor of Medicine, Cardiovascular Division, Miller School of Medicine, University of Miami, Miami, Florida

SALOMON COHEN, MD
School of Medicine, Universidad Anáhuac, Huixquilucan, Edo, Mexico

SARA D. COLLINS, MD
Division of Cardiology, Department of Internal Medicine, Washington Hospital Center, Washington, District of Columbia

ROBERTO J. CUBEDDU, MD
Interventional Cardiology and Structural Heart Disease, Massachusetts General Hospital, Harvard Medical School, Boston, Massachusetts

FRANCESCA DEL FURIA, MD
Cardiology Department, Cittadella General Hospital, Padua, Italy

RAQUEL DEL VALLE-FERNÁNDEZ, MD
Fellow in Structural and Congenital Heart Disease, Lenox Hill Heart and Vascular Institute, New York, New York

NABIL DIB, MD, MSc
Director, Cardiovascular Research, Catholic Health Care West (CHW) Mercy Gilbert and Chandler Medical Centers, Phoenix, Arizona; Director, Clinical Cardiovascular Cell Therapy; Associate Professor of Medicine, San Diego Medical Center, University of California, San Diego

CARLO DI MARIO, MD, PhD, FRCP
Professor of Interventional Cardiology, Cardiology Department, Royal Brompton Hospital, London, United Kingdom

JONATHAN H. DINSMORE, PhD
Children's Hospital Boston, Boston, Massachusetts

ESTHER FALCÃO, MD
School of Medicine, Federal University of Ceara, Fortaleza, Ceara, Brazil

ANA I. FLORES, MD
School of Medicine, Universidad Autonoma de Guadalajara, La Paz, B.C.S, Mexico

Videos for several of the articles in this issue can be accessed online at http://www.cardiology.theclinics.com/.

JOHN M. GALLA, MD
Division of Interventional Cardiology, Heart and Vascular Institute, Cleveland Clinic, Cleveland, Ohio

ANNAPOORNA S. KINI, MD, MRCP, FACC
Cardiac Catheterization Laboratory of the Cardiovascular Institute, Mount Sinai Hospital, New York, New York

YOUNG-HAK KIM, MD, PhD
Cardiac Center, Asan Medical Center, University of Ulsan College of Medicine, Seoul, Korea

GILLES LEMESLE, MD
Division of Cardiology, Department of Internal Medicine, Washington Hospital Center, Washington, District of Columbia

GABRIEL MALUENDA, MD
Division of Cardiology, Department of Internal Medicine, Washington Hospital Center, Washington, District of Columbia

CLAUDIA A. MARTINEZ, MD
Fellow in Structural and Congenital Heart Disease, Lenox Hill Heart and Vascular Institute, New York, New York

SAMEER MEHTA, MD, MBA
Voluntary Associate Professor of Medicine, University of Miami – Miller School of Medicine, Mercy Medical Center, Miami, Florida

NARBEH MELIKIAN, BSc(Hons), MD, MRCP
Clinical Lecturer in Cardiology and Interventional Cardiologist, Cardiology Department, King's College London British Heart Foundation Centre of Excellence and King's College Hospital, London, United Kingdom

PEDRO R. MORENO, MD, FACC
Director, Interventional Cardiology Research, Associate Professor of Medicine, Zena and Michael A. Wiener Cardiovascular Institute and The Marie-Josee and Henry R. Kravis Cardiovascular Health Center, The Mount Sinai School of Medicine, New York, New York

ESTEFANIA OLIVEROS, MD
School of Medicine, Central University of Venezuela, Caracas, Venezuela

IGOR F. PALACIOS, MD
Director of Interventional Cardiology, Interventional Cardiology and Structural Heart Disease, Massachusetts General Hospital, Harvard Medical School, Boston, Massachusetts

SEUNG-JUNG PARK, MD, PhD
Cardiac Center, Asan Medical Center, University of Ulsan College of Medicine, Seoul, Korea

CARLOS E. RUIZ, MD, PhD
Director, Structural and Congenital Heart Disease, Lenox Hill Heart and Vascular Institute, Black Hall, New York, New York

KUNAL SARKAR, MBBS
Cardiac Catheterization Laboratory of the Cardiovascular Institute, Mount Sinai Hospital, New York, New York

FAISAL SHAMSHAD, MD
Columbia University Division of Cardiology at Mount Sinai Medical Center, East Brunswick, New Jersey

SAMIN K. SHARMA, MD, FACC
Cardiac Catheterization Laboratory of the Cardiovascular Institute, Mount Sinai Hospital, New York, New York

JOSEPH SWEENY, MD
Cardiac Catheterization Laboratory of the Cardiovascular Institute, Mount Sinai Hospital, New York, New York

RON WAKSMAN, MD
Division of Cardiology, Department of Internal Medicine, Washington Hospital Center, Washington, District of Columbia

PATRICK L. WHITLOW, MD
Director of Interventional Cardiology, Heart and Vascular Institute, Cleveland Clinic, Cleveland, Ohio

Contents

Vulnerable Plaque: Definition, Diagnosis, and Treatment   1

Pedro R. Moreno

> This article provides a systematic approach to vulnerable plaques. It is divided into 4 sections. The first section is devoted to definition, incidence, anatomic distribution, and clinical presentation. The second section is devoted to plaque composition, setting up the foundations to understand plaque vulnerability. The third section relates to invasive plaque imaging. The fourth section is devoted to therapy, from conservative pharmacologic options to aggressive percutaneous coronary intervention alternatives.

Physiologic Lesion Assessment During Percutaneous Coronary Intervention   31

Narbeh Melikian, Francesca Del Furia, and Carlo Di Mario

> The 2-dimensional silhouette image provided by coronary angiography has well-recognized limitations. Angiographic images do not accurately represent the true complexity of the luminal morphology in coronary disease and give no indication of the functional influence of luminal changes on coronary blood flow. These limitations are more pronounced in angiographically intermediate stenoses and in patients in whom there is a clear discrepancy between the clinical picture and angiographic findings. In such cases there is often poor concordance between the estimated percentage angiographic stenosis and the corresponding intravascular ultrasound image or noninvasive functional data. The validation and clinical availability of robust and accurate physiologic indices, which can be used as an adjunct to diagnostic angiography in the cardiac catheterization laboratory, have been pivotal in promoting ischemia-driven coronary revascularization. Deferral or revascularization based on such physiologic indices is associated with improved clinical outcome as well as more favorable health economic data. Although there are several clinical indices, fractional flow reserve remains the "gold standard," with indications for physiologic assessment of angiographic intermediate stenoses, including left main stem stenoses and ostial disease as well as serial lesions. The availability of such indices is an important step in streamlining management of patients undergoing cardiac catheterization by allowing routine provision of an "all-in-one" ischemia-driven revascularization service.

Coronary Bifurcation Lesions: A Current Update   55

Samin K. Sharma, Joseph Sweeny, and Annapoorna S. Kini

> Coronary bifurcations are prone to develop atherosclerotic plaque because of turbulent blood flow and high shear stress. When compared with nonbifurcation coronary interventions, bifurcation interventions have historically reported a lower rate of procedural success, higher procedural costs, longer hospitalization, and higher clinical and angiographic restenosis. Treating bifurcation lesions is challenging, but a simple algorithm based on the side branch size, stenosis, and angulation can be used. The ongoing development of novel drug-eluting stent devices designed specifically for

coronary bifurcations and the large randomized clinical trials being conducted to address their utility will add to the already present literature regarding treatment of coronary bifurcation lesions.

John M. Galla and Patrick L. Whitlow

Chronic total coronary occlusions (CTOs) are a frequent finding in patients with coronary disease and remain one of the most challenging target lesion subsets for intervention. CTOs have been reported in approximately one-third of patients undergoing diagnostic coronary angiography. By nature of their complexity, CTO percutaneous interventions (PCIs) are associated with lower rates of procedural success, higher complication rates, greater radiation exposure, and longer procedure times compared with interventions in non-CTO stenoses. Despite these obstacles, reported benefits of successful CTO PCI include a reduction in symptoms and improvement in both ventricular function and survival. This article examines the technical challenges, procedural complications, and possible outcomes associated with CTO PCI.

Seung-Jung Park and Young-Hak Kim

Because of the long-term benefit of coronary artery bypass graft (CABG) surgery in medical therapy, CABG has been the standard treatment of unprotected left main coronary artery (LMCA) stenosis. However, with the advancement of techniques and equipment, the percutaneous interventional approach for implantation of coronary stents has been shown to be feasible for patients with unprotected LMCA stenosis. The recent introduction of drug-eluting stents (DESs), together with advances in periprocedural and postprocedural adjunctive pharmacotherapies, has improved outcomes of percutaneous coronary interventions (PCIs) for these complex coronary lesions. This review evaluates the current outcomes of PCI with DES in research conducted in several countries.

Gilles Lemesle, Gabriel Maluenda, Sara D. Collins, and Ron Waksman

In in-stent restenosis, drug-eluting stents are superior compared with bare metal stents. However, there are concerns about safety because of the reports of increased risk of late and very late stent thrombosis. Stent thrombosis remains a major pitfall in contemporary percutaneous coronary intervention, leading to high rates of death and nonfatal myocardial infarction. A new standardized definition of stent thrombosis was established to provide consistency in the reporting of this complication and to enable accurate and reliable data to be described for both types of stents, bare metal and drug-eluting. This new consensual definition reflects a large amount of new data reported in the literature. New generations of drug-eluting stents with novel polymers, antiproliferative drugs, and improved platforms are now approved and available for use. In this article, the authors provide a critical appraisal of the safety of different drug-eluting stents based on the published clinical data focusing on late and very late stent thrombosis.

Sameer Mehta, Carlos E. Alfonso, Estefania Oliveros, Faisal Shamshad, Ana I. Flores, Salomon Cohen, and Esther Falcão

ST-elevation myocardial infarction (STEMI) interventions have significantly reduced mortality and morbidity from acute myocardial infarction. Compulsive management of thrombus is a fundamental requirement of these interventions. A pragmatic thrombus-guided management strategy is reviewed along with additional novel therapeutic adjuncts for STEMI interventions.

The last decade has been accompanied by great optimism and interest in the concept of cell or tissue regeneration in the postinfarction myocardium. However, despite the promise, progress was slow. Data derived from multiple controlled studies in hundreds of patients postmyocardial infarction have shown hints of potential benefit but not of the magnitude anticipated. The complexity and hurdles to repair the damaged myocardium have been more daunting than originally estimated. In the end analysis, progress will be made incrementally. The promise for cell therapy continues to be significant, but so are the challenges ahead. This article takes a fresh look at the progress in myocardial regeneration. The authors look at the postmyocardial environment for cues that may guide repair and they look closely at the clinical data for evidence of cardiac regeneration. This evidence is used for suggestions on how to best proceed with future work.

Over the past 25 years we have witnessed the development of transcatheter techniques for treatment of valvular heart disease. For several years, percutaneous balloon valvuloplasty has been used to treat stenotic valvular disease, including pulmonary stenosis, rheumatic mitral stenosis, tricuspid stenosis, and, sometimes, congenital aortic stenosis. However, major advancements in transcatheter valve repair and replacement have revolutionized progress. Preliminary results of ongoing studies show promise in the percutaneous treatment of mitral regurgitation. This article covers established percutaneous techniques for treatment of mitral stenosis and reviews major recent advancements in the percutaneous treatment of mitral regurgitation.

In the 7 years since the first implant, more than 7000 transcatheter aortic valve implantations (TAVI) have been performed worldwide. This article describes the latest available information on this field and the upcoming technological expectations.

Several new-generation percutaneous support devices are available or are in different stages of development for use in high-risk percutaneous coronary intervention (PCI), cardiogenic shock, and for other indications. Preliminary studies have demonstrated the feasibility and safety of these devices and the beneficial effect on hemodynamic parameters. In this article, the authors discuss (1) the percutaneous circulatory support devices presently available and routinely used in the catheterization laboratory, (2) the technical aspects involved with insertion and removal, and (3) relevant data from randomized trials, meta-analyses, and registries about the benefits of their use in patients with cardiogenic shock complicating ST segment elevation myocardial infarction and in those with significant left ventricular systolic dysfunction undergoing complex PCI.

Cardiology Clinics

VISIT OUR WEB SITE!
The Clinics are available online!
Access your subscription at:
www.theclinics.com

Foreword

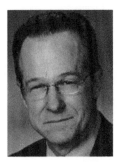

Michael H. Crawford, MD
Consulting Editor

In 2006 Dr Samin Sharma was Guest Editor of the May issue of *Cardiology Clinics* on Interventional Cardiology. That issue broadly defined the status of a variety of procedures in this field, including intravascular ultrasound, distal protection devices, drug-eluting stents, circulatory support devices, and vascular closure devices. This field continues to rapidly advance; therefore, I was delighted that Dr Sharma agreed to guest edit another issue on advanced applications in interventional cardiology. Some of the previous topics, such as drug-eluting stents, are updated, but the emphasis now is on late stent thrombosis. Also, advances in left ventricular support devices, coronary bifurcation lesions, and chronic total occlusions are updated. Most of the issue, however, is devoted to new topics such as left main stenosis, transcatheter valve replacement, stem cell therapy, percutaneous mitral valve procedures, and adjunctive therapy for ST elevation myocardial infarction. The topic authors are interventional experts who have done an outstanding job of synthesizing current scientific data and its application to practical problems.

Since the last issue, efforts by United States federal health care agencies to curtail unnecessary procedures by fostering comparative effectiveness research have intensified. Also, the American College of Cardiology/American Heart Association guidelines committees have embarked on a new paradigm called "effectiveness criteria," and one of the first of these efforts was on coronary artery revascularization. In this milieu cardiologists are going to need all the evidence they can muster to defend their therapeutic decisions, especially regarding relatively expensive procedures in the cardiac interventional laboratory. This issue of *Cardiology Clinics* will help keep those who perform and recommend invasive approaches to cardiovascular disease management at the forefront of the science and the expert opinions in these treatment areas.

Michael H. Crawford, MD
Division of Cardiology
Department of Medicine
University of California
San Francisco Medical Center
505 Parnassus Avenue
Box 0124, San Francisco
CA 94143-0124, USA

E-mail address:
crawfordm@medicine.ucsf.edu (M.H. Crawford)

doi:10.1016/j.ccl.2009.11.001

Preface

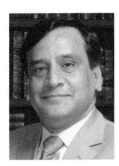
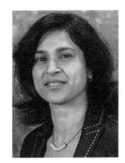

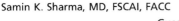

Samin K. Sharma, MD, FSCAI, FACC   Annapoorna S. Kini, MD, MRCP, FACC
Guest Editors

This issue of *Cardiology Clinics* is devoted to the topic of advanced interventional cardiology technique. Percutaneous coronary intervention in 2009 has emerged swiftly from the dark days of adverse publicity in 2006–2007 which were created partly by neutral results of a few randomized trials (Open Artery Trial [OAT] and Clinical Outcomes Utilizing Revascularization and Aggressive Drug Evaluation [COURAGE] trials) and concerns of very late drug-eluting stent thrombosis from various registries and randomized trials (Basel Stent Cost-effectiveness Trial-Late Thrombotic Events [BASKET LATE] trial and Swedish Coronary Angiography and Angioplasty registry [SCAAR] and Global Registry of Acute Coronary Events [GRACE] registries). In the past 2 years, publications of well-designed randomized trials have reinforced the efficacy of percutaneous interventional techniques even compared with cardiac surgery.

This issue comprises 11 selected topics in interventional cardiology, written by top experts in their field, to provide the most updated view of the rapidly changing field of interventional cardiology. Special focus and attention are placed on technical details of performing the interventional procedures. This issue starts with an update on the recognition and treatment of vulnerable plaque followed by the role of physiologic assessment in catheter laboratories, especially fractional flow reserve, highlighted by a few recent randomized trials (Deferral Versus Performance of Percutaneous Transluminal Coronary Angioplasty in

Patients Without Documented Ischemia [DEFER] and Fractional Flow Reserve Versus Angiography for Multivessel Evaluation [FAME] trials). Treatment of various complex lesions requires technical skills and intricate procedural steps. All of them are highlighted for bifurcation, chronic total occlusion, and left main lesions. Evolving strategies for treating acute myocardial infarction with interventional devices, adjunctive pharmacotherapy, and stem cell therapy are presented in depth. Another exciting area of interventional cardiology—percutaneous valve replacement—and an update on percutaneous aortic and mitral valve techniques are presented. Also included is an article focusing on late drug-eluting stent thrombosis. Lastly, use of a left ventricular assist device to provided extra confidence to interventionalists in performing complex percutaneous coronary intervention with severe left ventricular dysfunction is elaborated. Several of the articles have video components, which may be viewed in the online version of this issue available at http://www.cardiology.theclinics.com/.

We are thankful to all the authors whose contributions have made this *Cardiology Clinics* issue a valuable resource for interventional cardiologists and a future reference manual for technical details. We are also grateful to the staff of Mount Sinai Hospital, whose hard work and dedication have made our cardiac catheterization laboratory the number one catheterization laboratory in the country in terms of volume and safety, truly making Andreas Gruentzig's dream of performing catheter-based

Cardiol Clin 28 (2010) xi–xii
doi:10.1016/j.ccl.2009.11.002

percutaneous interventions with safety for all vascular disease states in alert, awake patients a reality.

Samin K. Sharma, MD, FSCAI, FACC
Director, Cardiac Catheterization Laboratory
and Intervention, Mount Sinai Hospital
Box 1030, One Gustave L. Levy Place
New York, NY 10029-6754, USA

Annapoorna S. Kini, MD, MRCP, FACC
Associate Director,
Cardiac Catheterization Laboratory
Mount Sinai Hospital
5 East 98th Street, 3rd Floor
New York, NY 10029, USA

E-mail addresses:
samin.sharma@mountsinai.org (S.K. Sharma)
annapoorna.kini@mountsinai.org (A.S. Kini)

Vulnerable Plaque: Definition, Diagnosis, and Treatment

Pedro R. Moreno, MD, FACC

KEYWORDS

- Vulnerable • Plaque • Atherosclerosis
- Thrombosis • Rupture • Neovascularization

Cardiovascular disease is by far the main cause of death in the world. In the United States, every 30 seconds 1 person experiences a heart attack, and the incidence is increasing. Nevertheless, coronary atherosclerosis is a condition that can be asymptomatic for decades. The transition from asymptomatic, nonobstructive disease to symptomatic, occlusive disease is related to atherothrombosis.[1] These asymptomatic, nonobstructive plaques prone to develop acute thrombosis are also called vulnerable plaques.[2] Specific morphologic and histologic features characterize these lesions. Most importantly, these features can be identified by novel imaging techniques. Therefore, detecting vulnerable plaques may prevent the clinical manifestations of atherothrombosis, and reduce heart attacks.[3]

First highlighted by pioneers in the field more than 25 years ago,[4–6] the vulnerable plaque has evolved as an elusive target. The difficulties involved in diagnosis, natural history, and therapy are great, and it is easy to understand why the vulnerable plaque hypothesis remains controversial.[7] Some of the pioneers in the field are now considering the "vulnerable patient" as a term to ease the frustration caused by decades of failure in diagnosis and therapy.[8] Nevertheless, the evidence brings us back to reality, and the concept of the "vulnerable patient" is now being brought into focus again at the plaque level.[9]

This article provides a systematic approach to vulnerable plaques. It is divided into 4 sections. The first section is devoted to definition, incidence, anatomic distribution, and clinical presentation. The second section is devoted to plaque composition, setting up the foundations to understand plaque vulnerability. The third section relates to invasive plaque imaging. The fourth section is devoted to therapy, from conservative, pharmacologic options to aggressive percutaneous coronary intervention (PCI) alternatives.

CLINICAL CHARACTERISTICS
Definition and Clinical Evidence

The vulnerable plaque is defined as a nonobstructive, silent coronary lesion that suddenly becomes obstructive and symptomatic, as shown in **Fig. 1**. The clinical evidence of this disease was developed by Ambrose and Fuster in 1988, when they identified that most lesions that evolved into acute myocardial infarction were nonobstructive, with mean diameter stenosis of 48%.[6]

Incidence

Following the Ambrose and Fuster criteria, the number of nonobstructive lesions that rapidly progress to symptomatic, occlusive disease in patients treated with PCI was redefined in 3 recent studies. The first study included 1228 patients. The incidence of vulnerable plaques requiring additional PCI was 12.4% in the first year, and 5% to 7% per year from years 2 to 5 after the initial procedure.[10] The second study included 3747 patients. The incidence of vulnerable plaques requiring additional PCI ranged from 4.4% to

Dr Moreno is a founder and stock option holder at InfraReDx, INC. He is also an advisor for Prescent Technologies and Abbott Vascular.
Zena and Michael A. Wiener Cardiovascular Institute and The Marie-Josee and Henry R. Kravis Cardiovascular Health Center, The Mount Sinai School of Medicine, Box 1030, New York, NY 10029, USA
E-mail address: pedro.moreno@msnyuhealth.org

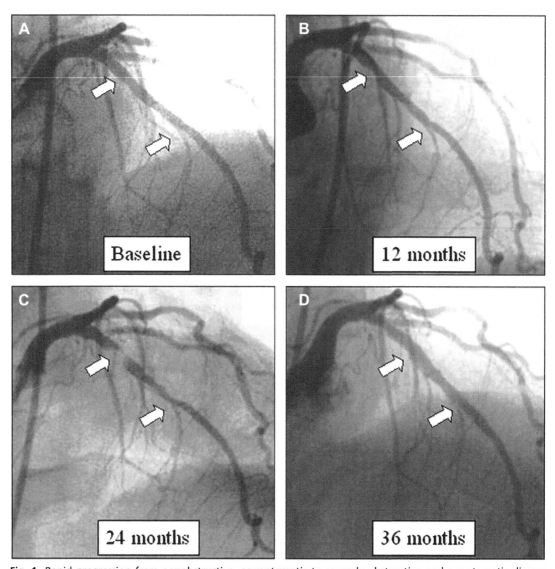

Fig. 1. Rapid progression from nonobstructive, asymptomatic to severely obstructive and symptomatic disease fulfilling the clinical definition of vulnerable plaques. Sequential coronary angiograms of the left anterior descending coronary artery performed with 12 months intervals. (*A*) Baseline angiogram showing 10% to 20% stenosis in the left anterior descending (LAD) coronary artery in the proximal and mid segments, highlighted by the arrows. (*B*) Progression to 30% to 40% stenosis in both segments, 12 months after the baseline angiogram. (*C*) Further progression to severe, 95% stenosis in the proximal segment and 50% stenosis in the mid segment, 24 months after the baseline angiogram. At that time, the patient was treated with a single drug-eluting stent covering both lesions (angiogram not shown). (*D*) 10% to 20% stenosis in the same segments 12 months after local therapy with stent, and 36 months after baseline angiogram. (*Courtesy of* the Cardiac Catheterization Laboratory at Mount Sinai Medical Center, New York, USA.)

12.8% according to the number of vessels involved.[11] The third study included 1059 patients who underwent computed tomography angiography (CTA). The incidence of vulnerable plaques ranged from 11% to 22%,[12] and was directly related to positive remodeling, and low attenuation ("soft") morphology on CT. On the other hand, the absence of these 2 features provided a strong negative predictive value, with an acute coronary syndrome (ACS) incidence of 0.5%. As Dr E Braunwald wrote, "The development of an acute coronary event can be excluded in >80% of patients with known or suspected coronary artery disease."[3]

Clinical Presentation

Vulnerable plaques presented as ACS in 68.5% of the cases, the majority presenting with unstable angina pectoris and 9.3% presenting with ST segment elevation myocardial infarction (STEMI).[11] Of note, these studies excluded death and therefore fatal events are probably underestimated.

Anatomic Distribution

Ambrose and Fuster identified the proximal anatomic location as the only independent predictor for progression to acute myocardial infarction (MI).[6] This observation was confirmed by Wang and colleagues,[13] who identified the proximal segment to be responsible for 80% of MI in all 3 major vessels. As a result, proper evaluation and treatment of high-risk plaques in the proximal segments of the coronary tree could prevent 80% of acute MIs.

> The incidence of vulnerable plaques evolving into clinical events ranges from 4% to 13% per year in patients with single vessel disease. On CTA, positive remodelling and soft plaque gives a 22% risk for ACS in 2 years. Most lesions are usually located in the proximal segment of the coronary arteries, and 69% present with ACS.

After reviewing the clinical characteristics, the next section provides the basis for understanding the pathophysiology of the disease and provides a foundation for critical evaluation of novel imaging techniques that claim effectiveness in the diagnosis of high-risk, vulnerable plaques.

PLAQUE COMPOSITION

Plaque rupture is the most common cause of atherothrombosis, responsible for 70% to 75% of all events, as shown in **Fig. 2**.[14] The second cause of atherothrombosis is plaque erosion, a significant substrate for coronary thrombosis and sudden cardiac death in premenopausal female patients.[15] Opposite to plaque rupture, erosion occurs in plaques with no specific features suitable for detection. They are characterized by a thick, smooth muscle cell rich fibrous cap, reduced necrotic core areas, and low degree of inflammation,[15] as shown in **Fig. 3**. Plaque erosion is associated with cigarette smoking, suggesting that thrombosis in these patients may be related to a systemic, prothrombogenic pathway rather than a local, atherothrombotic mechanism.

The preceding lesion for plaque rupture is also known as the thin-cap fibroatheroma (TCFA), the hallmark of vulnerable plaques,[16] as shown in **Fig. 4**. The classical histologic patterns of TCFA include but are not limited to: (1) thin fibrous cap;

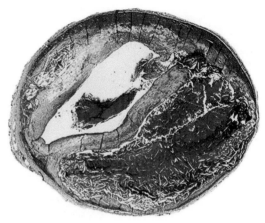

Fig. 2. Cross-sectioned coronary artery containing a ruptured plaque at the shoulder of the fibrous cap with a nonocclusive thrombus superimposed. The large necrotic core can be identified by cholesterol crystals and extensive IPH secondary to plaque rupture. Trichrome stain, rendering thrombus red, collagen blue, and lipid colorless. (*Courtesy of* Dr K-Raman Purushothaman, Mount Sinai Hospital, New York, USA.)

(2) large necrotic core with increased free/esterified cholesterol ratio; (3) increased plaque inflammation; (4) positive vascular remodeling; (5) increased vasa-vasorum neovascularization; and (6) intraplaque hemorrhage.

Thin Fibrous Cap

Autopsy studies have shown that ruptured plaques are characterized by a thin fibrous cap, measuring 23 ± 19 μm in thickness. Of ruptured caps, 95%

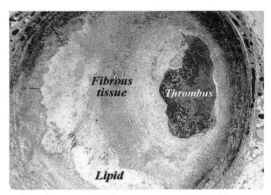

Fig. 3. Plaque erosion. Cross section of a coronary artery containing a stenotic atherosclerotic plaque with an occlusive thrombosis superimposed. The endothelium is missing at the plaque-thrombus interface, but the plaque surface is otherwise intact. Trichrome stain, rendering thrombus red, collagen blue, and lipid colorless. (*Courtesy of* Dr Erling Falk, Aarhus, Denmark.)

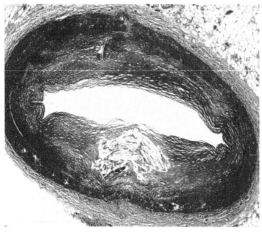

Fig. 4. TCFA, characterized by a thin fibrous cap and a large necrotic core. Trichrome stain. (*Courtesy of Dr K-Raman Purushothaman, Mount Sinai Hospital, New York, NY, USA.*)

than 50% of TCFAs showed a lack of calcification, or only speckled calcification on postmortem analysis.[25] In contrast, 65% of acute ruptures demonstrated speckled calcification, with the remainder showing fragmented or diffuse calcification.[25] The authors' group evaluated the incidence of calcification in human aortic TCFA (n = 42) and compared with non-TCFA (n = 128) plaques using von Kossa staining.[26] The incidence of calcification was lower in TCFA (62% vs 82%; $P = .006$), suggesting that calcification is an equivocal variable in TCFA, and may not be used as a surrogate for vulnerable plaques.[27,28]

> Invasive technology may also quantify necrotic core areas, which should be 24% or more of total plaque area. It should also provide free cholesterol and tissue factor content, independent from the degree of calcification.

measured 64 μm or less in the coronary[17] and 60 μm or less in the aorta.[18] As a result, the first and probably most important histologic feature of TCFA is a fibrous cap 65 μm or less in thickness. These thin caps are unable to withstand the circumferential stress. As caps become thinner, the stress increases in an exponential pattern.[19,20]

> Invasive technology aiming to detect TCFA should have a radial resolution less than 65 μm, and the ability to quantify the stress/strain relationship in the fibrous cap.

Large Necrotic Core with Increased Free/Esterified Cholesterol Ratio

Oxidized low-density lipoprotein (LDL) is taken up by macrophages, leading to cell death and extracellular lipid accumulation within the plaque, which forms the necrotic core.[21] Coronary plaques with necrotic cores larger than 50% of the total plaque area are at risk for rupture and thrombosis.[22] More recently, other studies in coronary arteries show lower necrotic areas, down to 24% and 34% in TCFAs and ruptured plaques, respectively.[16]

Necrotic cores with increased free/esterified cholesterol ratio favors plaque rupture.[23] Most importantly, tissue factor activity within the necrotic core is currently considered the major source of thrombin generation leading to arterial thrombosis in humans.[24] The degree of calcification in the necrotic core is variable in TCFA. In a series of sudden coronary death cases, more

Increased Plaque Inflammation

Macrophages and T cells play a major active role in the pathophysiology of TCFA. These cells are capable of degrading extracellular matrix by phagocytosis or secretion of proteolytic enzymes; thus, enzymes such as plasminogen activators and matrix metalloproteinases (MMPs), including collagenases, elastases, gelatinases, and stromelysins, weaken the already thin fibrous cap and predispose it to rupture.[29] Macrophages also express tissue factor.[24] This link was documented by Hutter and colleagues,[30] who showed correlations between macrophage density, apoptosis, and tissue factor expression in human and mouse atherosclerotic lesions. Of clinical relevance, multiple studies have shown that macrophage content is increased in plaques from patients with ACS when compared with plaques from patients with stable angina.[14] Therefore, plaque inflammation is a pivotal feature of plaque vulnerability.

> Invasive technology aiming to detect TCFA should have the resolution to identify and quantify macrophages in the fibrous cap and shoulders of the atherosclerotic plaque.

Degree of Vascular Remodeling

The eccentric growth of atheroma away from the lumen was described by Glagov and colleagues in 1987,[31] as shown in **Fig. 5**. Varnava and colleagues[32] studied the relationship between

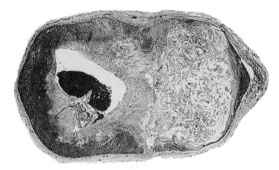

Fig. 5. Large human thrombotic left main coronary plaque with extensive remodeling containing a large necrotic core. (*Courtesy of* Dr K-Raman Purushotha-man, Mount Sinai Hospital, New York, NY, USA.)

Remodeling is triggered by an inflammatory process at the base of the plaque with digestion of the internal elastic lamina, involving the tunica media and the adventitia.[18,33,34] The clinical rele-vance of remodeling was pioneered by Schoen-hagen and colleagues[35] using intravascular ultrasound (IVUS), as shown in **Fig. 6**. Remodeling was higher at target lesions in patients with ACS than in patients with stable angina (51.8% vs 19.6%), whereas negative remodeling was more frequent in stable angina (56.5% vs 31.8%) ($P = $ .001), confirming the histopathological associa-tions between plaque remodeling and vulnerability.[35]

remodeling and plaque vulnerability. Of 108 coro-nary plaques analyzed, 64 (59%) had undergone no remodeling or positive remodeling, and 44 (41%) had undergone negative remodeling (vessel shrinkage). Lesions with positive remodel-ing had a larger lipid core and a higher macro-phage content, explaining the common link between compensatory remodeling and plaque rupture.

> Invasive technology aiming to detect TCFA should provide exact measurements to quantify the degree of vascular remodeling.

Of clinical relevance, Corti and colleagues[36] were first to document the same eccentric pattern for plaque regression after aggressive lipid therapy. More recently, multiple studies have confirmed this observation,[37] as shown in **Fig. 7**.

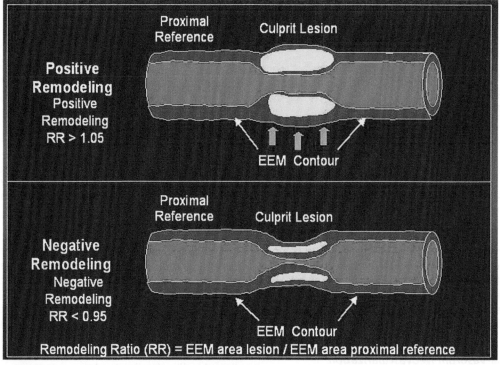

Fig. 6. Remodeling cartoon explaining the direction of positive and negative remodeling. See text for details. (*Adapted from* Schoenhagen P, Ziada KM, Kapadia SR, et al. Extent and direction of arterial remodeling in stable versus unstable coronary syndromes: an intravascular ultrasound study. Circulation 2000;101(6):598–603; with permission.)

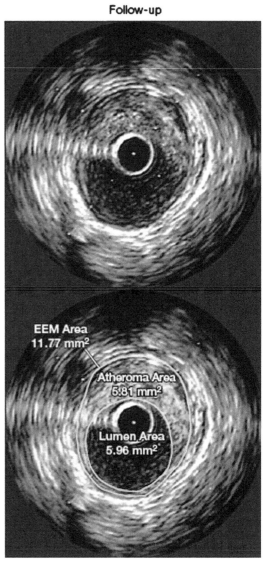

Fig. 7. The top panels show the baseline and follow-up IVUS images of a single coronary cross section after 24 months of rosuvastatin treatment. The 2 bottom panels illustrate measurements superimposed on the same cross sections, demonstrating the reduction in atheroma area. EEM, external elastic membrane. (*Reproduced from* Nissen SE, Nicholls SJ, Sipahi I, et al. Effect of very high-intensity statin therapy on regression of coronary atherosclerosis: the ASTEROID trial. JAMA 2006;295(13):1556–65; with permission.)

Considering that lipid is the main plaque component that can reverse with therapy, this eccentric pattern of plaque regression suggests an effective reverse lipid transport system through the deeper layers of the vessel wall, probably mediated by vasa-vasorum neovascularization.[14,38]

Vasa-Vasorum Neovascularization

Neovascularization is the process of generating new blood vessels to nurture the atherosclerotic plaque. Angiogenesis, the predominant form of neovascularization in atherosclerosis,[39] is mediated by progenitor or endothelial cells sprouting to form new capillaries. Atherosclerotic neovascularization evolves in early atherogenesis as a defense mechanism against hypoxia, generated by thickening of the tunica intima.[40] In advanced disease, neovessels may play a defensive role, allowing for lipid removal from the plaque through the adventitia, leading to plaque regression.[1] The adventitial vasa vasorum is the main source of neovascularization in atherosclerotic lesions, as shown in **Fig. 8**.

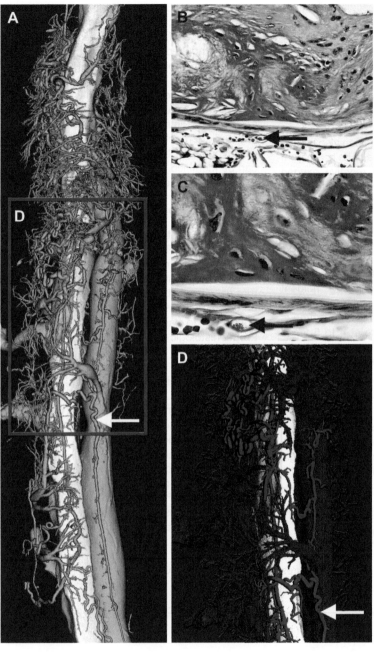

Fig. 8. (A) Volume-rendered high-resolution, 3-dimensional micro-CT image of the descending aorta vasa vasorum. (B) and (C) Corresponding histologic cross sections demonstrate atherosclerotic lesions in the inferior vena cava (black arrow). (D) Highlighted differentiated arterial (red) and venous (blue) vasa vasorum. (Masson trichrome stain, bar 500 μm). (Reproduced from Langheinrich AC, Michniewicz A, Sedding DG, et al. Correlation of vasa vasorum neovascularization and plaque progression in aortas of apolipoprotein E(-/-)/low-density lipoprotein(-/-) double knockout mice. Arterioscler Thromb Vasc Biol 2006;26(2):347–52; with permission.)

Neovessels may also serve as a pathway for leukocyte recruitment to high-risk areas of the plaque, including the cap and shoulders.[41–43] More recently, the authors' group documented histologic evidence for atherosclerotic neovascularization as a pathway for macrophage infiltration in advanced, lipid-rich plaques.[44] Moreover, ruptured plaques exhibited the highest degree of neovascularization,[45] mostly in diabetic patients with complex morphology including sprouting, red blood cell (RBC) extravasation, and perivascular inflammation.[46]

> Invasive technology detecting TCFA should quantify vasa-vasorum neovascularization in the adventitia, tunica media and within the atherosclerotic plaque.

In summary, plaque neovascularization, following what seems to be a defensive mission to provide oxygen and remove lipid from the atherosclerotic lesion, may eventually fail, leading to extravasation of RBCs, perivascular inflammation, and intraplaque hemorrhage.

Intraplaque Hemorrhage

Extravasation of RBCs into the plaque leads to intraplaque hemorrhage (IPH). The erythrocyte membrane is rich in cholesterol, promoting lipid core accumulation and increasing plaque vulnerability for rupture.[47,48] After RBC membrane lysis, extracorpuscular hemoglobin (Hb) can also induce oxidative tissue damage by virtue of its heme iron, with subsequent production of reactive oxygen species. The primary defense mechanism against free Hb is haptoglobin (Hp), which rapidly and irreversibly binds to free Hb, forming an Hp-Hb complex. In the plaque, the only route for clearance of the Hp-Hb complex is via the macrophage.[49] Clearance of the Hp-Hb complex may be genotype-dependent.[49–53] Multiple independent epidemiologic studies examining incident cardiovascular disease have demonstrated that diabetic patients with the Hp 2-2 (homozygous for the Hp 2 allele) genotype are at 4 to 5 times the risk of cardiovascular events compared with individuals with the Hp 1-1 (homozygous for the Hp 1 allele) genotype.[50,54–56]

Invasive technology detecting TCFA should identify IPH, iron deposition, RBC membranes, and hemosidering deposits in macrophages. In diabetic patients, haptoglobin genotyping may offer additional prognostic value.

Summary of Plaque Composition

Atherosclerotic plaques at high risk for rupture and thrombosis are composed of several features including large lipid core, thin fibrous cap, macrophage infiltration, positive remodeling, vasa-vasorum neovascularization, and increased IPH. These concepts apply only for lesions at risk for plaque rupture and thrombosis (TCFA). Plaques at risk for erosion and thrombosis do not exhibit any specific morphologic feature, limiting their detection by any imaging technique. This finding is a significant limitation of the individual, lesion-oriented approach to the high-risk, vulnerable plaque hypothesis. Nevertheless, even if only TCFAs can be identified and treated, a significant reduction of clinical events will be achieved.

INVASIVE PLAQUE IMAGING

Considering that most atherosclerotic plaques (TCFA and non-TCFA) have a certain degree of fibrous cap thickness, necrotic core area, macrophage area, positive remodeling, and vasa-vasorum neovascularization, the presence or absence of these features (sensitivity and specificity) is not enough to classify them as vulnerable plaques. Proper histologic validation should be confirmed in animal models of TCFA before being introduced in human coronary arteries,[57] with the ultimate test being a natural history study.

Seven novel intracoronary techniques to detect TCFA are clinically relevant, including IVUS, virtual histology (VH), palpography, optical coherence tomography (OCT), intravascular magnetic resonance imaging (MRI), angioscopy, and spectroscopy. A summary of these techniques, the component detected, and the resolution/accuracy [58] is presented in **Table 1**. All these techniques are already available in the catheterization laboratory. This section of this article presents these techniques following the principles of plaque composition, using a summarized evidence-based approach.

Table 1
Summary of invasive imaging technologies

Technology	Component Detected	Resolution/Accuracy (μm)
IVUS	Remodeling, calcium	100–250
IVUS-VH	Necrotic core, calcium, collagen	480
OCT	Necrotic core, fibrous cap thickness, macrophages	5–20
IVUS-elastography	Plaque strain	100–250
Intravascular MRI	Necrotic core	250
Angioscopy	Surface appearance of the plaque	N/A
Spectroscopy	Necrotic core	N/A
Thermography	Metabolic activity of the plaque	0.05°C accurate

Abbreviation: N/A, not applicable.

The interventionalist must develop a critical approach to evaluate these novel techniques, understanding their potential but most importantly discerning their multiple limitations before considering them for clinical use.

IVUS

IVUS allows for proper cross-sectional and linear imaging of atherosclerotic plaques in vivo. IVUS allows for identification of hemodynamically significant lesions that may be underestimated by angiography, and the proper apposition of stent struts after deployment; these are the most common indications for IVUS in clinical practice. In addition, IVUS provides the degree of calcification, plaque density, and most importantly, the degree of arterial remodeling. As a result, IVUS is a fundamental tool for the interventionalist interested in vulnerable plaque.

Several studies have reported the IVUS characteristics of culprit lesions,[59] and the presence of multiple ruptured plaques in patients with acute coronary events.[60]

The next section reviews the ability of IVUS to identify TCFA, which can be summarized as follows.

Fibrous cap thickness

Considering that the resolution of IVUS (between 100 and 250 μm) is greater that that needed to detect TCFA, thin fibrous caps are always underestimated. Ge and colleagues[61] carefully quantified IVUS-derived fibrous cap thickness in ruptured and nonruptured plaques from 144 consecutive patients with angina pectoris. IVUS-derived ruptured plaques showed thinner caps when compared with nonruptured plaques, with a mean cap thickness of 0.47 mm (470 μm), as shown in **Fig. 9**. However, when ruptured plaques are evaluated by histology, the mean cap thickness is about 20 times lower: 23 ± 19 μm in the coronary,[17] and 34 ± 16 μm in the aorta.[18] As discussed earlier, this significant overestimation of cap thickness by IVUS is related to its poor axial resolution (100–200 μm), an inherent limitation impossible to overcome. As a result, IVUS-related technology does not always easily detect TCFA, the more common form of high-risk, vulnerable plaque, and may actually provide controversial information.[62]

Necrotic core area

Peters and colleagues[63] evaluated the ability of IVUS to detect human coronary necrotic cores using in vitro video densitometry with a 30-MHz ultrasound catheter. The sensitivity of IVUS for necrotic core was 46% and the specificity was 97%. Several studies were then performed to try to improve these results, using an integrated backscatter approach.[64] Other studies by Sano and colleagues[65] showed encouraging results. Of clinical relevance, a 3-vessel prospective IVUS study evaluated the association between large echolucent areas (possible necrotic cores) and the risk of future coronary events in 106 patients, 80% with chronic stable angina.[66] Twelve patients had events 4 ± 3 months after IVUS evaluation. Most of these events (93%) occurred in plaques with large echolucent areas, suggesting a prognostic value for IVUS in predicting future coronary events.[66] More recently, the attenuation of the echo signal can be considered a surrogate for large necrotic cores, and may have clinical implications.[67,68] The authors conclude that the sensitivity and accuracy to identify necrotic cores by IVUS are an evolving target.

Plaque inflammation

Detection of macrophages within the fibrous cap requires a resolution within 10–20 μm. Considering that IVUS resolution is 10–20 times higher, it is impossible for IVUS to detect macrophages in atherosclerotic plaques.

Degree of positive remodeling

IVUS is an excellent tool to detect remodeling, a major feature of plaque vulnerability.[69] Ruptured plaques are larger in size when compared with fibrocalcific, nonruptured plaques.[18,59] However, the degree of arterial remodeling is so pronounced that even large plaques can appear as nonobstructive "mild" stenosis on angiography.[59]

Plaque neovascularization

IVUS has the potential to detect flow within the plaque, and therefore identify functional neovessels. Although the real-time IVUS is limited to evaluating plaque perfusion, recent developments with contrast agents have dramatically improved the quality of Doppler ultrasound. Intravascular injection of microbubbles (ie, small encapsulated air or gas bubbles) can boost the Doppler signal from blood vessels, as shown in **Fig. 10**.[70] To improve resolution, an IVUS prototype using "harmonic" imaging with transmitting ultrasound at 20 MHz (fundamental) and detecting contrast signals at 40 MHz (second harmonic) is being developed and may evolve as a clinical tool.[71]

VH

Considering the significant limitations of traditional IVUS imaging in identifying necrotic cores, Nair

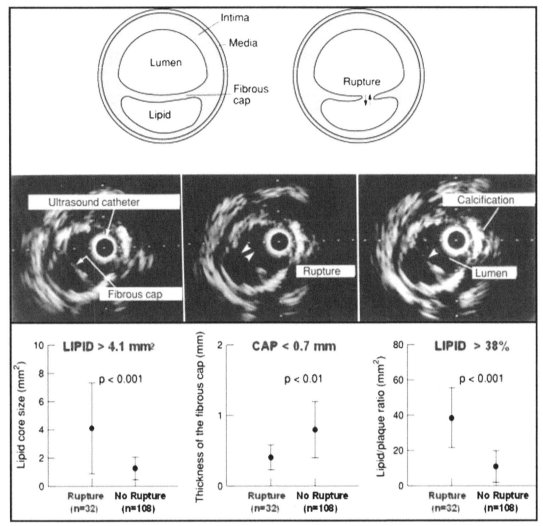

Fig. 9. IVUS images of ruptured plaques, highlighting the fibrous cap and a large echolucent area under the cap suggestive of large necrotic cores (*upper panel*). Lipid area, cap thickness, and lipid percent area in ruptured (*red*) versus non-ruptured (*black*) plaques (*lower panel*). (*Adapted from* Ge J, Chirillo F, Schwedtmann J, et al. Screening of ruptured plaques in patients with coronary artery disease by intravascular ultrasound. Heart 1999;81(6):621–7; with permission.)

and colleagues[72,73] at Cleveland Clinic decided to evaluate the ultrasound scattered reflection wave as a possible alternative to improve tissue characterization by IVUS. This backscattered reflection wave is received by the transducer, where it is converted into voltage. This voltage is known as the backscattered radiofrequency (RF) data. Using a combination of previously identified spectral parameters, a classification scheme was developed to construct an algorithm to test plaque composition ex vivo. Four major plaque components were tested, including fibrotic tissue, fibrofatty tissue, calcific-necrotic core, and calcium. A color was assigned for each of these components, and is displayed on the IVUS image.

Initial validation was performed using ex vivo human coronary specimens using a 30-MHz, 2.9-F, mechanically rotating IVUS catheter (Boston Scientific Corporation, Natick, MA, USA). The Movat-stained histologic images identified homogeneous regions representing each of the 4 plaque components, as shown in **Fig. 11**. The unit of analysis (also called the box) was initially composed of 64 backscattered RF data samples in length (480 μm).[73] In 2007, the unit of analysis was composed of 32 backscattered RF data samples in length (240 μm) (DG Vince, personal communication, 2007). The algorithm developed is then validated ex vivo, with sensitivities and specificities between 79% and 93% for all

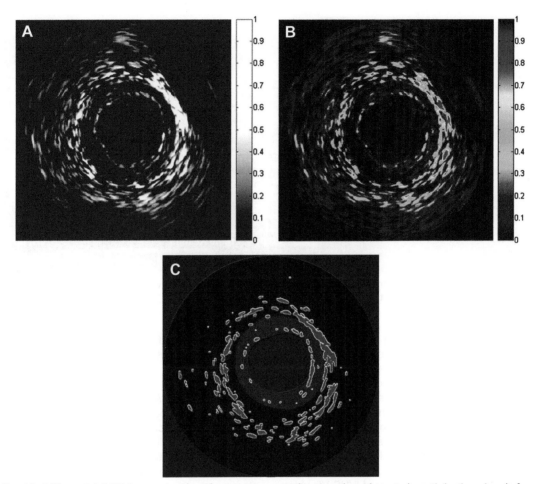

Fig. 10. Differential IVUS images to identify vasa vasorum, showing the subtracted postinjection signals from baseline signals. (*A*) Black and white (signal intensity of **Fig. 1**A–C). (*B*) color-coded panel A. (*C*) Thresholded to show most significant areas of enhancement. (*Adapted from* Vavuranakis M, Kakadiaris IA, O'Malley SM, et al. Images in cardiovascular medicine. Detection of luminal-intimal border and coronary wall enhancement in intravascular ultrasound imaging after injection of microbubbles and simultaneous sonication with transthoracic echocardiography. Circulation 2005;112(1):e1–2; with permission.)

4-plaque components.[73] The initial work was performed with a 30-MGz catheter, then the 20-MGz (Eagle Eye Gold, Volcano, San Diego, CA, USA) device, which is approved by the US Food and Drug Administration.[74] Recent correlation studies in experimental animal models showed encouraging results.[75] The catheter was upgraded with a 45-MGz transducer, currently available for clinical practice. Recent data showed relevant information regarding plaque stabilization in patients receiving aggressive statin therapy.[76] Despite these findings about IVUS-VH, the interventionalist needs objective information regarding the ability of to detect TCFA, which can be summarized as follows.

Fibrous cap thickness

Considering that the resolution of IVUS-VH is greater that that needed to detect TCFA, IVUS-VH is limited in cap thickness evaluation. This point was addressed in Nair and colleagues' initial publication, when they comment on the limitations: "The window size currently applied for selection of regions of interest and eventual tissue map reconstructions is 480 μm in the radial direction. Therefore, detection of thin fibrous caps (≤65 μm below the resolution of IVUS) would be compromised, restricting the detection of vulnerable atheromas."[73] Despite this inherent limitation, investigators proposed a classification of "VH-TCFA."[77,78] As a result, lesions with fibrous cap thickness greater than 65 μm will be incorrectly classified as TCFAs, and the total number per patient will be overestimated.

Necrotic core area

IVUS-derived VH was initially developed to identify calcific necrotic cores. However, the incidence

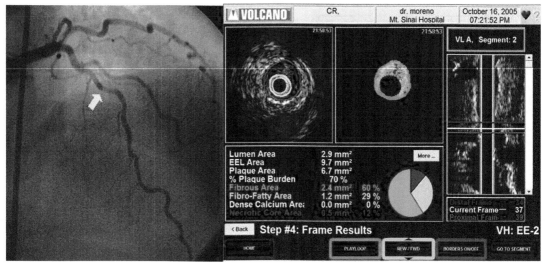

Fig. 11. Color-coded reproduction of IVUS-VH plaque composition displayed in vivo in the cardiac catheterization laboratory at Mount Sinai Hospital, New York, USA.

and degree of calcification in necrotic cores are variable, and therefore necrotic cores without calcification may not be properly identified.[28] Most importantly, most advanced atherosclerotic lesions display a certain degree of necrotic core. As a result, when validating necrotic core using IVUS-VH, not only the presence/absence of the necrotic core is important (sensitivity/specificity)[79] but also the area. IVUS-VH routinely reports necrotic core area in mm², which provides an opportunity for direct validation of IVUS-VH using planimetry in histologic specimens. However, no proper validation of these areas (linear regression analysis) has been published in patients. Only presence/absence studies have been carried out, showing good sensitivity and specificity. As discussed earlier in this article, multiple pathologic studies have established the concept that necrotic core areas from patients with ACS are larger when compared with necrotic core areas from patients with chronic stable angina.[14,16,80] Conversely, fibrous plaque areas (collagen) have been found to be significantly lower in ACS patients.[24] In a human study by Surmely and colleagues[81] necrotic core areas were significantly lower in patients with ACS (6.8 ± 6 vs 11 ± 8%, $P = .02$). In addition, fibrous areas were higher in patients with ACS (66 ± 11 vs 61 ± 9%, $P = .03$). These investigators concluded that plaque composition obtained by IVUS-VH is in contradiction with previously published histopathological data. Contrary to this observation, Rodriguez-Granillo and colleagues[82] have identified larger necrotic areas in ruptured plaques and in nonculprit[83] lesions from patients with ACS. In addition, recent studies

have shown a significant reduction in necrotic core area in coronary lesions aggressively treated with statin therapy.[76]

Plaque inflammation
As discussed earlier, detection of macrophages within the fibrous cap requires a resolution within 10 to 20 μm. Considering that IVUS-VH resolution is at least 10 to 20 times higher, it is impossible for VH to detect macrophages in the fibrous cap of the plaque.

Degree of positive remodeling
IVUS is an excellent tool to detect remodeling, and IVUS-VH preserves this advantage. Recent studies evaluated IVUS-VH necrotic core areas in plaques with positive and negative remodeling, and found lower necrotic core areas in positively remodeled plaques.[59] Other investigators[84] confirmed these data. However, Rodriguez-Granillo and colleagues[85] published opposing data showing larger IVUS-VH necrotic core areas in positively remodeled plaques, with an impressive correlation ($r = 0.83$; $P<.0001$).

The PROSPECT Trial was the first prospective natural history study designed to evaluate the prognostic value of IVUS-VH derived plaque composition in nonobstructive segments in patients with ACS. After successful PCI of the culprit lesion, 700 patients underwent 3-vessel IVUS-VH to evaluate plaque composition and severity of nonculprit lesions that were left alone for medical therapy. The final results were presented by Dr Gregg Stone at the Transcatheter Cardiovascular Therapeutics meetings in San

Francisco, CA, USA (September 24, 2009). On average, 22.1% of lesions were VH-TCFA. The incidence of 1 or more VH-TCFA was 51.2% per patient. The clinical results can be summarized as follows:

- 20.4% of all patients developed a major adverse cardiac event (MACE) event by 3 years. Culprit lesions exhibited a MACE rate of 12.9%, nonculprit lesions a MACE rate of 11.6% by 3 years.
- Presentation by cardiac death, cardiac arrest, and MI occurred less frequently with a combined MACE rate of 4.9% at 3 years.
- The combination of IVUS ≥70% plaque burden and VH-TCFA plaque morphology identified lesions at especially high risk, with a lesion hazard ratio of 10.8.

Although not peer-reviewed or published at the time of writing, these results suggest that nonculprit lesions with large plaque burden and VH-TCFA morphology need further evaluation to reduce the risk of future coronary events. A PROSPECT II study randomizing these lesions to stenting or not along with aggressive medical therapy may be considered if funding is available.

Palpography

The stress-strain relationship on coronary lesions may play a significant role in plaque rupture, and can be identified by another IVUS-derived technique called elastography or palpography.[19] Changes in blood pressure (stress) can induce deformation on the fibrous cap (strain) that can be quantified and displayed in a color-coded scale.[78] Studies at the Thoraxcenter, Rotterdam, The Netherlands[86] have documented high sensitivity and specificity of this technique, with a deformation of more than 2%, reflecting increased macrophage infiltration and reduced smooth muscle cell and collagen content. This specific technique was not designed to evaluate any of the other components of TCFA. As a result, fibrous cap thickness, necrotic core, degree of remodeling, neovascularization, and IPH are not suitable for evaluation by palpography.

Optical Coherence Tomography

OCT is promising for identifying TCFA. It is catheter-based, measures back-reflected infrared light, and provides the highest resolutions of all invasive modalities (5–20 μm).[87] Excellent histopathological correlations have been performed, for human coronary tissue and for animal models, highlighting a sensitivity and specificity of 92%

and 94%, respectively, for lipid-rich plaque, 95% and 100% for fibrocalcific plaque, and 87% and 97% for fibrous plaque.[87] Superb resolution allows for detailed imaging, as shown in **Fig. 12**. The major limitation of OCT is the need to displace blood in the vessel with saline flush, making this technique difficult in the evaluation of long segments. However, recent advances using optical frequency domain imaging allows for high-speed comprehensive imaging, scanning up to 5 cm with 1 single saline flush.[88]

Fibrous cap thickness
OCT is the only imaging tool that can identify plaques with cap thickness 65 μm or less. Fibrous cap thickness was lowest in patients with acute MI, intermediate in patients with ACS, and highest in patients with chronic stable angina,[89] as shown in **Fig. 13**.

Necrotic core area
Lipid pool and necrotic core are signal-poor, and therefore are poorly delineated with respect to the surrounding tissue. The lipid-rich plaque can be recognized, therefore, by the presence of large areas of ill-defined, signal-poor regions, which are evident to the naked eye, as seen in **Fig. 12**C. On the other hand, when the cap is thick and the signal is strong, the operator can tell that the signal is coming from a fibrous plaque mostly composed of collagen, as illustrated in **Fig. 12**A. Predictive values for collagen were between 89% and 93%.[90]

Plaque inflammation
OCT resolution allows for proper identification of macrophages in the atherosclerotic plaques.[87] The first correlation in vitro was performed by Tearney and colleagues,[91] who identified multiple strong back-reflections from caps with abundant macrophage infiltration, resulting in a high OCT signal variance. This signal variance was then processed using logarithmic transformation. In vivo studies then showed increased macrophage density in ruptured plaques from patients with ACS (at culprit and nonculprit lesions) when compared with nonruptured plaques from patients with chronic stable angina.[92]

Degree of positive remodeling
OCT has limited penetration, and requires a bloodless field to obtain good images. As a result, OCT may not properly quantify remodeling.

Plaque neovascularization and IPH
OCT is the gold standard to quantify neovascularization and the effects of novel antiangiogenic therapies in other common diseases like age-related

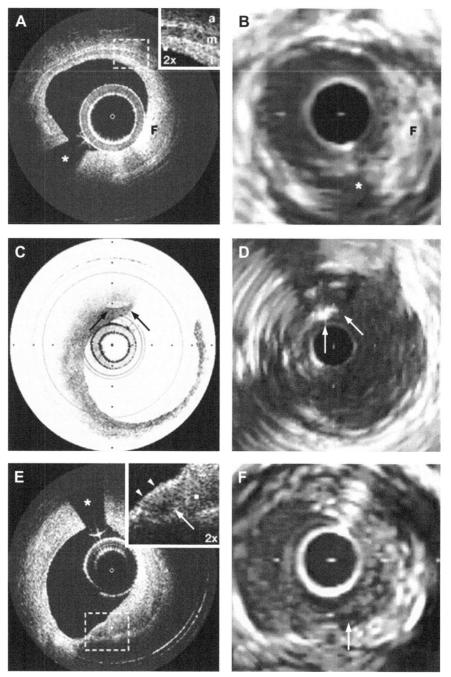

Fig. 12. In vivo OCT images of different coronary plaque types compared with intravascular ultrasonography of the corresponding sites. (*A*) Fibrous plaque: from 9 o'clock to 2 o'clock, the 3-layer structure of a typical intimal hyperplasia is shown and a magnified area is shown in the box. A homogeneous, signal-rich pattern indicates fibrous plaque (*F*), which is partly obscured by a guide wire artifact (*). (*B*) Fibrous plaque: the IVUS image corresponding to A. (*C*) Calcific plaque: a signal-poor region surrounded by sharp borders represents calcific plaque, which is clearly delineated (*arrows*). (*D*) Calcific plaque: on the corresponding IVUS image calcium is easily identified but the strong signal obscures the structure in front of the calcium deposit and a back-shadow artifact obscures that behind the deposit. (*E*) Lipid-rich plaque: a signal-poor region (arrow in inset) surrounded by diffuse borders and separated by a thin cap (*arrow heads* in inset) is consistent with TCFA. (*F*) Lipid-rich plaque: the corresponding IVUS image suggests a superficial echolucent region. a, adventitia; i, intima; m, media. (*Adapted from* Low AF, Tearney GJ, Bouma BE, et al. Technology Insight: optical coherence tomography–current status and future development. Nat Clin Pract Cardiovasc Med 2006;3(3):154–62; with permission.)

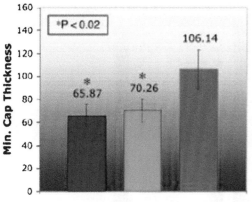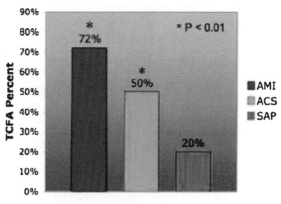

Fig. 13. In-vivo quantification of fibrous cap thickness by OCT. Cap thickness was lowest in patients with acute myocardial infarction (*red*), intermediate in patients with ACS (*green*), and highest in patients with chornic stable angina (*blue*). As a result, the incidence of TCFA is highest in acute myocardial infarction and lowest in chronic stable angina. (*Data from* Jang IK, Tearney GJ, MacNeil B, et al. In vivo characterization of coronary atherosclerotic plaque by use of optical coherence tomography. Circulation 2005;111(12):1551–5.)

macular degeneration, extrafoveal choroidal neovascularization, and proliferative diabetic retinopathy.[71] However, at the time of this report, no studies have tested OCT in the evaluation of atherosclerotic neovascularization or IPH. Nevertheless, it is likely that OCT reproduces its resolution and clinical value in ophthalmology if it is tested to quantify atherosclerosis neovascularization in the cardiac catheterization laboratory.

Intravascular MRI

MRI allows for 3-dimensional evaluation of vascular structures with outstanding depiction of various components of the atherothrombotic plaque, including lipid, fibrous tissue, calcium, and thrombus formation.[93,94] In addition, combining MRI with cellular and molecular targeting provides important data on the biologic activity of high-risk, vulnerable plaques, especially for carotid and aortic lesions.[95] Whereas the conventional MRI resolution is approximately 460 μm, the intravascular MRI (ivMRI) resolution is improved to 250 μm. A catheter was developed and tested in human coronaries in vivo in the United States and Europe, with more than 100 patients enrolled. The ability of ivMRI to detect TCFA can be summarized as follows.

Fibrous cap thickness and necrotic core
The resolution of ivMRI is higher than 65 μm. As a result, ivMRI is limited in the identification of TCFA. To overcome this limitation, TCFA was then defined as the presence of an increased lipid fraction within the superficial band (0–100 μm).[96] Conversely, the absence of lipid within the superficial band may indicate a thick fibrous cap, which

is associated with more stable lesions.[96] With the aid of a partially inflated balloon, the MRI catheter obtains color-coded images in 4 quadrants, as shown in **Fig. 14**. Results of histologic in addition to the aortic data resulted in a sensitivity of 100% and a specificity of 89%.[96]

Plaque inflammation
With the advantage of molecular targeting, MRI can image macrophages using different pathways.[97,98] The ultrasmall superparamagnetic particles of iron oxide compounds (USPIOs, SPIOs), also called magnetic nanoparticles, are internalized by macrophage receptors and can be properly imaged by MRI, as shown in **Fig. 15**. The combination of MRI and [18]fluorodeoxyglucose positron emission tomography successfully image metabolic activity of plaque macrophages in patients with symptomatic carotid atherosclerosis, as shown in **Fig. 16**.[99,100] Contrast agents including gadolinium-containing immunomicelles can also identify inflammatory cells in atherosclerosis.[101] Imaging interleukin 2 [102] and apoptosis [103] may also provide an estimation of macrophage content in atherosclerotic plaques.

Degree of positive remodeling
The current stage of ivMRI does not provide this degree of delineation, and therefore cannot quantify remodeling.

Plaque neovascularization
Molecular imaging can target angiogenic molecules like the integrin $\alpha_v\beta_3$, $\alpha_v\beta_5$, and growth factors like basic fibroblast growth factor at the endothelial cell level.[104] Winter and colleagues[105] successfully imaged atherosclerotic neovessels

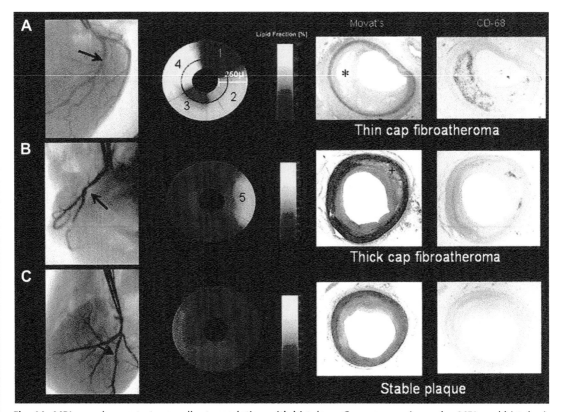

Fig. 14. MRI scan demonstrates excellent correlation with histology. Coronary angiography, MRI, and histologic cross sections of 3 intermediate coronary lesions are shown. An arrow on the angiogram marks the site of inter-rogation. The corresponding MRI is shown in the second column, whereas corresponding histologic sections of the interrogated sections are shown in the third and fourth columns (Movat's pentachrome and anti-CD68 anti-body staining, respectively). (*A*) TCFA (*left* to *right*) in the proximal left anterior descending artery; the MRI display shows the presence of a high lipid content within 3 quadrants (2 to 4). Quadrant 1 has little lipid within the wall, as indicated by the lack of foam cells by Movat's staining or macrophages by CD68 staining. Quadrant 2 has moderately increased lipid concentrations, as noted by an approximate lipid fractional index of 60%. Quad-rant 3 has increased lipid only in the deep layer, whereas quadrant 4 has high lipid fractional indexes (±100%) within the superficial and deep layers. Approximately 75% of the arterial circumference is lipid-rich. The MRI display corresponds well with subsequent histology, as the Movat's section shows a large necrotic core (*) and a thin fibrous cap, and the adjoining immunohistochemical staining shows markedly positive staining for CD68 in the area corresponding to quadrant 4 of the MRI display. (*B*) TCFA in the right coronary artery. The MRI display shows no lipid content within the superficial layer (*blue*); however, a mild degree of increased lipid concentration is observed within the deep band more than 100 μm from the lumen in quadrant 5 only. The lipid fractional index is about 50%. The corresponding histologic section shows a TCFA with a small, deep necrotic core (+), confirmed by the anti-CD68 staining, corresponding with the MRI image. Because there is little to no lipid within the super-ficial layer, this lesion is considered a thick fibroatheroma. (*C*) Stable lesion. A mild stenosis by angiography is seen in the intermediate branch of the left coronary artery. The MRI display of the lesion shows no increased lipid concentration in the shallow or the deep bands of any quadrant, indicating the presence of a fibrous lesion (hence, blue display). This diagnosis was confirmed by histology as adaptive intimal hyperplasia, and the corre-sponding anti-CD68 staining was negative for foam cells or a necrotic core. (*Reproduced from* Schneiderman J, Wilensky RL, Weiss A, et al. Diagnosis of thin-cap fibroatheromas by a self-contained intravascular magnetic reso-nance imaging probe in ex vivo human aortas and in situ coronary arteries. J Am Coll Cardiol 2005;45(12):1961–9; with permission.)

using $\alpha_v\beta_3$-targeted, paramagnetic nanoparticles in hypercholesterolemic rabbits, as seen in **Fig. 17**. Other molecular targets like the fibronectin extra-domain B, have been found predominantly around the vasa vasorum.[106] Vascular cell

adhesion molecule 1 (VCAM-1), a critical compo-nent of the leukocyte-endothelial adhesion cascade, was successfully targeted using phage display-derived peptide sequences and multi-modal nanoparticles for MRI and fluorescence

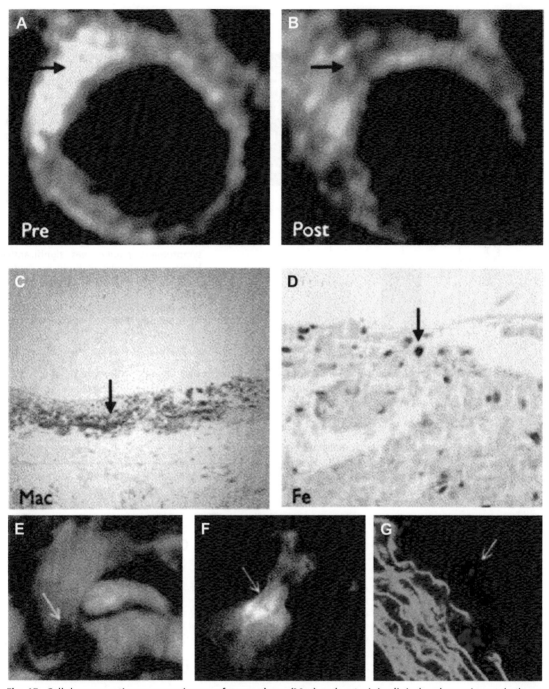

Fig. 15. Cellular magnetic resonance image of macrophage (Mac) endocytosis in clinical and experimental atherosclerosis using magnetic nanoparticles. (*A*) Dextranated magnetic nanoparticle injection (ferumoxtran, 2.6 mg/kg) produces focal signal loss within a carotid plaque of a neurologically symptomatic patient (*top*, pre and post images, *arrow*). Histologic examination of the carotid endarterectomy specimen demonstrates colocalization of macrophages (*C*, anti-CD68 macrophage antibody, original magnification ×100), and iron (Fe) (*D*, Perls iron stain, neutral red counterstain; original magnification ×400). (*B*) Multimodality magnetic resonance image and NIR fluorescent imaging of murine atherosclerosis using a magnetofluorescent nanoparticle. (*E*) In vivo 9.4-T electrocardiogram and respiratory-gated magnetic resonance image of an apolipoprotein E−/−-deficient mouse. Injection of a clinical-type NIR fluorescent dextranated magnetic nanoparticle (15 mg/kg of iron, 24 hour circulation time) produces focal signal loss (*arrow*) in the aortic root, a known site of atherosclerosis in the apolipoprotein E−/− mouse. (*F*) Fluorescence reflectance imaging of the resected aorta confirms a focal NIR fluorescent signal within the aortic root (*arrow*). (*G*) On fluorescence microscopy, the NIR magnetofluorescent nanoparticle accumulates in intimal macrophages (*red, arrow*) within aortic root plaque sections (original magnification ×200). In contrast, smooth muscle cells (stained here with a spectrally distinct α-actin fluorescent antibody, *green*) modestly colocalize with the magnetofluorescent nanoparticle. (*From* Jaffer FA, Weissleder R. Molecular imaging in the clinical arena. JAMA 2005;293:855–62; with permission.)

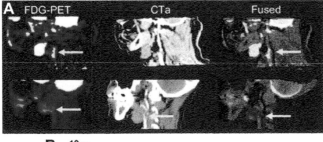

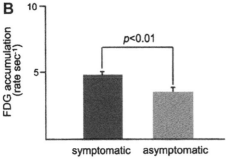

Fig. 16. Positron emission tomography (PET) images from patients with unstable carotid disease after administration of fluorine-18-labeled deoxyglucose (FDG). (*A*) FDG-PET (*left column*), CTA (*middle column*), and fused (*right column*) images from patient with symptomatic carotid stenosis (*top row*) and contralateral asymptomatic carotid stenosis (*bottom row*). The yellow arrows highlight areas of FDG uptake corresponding to stenotic carotid plaque. (*B*) A graph showing FDG accumulation rate in symptomatic versus asymptomatic carotid plaques. Note that FDG uptake into symptomatic plaque was significantly higher. (*From* Davies JR, Rudd JH, Weissberg PL, et al. Radionuclide imaging for the detection of inflammation in vulnerable plaques. J Am Coll Cardiol 2006; 47(Suppl 8):C57–68; with permission.)

molecular imaging in apolipoprotein E-knockout mice, adding an additional method to interrogate angiogenesis in atherosclerotic plaques.[107]

IPH
Human carotid IPH was evaluated by Takaya and colleagues,[108] as shown in **Fig. 18**. Of clinical relevance, IPH detected by MRI is associated with a significant increase in subsequent cerebrovascular events (hazard ratio, 5.2; $P = .005$).[109] Other investigators have confirmed these findings,[110] highlighting the value of MRI-detected IPH in complex atherosclerosis.

Angioscopy

The color of atherosclerotic plaques can provide information about plaque composition. White,

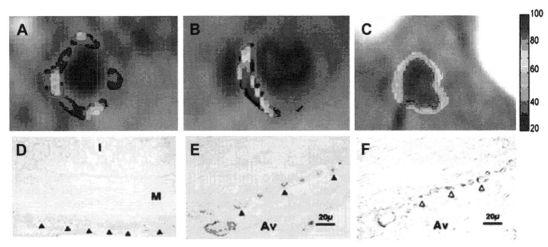

Fig. 17. Molecular MRI of arterial neovessels in cholesterol-fed rabbits. Percent enhancement of adventitial signal (false-colored from *blue* to *red*) is shown in aortic segments at renal artery (*A*), mid-aorta (*B*), and diaphragm (*C*) 2 hours after $\alpha_v\beta_3$-targeted gadolinium-loaded nanoparticles. Immunohistochemistry of $\alpha_v\beta_3$-integrin (*D*) demonstrates thickened intima (I) and $\alpha_v\beta_3$-integrin staining in adventitial neovessels (*black arrow heads*). Immunostaining in aorta from cholesterol-fed animal in *A* at 600× delineates neovascular $\alpha_v\beta_3$-integrin (*E, solid arrows*) and platelet and endothelial cell adhesion molecule (*F, open arrows*) expression at the interface between media (M) and adventitia (Av). (*From* Winter PM, Morawski AM, Caruthers SD, et al. Molecular imaging of angiogenesis in early-stage atherosclerosis with alpha(v)beta3-integrin-targeted nanoparticles. Circulation 2003;108(18):2270–4; with permission.)

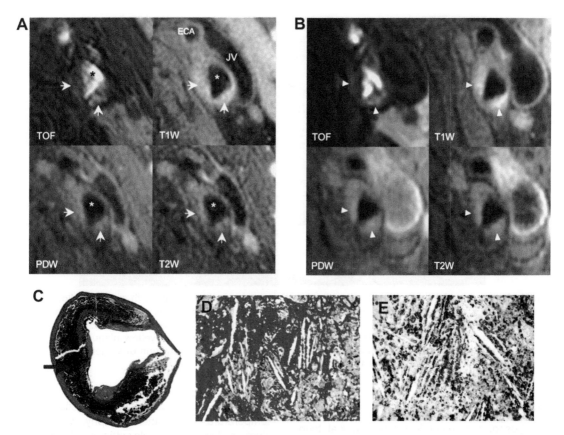

Fig. 18. (*A*) Signal intensity of type II hemorrhage at baseline examination. Type II hemorrhage is identified by hyperintense signals on TOF, T1W, PDW, and T2W images of left internal carotid artery (*arrow*). Asterisks show location of lumen. (*B*) Images from 18-month follow-up scan showed a similar signal intensity pattern in the same regions (*arrowheads*). (*C*) Matched Mallory's trichrome-stained section from excised CEA specimen. (*D*) High-power (×400) field taken from region (*arrow* in *C*) deep within necrotic core showing hemorrhagic debris and cholesterol clefts. (*E*) Glycophorin A immunostaining of the same region (×400) in an adjacent section shows extensive staining of hemorrhagic debris, indicating the presence of erythrocyte membranes. JV, jugular vein; ECA, external carotid artery. (*From* Takaya N, Yuan C, Chu B, et al. Presence of intraplaque hemorrhage stimulates progression of carotid atherosclerotic plaques: a high-resolution magnetic resonance imaging study. Circulation 2005;111(21):2768–75; with permission.)

yellow, and glistening yellow plaques have been quoted and studied in patients with coronary artery disease (CAD). Of significant clinical value, Uchida and colleagues[111] evaluated these 3 different types of plaques in a prospective, 3-vessel angioscopic study including 157 patients with chronic stable angina. White plaques were associated with a low incidence of ACS (3.3%), and yellow and glistening yellow were associated with a higher incidence of ACS (7.6% and 68%, respectively), including death in 22% of the glistening yellow cases.[111] Using light microscopy in the autopsy cases, white plaques were associated with thick caps (400 μm), yellow plaques with thinner caps (80 μm), and glistening yellow with the thinnest caps (10–20 μm).[111] In another study, Asakura and colleagues[112] performed 3-vessel angioscopy in patients 1 month after MI. Yellow

plaques were detected in 90% of 21 culprit lesions. Yellow plaques were equally prevalent in the infarct-related and noninfarct-related coronary arteries (3.7 ± 1.6 vs 3.4 ± 1.8 plaques/artery), suggesting a diffuse rather than a localized process in patients with MI. To evaluate the predictive value of yellow plaques in clinical practice, Ohtani and colleagues[113] performed culprit vessel angioscopy in 552 patients with chronic stable angina, ACS, and acute MI. Yellow color intensity was also graded. The number of yellow plaques varied from 0 to more than 5, as seen in **Fig. 19**. After 5 years, 7.1% of patients developed ACS. The mean number of yellow plaques was higher in the patients with an ACS event than those without the event (3.1 ± 1.8 vs 2.2 ± 1.5; P = .008). However, the yellow color intensity scale was similar and not predictive.

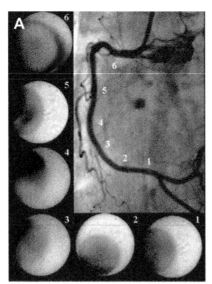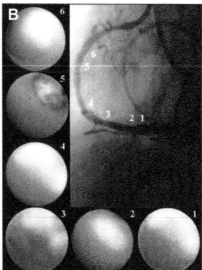

Fig. 19. A representative case with no yellow plaque (*A*) and a representative case with multiple yellow plaques (*B*). (*A*) No yellow plaque was detected in the right coronary artery; number of yellow plaques: 0, maximum color grade of yellow plaques: 0. (*B*) Three yellow plaques were detected in the right coronary artery; maximum color grade of yellow plaques: 3. (*From* Ohtani T, Ueda Y, Mizote I, et al. Number of yellow plaques detected in a coronary artery is associated with future risk of acute coronary syndrome: detection of vulnerable patients by angioscopy. J Am Coll Cardiol 2006;47(11):2194–200; with permission.)

Spectroscopy

Spectroscopy is a nondestructive optical technology able to analyze chemical composition of plaque components.[114] After irradiation of tissue with a laser beam, scattered photons are then acquired to identify specific features of plaque vulnerability.[114] Two different modalities are currently being evaluated for intravascular detection of high-risk, vulnerable plaques: near-infrared (NIR) and Raman spectroscopy. Both techniques have good correlations with histologic analysis of coronary and aortic tissue.[115–117] However, the complexity of signal analysis may force the investigators to focus on only 1 or 2 features of plaque vulnerability. NIR focused on lipid cores, and developed a catheter providing a bright yellow image reflecting lipid cores, as shown in **Fig. 20**. The validity and safety of this catheter was properly evaluated in a multicenter study, with encouraging results.[118] Validation studies are needed,[119] and multiple prospective trials are ongoing in the United States and Europe. NIR combined the LipiScan catheter with IVUS, and will test the ability of aggressive medical therapy to modify plaque composition in more than 600 patients in a study led by Dr Patrick Serruys in Europe. This test provides the first combined imaging catheter and is promising for this technique. Proof is needed that spectroscopy will stand as a useful, clinical tool in the catheterization laboratory.

Another technique evaluating changes in temperature, called thermography, was extensively evaluated in multiple settings with promising results.[120] Despite these evaluations, the cooling effect of the blood and other limitations significantly reduced enthusiasm for thermography to become a useful tool for intravascular detection of high-risk plaques.

Summary of Intracoronary Imaging

The development of new technologies for the purpose of detection of high-risk plaques is progressing rapidly. Although individual devices have reached a certain degree of technological sophistication, a combination of these modalities may have a better future (ie, OCT/Backscattered IVUS[121]; IVUS/Raman spectroscopy[122]). The recently completed Prospect trial performed 3-vessel coronary imaging in patients with ACS, and will provide prognostic information related to invasive plaque imaging in CAD. If the event rate at follow-up is higher than expected with pharmacologic therapy, the scientific community will need to consider additional therapeutic strategies. As a result, a comprehensive approach regarding invasive therapy is becoming mandatory for the interventionalist interested in the prevention of recurrent coronary events. The next section of this article summarizes current and future therapies for high-risk, vulnerable plaques.

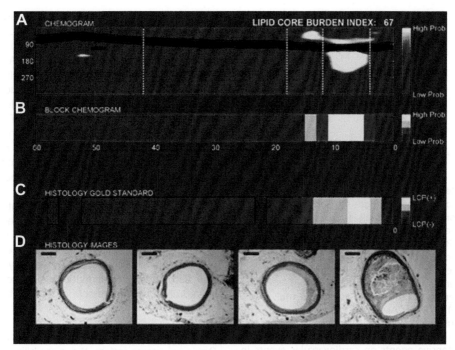

Fig. 20. (*A*) Chemogram image indicating artery wall lipid content (x axis = pullback in millimeters; y axis = rotation in degrees). Each pixel is marked with red for low probability and yellow for high probability of lipid core plaque of interest (LCP). The lipid core burden index (*top right*) indicates amount of lipid in scanned artery on a 0 to 1000 scale. (*B*) Summary (block chemogram) of LCP presence at 2-mm intervals in 4 probability categories. (*C*) Map of histologic classifications (*yellow*, LCP; *light orange*, small or thick-capped fibroatheroma; *dark orange*, intimal xanthoma and pathologic intimal thickening; *red*, all other types). (*D*) Movat cross sections from locations along the artery (*dotted lines*). Black bars denote 1 mm. Image interpretation: The chemogram shows prominent lipid core signal at 2 to 16 mm, occupying 180°. The block chemogram shows that the strongest LCP signals extend 5 to 11 mm. The NIR spectroscopy signals at 18 and 42 mm correctly indicate absence of LCP. MI, myocardial infarction. (*From* Waxman S, Dixon SR, L'Allier P, et al. In vivo validation of a catheter-based near-infrared spectroscopy system for detection of lipid core coronary plaques: initial results of the SPECTACL study. JACC Imaging 2009;2(7):858–68; with permission.)

THERAPY
Systemic Therapy

Systemic pharmacologic therapy is the cornerstone of plaque stabilization, with documented reductions in lipid content, inflammation, and vasa-vasorum neovascularization.[123] Intensive statin therapy has demonstrated a significant decrease in coronary events in patients with stable disease and in patients with ACS.[124,125] In the ASTEROID trial[37] aggressive therapy with rosuvastatin 40 mg/d led to an absolute regression of atheroma volume, as shown in **Fig. 21**. Another potent antiatherogenic therapy is increasing high-density lipoprotein (HDL). Studies using bezafibrate, a peroxisome proliferator-activated receptor (PPAR)-α agonist, and fenofibrate have demonstrated reduced events and plaque regression, respectively.[126,127] These beneficial effects may be caused not only by HDL augmentation and reverse cholesterol transport[128] but also by recruitment of endothelial progenitor cells into damaged endothelium.[129]

Despite the value of systemic therapy, patients still return with recurrent events and therefore prove resistant to systemic therapy. For example, the combination of angiotensin-converting enzyme inhibitors, β-blockers, aspirin, and high doses of atorvastatin (80 mg/d), still yield a 22% recurrent event rate within 2 years, as shown in the PROVE IT trial.[130] As a result, even the best combination of systemic therapy available today does not successfully prevent all episodes of plaque rupture and thrombosis. Therefore, new therapies are urgently needed as coadjutants to systemic therapy in high-risk patients. Classified as regional and local therapies, these new options are under investigation, and will need prospective, placebo-controlled randomized trials before being considered for clinical use.

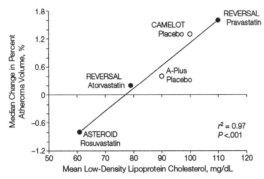

Fig. 21. Relationship between mean LDL cholesterol levels and median change in percent atheroma volume for several IVUS trials. There is a close correlation between these 2 variables ($r^2 = 0.97$). REVERSAL indicates Reversal of Atherosclerosis With Aggressive Lipid-Lowering (Nissen SE, Tuzcu EM, Brown BG, et al. Effect of intensive compared with moderate lipid-lowering therapy on progression of coronary atherosclerosis: a randomized controlled trial. JAMA 2004;291:1071–80); CAMELOT, Comparison of Amlodipine versus Enalapril to Limit Occurrences of Thrombosis (Nissen SE, Tuzcu EM, Libby P, et al. Effect of antihypertensive agents on cardiovascular events in patients with coronary disease and normal blood pressure: the CAMELOT study: a randomized controlled trial. JAMA 2004;292:2217–26); A-Plus, Avasimibe and Progression of Lesions on Ultrasound (Tardif JC, Gregoire J, L'Allier PL, et al. Avasimibe and Progression of Lesions on Ultrasound (A-PLUS) Investigators. Effects of the acyl coenzyme A:cholesterol acyltransferase inhibitor avasimibe on human atherosclerotic lesions. Circulation 2004;110:3372–7); and ASTEROID, a study to evaluate the effect of rosuvastatin on intravascular ultrasound-derived coronary atheroma burden. (*From* Nissen SE, Nicholls SJ, Sipahi I, et al. Effect of very high-intensity statin therapy on regression of coronary atherosclerosis: the ASTEROID trial. JAMA 2006;295(13):1556–65; with permission.)

Regional Therapy

Regional therapy is defined as the intravascular treatment of coronary segments with therapeutic agents that will stabilize high-risk, vulnerable plaques. Regional therapy includes photodynamic therapy (PDT),[131] endoluminal phototherapy,[132,133] and cryotherapy.[134] Of these, PDT has gained more attention. PDT involves photosensitizing (light-sensitive) drugs, light, and tissue oxygen to treat targeted diseases, mostly in cancer.[135] Photosensitizing agents (porphyrins) are administered locally or parenterally. They are selectively absorbed and retained within tissues for targeted therapy. This differential selectivity offers selective therapeutic effects when the target tissue is exposed to light at an appropriate wavelength; the surrounding normal tissue is then spared from therapeutic injury.[132] Activation of the photosensitizer within tissue induces the production of free radicals, leading to selective cytotoxic effects, mostly apoptosis (DNA fragmentation), or delayed necrosis. The application of PDT to atherosclerotic plaques was successfully performed in vivo by Waksman and colleagues[136] in hypercholesterolemic rabbits. PDT induced a significant reduction (92% ± 6%) in the population of nuclei of all cell types in plaques relative to controls ($P<.01$). This effect was partly caused by reduction of smooth muscle cells and macrophages. These results suggest that PDT can almost eliminate macrophages from atherosclerotic plaques, and may provide a therapeutic alternative for high-risk, vulnerable plaques refractory to aggressive systemic therapy. The other 2 therapies, endoluminal phototherapy and cryotherapy, are also under investigation but experience is limited and beyond the scope of this article.

Local Therapy

Coronary stents offers the possibility of stabilizing vulnerable plaques, thickening the fibrous cap through the formation of neointimal hyperplasia. Davies[137] predicted local: "The time for prophylactic angioplasty has not come yet, but it may." [137] Libby[138] said: "If we could identify potentially unstable atheroma before they are evident, clinically we might even contemplate angioplasty or stenting on non-significant stenosis to induce smooth muscle cell proliferation and reinforce the plaque fibrous cap." These concepts were reinforced by Serruys in 2006,[78] and more recently in 2009 by Braunwald[3]: "The clinical application of vulnerable plaques at risk of future rupture (namely, locking the barn door before the horse is stolen) would require the development of measures for the prevention of plaque rupture that are more potent than those currently employed, in what we currently refer to as intensive prevention. Perhaps stenting or surgically bypassing these plaques could be considered in some patients."

Balloon-expandable stents are successfully used in rupture-thrombotic lesions, and may also stabilize TCFA. However, considering the highly controversial concept of stenting vulnerable plaques, the risk/benefit must be evaluated in experimental animal models. In addition, drug-eluting stents (DES) are associated with impaired healing that may contribute to stent thrombosis. To evaluate all these parameters, the authors developed an experimental animal model of spontaneous vulnerable plaques in New Zealand hypercholesterolemic rabbits followed for 4 years.[139] These

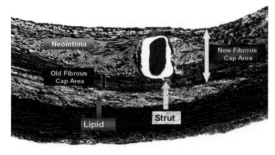

Fig. 22. Histologic section illustrating different components of TCFA 28 days after stent deployment. The strut compresses the old, thin fibrous cap (*blue arrow*). A cellular neointimal layer has been laid down, creating a new, thick fibrous cap (*yellow arrow*). Elastic-trichrome stain; 20× field.

animals developed atherosclerotic plaques similar to humans. Twenty-seven animals were randomized to metallic stents (6), DES (10), and controls (11).[140] Only struts deployed on vulnerable plaques were evaluated, as shown in **Fig. 22**. Fibrous cap thickness, stent-induced fibrous cap rupture (**Fig. 23**), and peristrut healing (**Fig. 24**) were also evaluated. Peristrut inflammation was defined as the presence of mononuclear round cells in hematoxylin and eosin (H&E) stained sections and scored as shown in **Fig. 24A**. Fibrin was defined as intensely eosinophilic amorphous (nonfibrillar) extracellular deposits on H&E stain, as shown in

Fig. 24B. Hemorrhage was defined as extravasated interstitial collections of RBCs with or without brown pigmented (hemosiderin laden) macrophages and scored as shown in **Fig. 24C**. Endothelialization was defined as the presence of endothelial cells covering struts and scored as shown in **Fig. 24D**.

Metallic, β-estradiol and everolimus stents increased fibrous cap thickness by 396%, 322%, and 270% respectively ($P<.0001$ for all comparisons), as shown in **Table 2**. Stent-induced fibrous cap rupture was present in 63% of stented lesions, increasing neointima in metallic ($P = .03$) but not in DES (not statistically significant). Peristrut inflammation, fibrin deposition, and hemorrhage were increased, and endothelialization decreased in DES when compared with metallic stents ($P<.05$), as shown in **Table 3**.

The results of this study provide histopathological evidence of fibrous cap thickening after stenting using bare metal and DES. These effects were obtained at the cost of increased cap damage and potentially iatrogenic, peristrut healing patterns including increased inflammation, fibrin deposition, hemorrhage, and decreased endothelialization. New self-expanding devices with thin struts are being clinically tested in humans to stabilize vulnerable plaques. Despite these and other results, there are some doubts that better understanding of vulnerable plaques will improve preventive therapy, particularly with stents. Atherosclerosis compromises the entire coronary

A   B

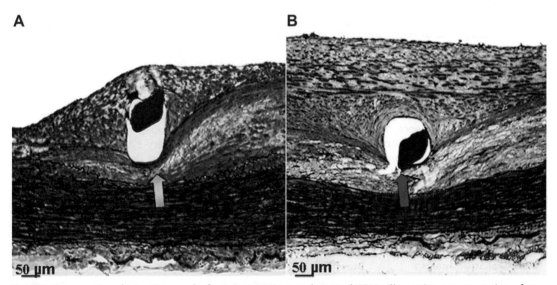

Fig. 23. Comparative photomicrographs from 2 separate metal stented TCFAs illustrating augmentation of neointimal proliferation following strut-induced fibrous cap rupture. (*A*) Fibrous cap compression without rupture (*cream arrow*) showed limited neointimal proliferation. (*B*) Strut-induced, torn fibrous cap rupture showing interruption and loss of continuity of the thin fibrous cap with direct apposition of strut to residual lipid core (*red arrow*), and increased neointimal proliferation.

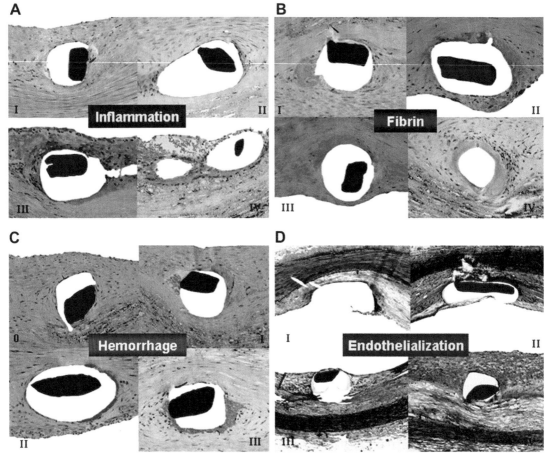

Fig. 24. Composite of micrographs displaying examples of numerical scoring (scale I to IV) applied to 4 categories (A–D) of strut-related healing patterns at 28 days post stent deployment: (A) inflammation; (B) fibrin deposition; (C) hemorrhage; (D) endothelialization. Score criteria common to A, B, and C categories record the extent of the perimeter of each strut affected as follows: score I, up to 1 quadrant around strut (or 25%); score II, up to 2 quadrants (50%); score III, up to 3 quadrants (75%); score IV, up to 4 quadrants (100%). Endothelialization (category D) was recorded as score I, up to 25% endothelial coverage; score II, up to 75% endothelial coverage; score III, up to 100% endothelial coverage; score IV, complete coverage with neointimal tissue.

system, and local therapy to reinforce TCFA may lead to a losing game of medical "whack-a-mole": fixing 1 trouble spot, then finding many others.[141] Furthermore, the controversy associated with late stent thrombosis is another disadvantage for the potential application of coronary stents in vulnerable plaques.[142] New stent design, including biodegradable material [143] and self-expanding delivery systems, may reduce the long-term risk of stent thrombosis and preserve

Table 2
Planimetric data comparing fibrous cap thickness in stenting and nonstented thin-cap fibroatheromas

Individual Strut Analysis	Metallic (n = 127)	Beta-Estradiol (n = 46)	Everolimus (n = 41)	Control (n = 122)
Old fibrous cap area (μm^2)	26 ± 3.9	24.4 ± 1.7	23 ± 1.9	27 ± 1.3
New fibrous cap area (μm^2)	107 ± 6.5[a]	87.6 ± 6.7[a,b]	72.8 ± 3.9[a,b]	27 ± 1.3

[a] $P<.0001$ in comparison with control group.
[b] $P<.05$ in comparison with metallic group.

Table 3
Planimetric data comparing potential iatrogenic peristrut healing patterns after metallic and drug eluting stents in thin-cap fibroatheromas

Vascular Healing	Metallic (n = 127)	Beta-Estradiol (n = 46)	Everolimus (n = 41)
Inflammation score	0.9 ± 0.1	1.1 ± 0.1[a]	1.1 ± 0.1[a]
Fibrin score	0.6 ± 0.1	1.1 ± 0.1[a]	1.1 ± 0.2[a]
Hemorrhage score	0.1 ± 0.0	0.1 ± 0.0	0.2 ± 0.1[a]
Endothelialization score	3.7 ± 0.1	3.2 ± 0.2[a]	3.6 ± 0.1

[a] $P<.05$ in comparison with metallic group.

the integrity of the fibrous cap, with further reinforcement by neointimal tissue. The prediction of how to treat vulnerable plaques resistant to aggressive medical therapy is controversial, but presents an opportunity for interventional cardiologists. Only prospective, randomized clinical trials will completely elucidate this issue.

SUMMARY AND FUTURE PREDICTIONS

Atherothrombosis continues to evolve in diagnosis, imaging, and therapy. The concept of a high-risk, vulnerable plaque with specific histologic features continues to be the focus of many investigators developing multiple imaging modalities for invasive diagnosis and therapy. This article provides a state-of-the-art review of these techniques. However, the concept of vulnerable plaques keeps evolving. That multiple lesions may exhibit the same morphology simultaneously in the same patient suggests that a single-plaque approach is narrow minded and difficult to prove in clinical practice. Nevertheless, the recently released results of the PROSPECT trial provide objective evidence for increased risk for large plaques with VH-TCFA morphology on IVUS. At the other end of the spectrum, a broader concept of disease burden is evolving, leading toward quantification by noninvasive imaging techniques. Regarding therapy, only randomized clinical trials will help to elucidate the risk/benefit of the proper approach, either invasive with local devices or noninvasive with aggressive systemic therapy.

REFERENCES

1. Moreno PR, Sanz J, Fuster V. Promoting mechanisms of vascular health: circulating progenitor cells, angiogenesis, and reverse cholesterol transport. J Am Coll Cardiol 2009;53(25):2315–23.
2. Schaar JA, Muller JE, Falk E, et al. Terminology for high-risk and vulnerable coronary artery plaques. Report of a meeting on the vulnerable plaque, June 17 and 18, 2003, Santorini, Greece. Eur Heart J 2004;25(12):1077–82.
3. Braunwald E. Noninvasive detection of vulnerable coronary plaques: locking the barn door before the horse is stolen. J Am Coll Cardiol 2009;54(1): 58–9.
4. Falk E. Plaque rupture with severe pre-existing stenosis precipitating coronary thrombosis. Characteristics of coronary atherosclerotic plaques underlying fatal occlusive thrombi. Br Heart J 1983;50(2):127–34.
5. Davies MJ, Thomas A. Thrombosis and acute coronary-artery lesions in sudden cardiac ischemic death. N Engl J Med 1984;310(18):1137–40.
6. Ambrose JA, Tannenbaum MA, Alexopoulos D, et al. Angiographic progression of coronary artery disease and the development of myocardial infarction. J Am Coll Cardiol 1988;12(1):56–62.
7. Nissen SE. The vulnerable plaque "hypothesis": promise, but little progress. JACC Imaging 2009; 2(4):483–5.
8. Ambrose JA, Srikanth S. Preventing future acute coronary events: is the target the so-called vulnerable plaque or the high-risk or vulnerable patient? Curr Opin Cardiol 2009;24(5):483–9.
9. Eijgelaar WJ, Heeneman S, Daemen MJ. The vulnerable patient: refocusing on the plaque? Thromb Haemost 2009;102(2):231–9.
10. Cutlip DE, Chhabra AG, Baim DS, et al. Beyond restenosis: five-year clinical outcomes from second-generation coronary stent trials. Circulation 2004;110(10):1226–30.
11. Glaser R, Selzer F, Faxon DP, et al. Clinical progression of incidental, asymptomatic lesions discovered during culprit vessel coronary intervention. Circulation 2005;111(2):143–9.
12. Motoyama S, Sarai M, Harigaya H, et al. Computed tomographic angiography characteristics of atherosclerotic plaques subsequently resulting in acute coronary syndrome. J Am Coll Cardiol 2009;54(1):49–57.

13. Wang JC, Normand SL, Mauri L, et al. Coronary artery spatial distribution of acute myocardial infarction occlusions. Circulation 2004;110(3):278–84.

14. Fuster V, Moreno PR, Fayad ZA, et al. Atherothrombosis and high-risk plaque part I: evolving concepts. J Am Coll Cardiol 2005;46(6):937–54.

15. Farb A, Burke AP, Tang AL, et al. Coronary plaque erosion without rupture into a lipid core. A frequent cause of coronary thrombosis in sudden coronary death. Circulation 1996;93(7):1354–63.

16. Virmani R, Burke AP, Farb A, et al. Pathology of the vulnerable plaque. J Am Coll Cardiol 2006;47(8 Suppl):C13–8.

17. Burke AP, Farb A, Malcom GT, et al. Coronary risk factors and plaque morphology in men with coronary disease who died suddenly. N Engl J Med 1997;336(18):1276–82.

18. Moreno PR, Purushothaman KR, Fuster V, et al. Intimomedial interface damage and adventitial inflammation is increased beneath disrupted atherosclerosis in the aorta: implications for plaque vulnerability. Circulation 2002;105(21):2504–11.

19. Schaar JA, van der Steen AF, Mastik F, et al. Intravascular palpography for vulnerable plaque assessment. J Am Coll Cardiol 2006;47(8 Suppl):C86–91.

20. Loree HM, Kamm RD, Stringfellow RG, et al. Effects of fibrous cap thickness on peak circumferential stress in model atherosclerotic vessels. Circ Res 1992;71(4):850–8.

21. Oliver MF, Davies MJ. The atheromatous lipid core. Eur Heart J 1998;19(1):16–8.

22. Davies MJ. The pathophysiology of acute coronary syndromes. Heart 2000;83(3):361–6.

23. Felton CV, Crook D, Davies MJ, et al. Relation of plaque lipid composition and morphology to the stability of human aortic plaques. Arterioscler Thromb Vasc Biol 1997;17(7):1337–45.

24. Moreno PR, Bernardi VH, Lopez-Cuellar J, et al. Macrophages, smooth muscle cells, and tissue factor in unstable angina. Implications for cell-mediated thrombogenicity in acute coronary syndromes. Circulation 1996;94(12):3090–7.

25. Burke AP, Weber DK, Kolodgie FD, et al. Pathophysiology of calcium deposition in coronary arteries. Herz 2001;26(4):239–44.

26. Moreno PR, PK, Fuster V, et al. Lack of association between aortic calcification and histologic signs of plaque rupture. J Am Coll Cardiol 2000;35:303A.

27. Moreno P. The role of calcification in plaque vulnerability and disruption. New York: Futura; 2002. 347–64.

28. Burke AP, Joner M, Virmani R. IVUS-VH: a predictor of plaque morphology? Eur Heart J 2006;27(16):1889–90.

29. Waxman S, Ishibashi F, Muller JE. Detection and treatment of vulnerable plaques and vulnerable patients: novel approaches to prevention of coronary events. Circulation 2006;114(22):2390–411.

30. Hutter R, Valdiviezo C, Sauter BV, et al. Caspase-3 and tissue factor expression in lipid-rich plaque macrophages: evidence for apoptosis as link between inflammation and atherothrombosis. Circulation 2004;109(16):2001–8.

31. Glagov S, Weisenberg E, Zarins CK, et al. Compensatory enlargement of human atherosclerotic coronary arteries. N Engl J Med 1987;316(22):1371–5.

32. Varnava AM, Mills PG, Davies MJ. Relationship between coronary artery remodeling and plaque vulnerability. Circulation 2002;105(8):939–43.

33. Tronc F, Mallat Z, Lehoux S, et al. Role of matrix metalloproteinases in blood flow-induced arterial enlargement: interaction with NO. Arterioscler Thromb Vasc Biol 2000;20(12):E120–6.

34. Burke AP, Kolodgie FD, Farb A, et al. Morphological predictors of arterial remodeling in coronary atherosclerosis. Circulation 2002;105(3):297–303.

35. Schoenhagen P, Ziada KM, Kapadia SR, et al. Extent and direction of arterial remodeling in stable versus unstable coronary syndromes: an intravascular ultrasound study. Circulation 2000;101(6):598–603.

36. Corti R, Fayad ZA, Fuster V, et al. Effects of lipid-lowering by simvastatin on human atherosclerotic lesions: a longitudinal study by high-resolution, noninvasive magnetic resonance imaging. Circulation 2001;104(3):249–52.

37. Nissen SE, Nicholls SJ, Sipahi I, et al. Effect of very high-intensity statin therapy on regression of coronary atherosclerosis: the ASTEROID trial. JAMA 2006;295(13):1556–65.

38. Moreno PR, Purushothaman KR, Zias E, et al. Neovascularization in human atherosclerosis. Curr Mol Med 2006;6(5):457–77.

39. Simons M. Angiogenesis: where do we stand now? Circulation 2005;111(12):1556–66.

40. Moreno PR, Purushothaman KR, Sirol M, et al. Neovascularization in human atherosclerosis. Circulation 2006;113(18):2245–52.

41. de Boer OJ, van der Wal AC, Teeling P, et al. Leucocyte recruitment in rupture prone regions of lipid-rich plaques: a prominent role for neovascularization? Cardiovasc Res 1999;41(2):443–9.

42. O'Brien KD, Allen MD, McDonald TO, et al. Vascular cell adhesion molecule-1 is expressed in human coronary atherosclerotic plaques. J Clin Invest 1993;92:945–51.

43. O'Brien KD, McDonald TO, Chait A, et al. Neovascular expression of E-selectin, intercellular adhesion molecule-1, and vascular cell adhesion molecule-1 in human atherosclerosis and their relation to intimal leukocyte content. Circulation 1996;93(4):672–82.

44. Moreno PR, Fuster V. New aspects in the pathogenesis of diabetic atherothrombosis. J Am Coll Cardiol 2004;44(12):2293–300.

45. Moreno PR, Purushothaman KR, Fuster V, et al. Plaque neovascularization is increased in ruptured atherosclerotic lesions of human aorta: implications for plaque vulnerability. Circulation 2004;110(14): 2032–8.

46. Moreno PR, Purushothaman KR, O'Connor WN, et al. Microvessel sprouting, red blood cell extravasation, and peri-vascular inflammation is increased in plaques from patients with diabetes mellitus. J Am Coll Cardiol 2005;45:430A.

47. Arbustini E, Morbini P, D'Armini AM, et al. Plaque composition in plexogenic and thromboembolic pulmonary hypertension: the critical role of thrombotic material in pultaceous core formation. Heart 2002;88(2):177–82.

48. Kolodgie FD, Gold HK, Burke AP, et al. Intraplaque hemorrhage and progression of coronary atheroma. N Engl J Med 2003;349(24):2316–25.

49. Levy AP, Moreno PR. Intraplaque hemorrhage. Curr Mol Med 2006;6(5):479–88.

50. Levy AP. Haptoglobin: a major susceptibility gene for diabetic cardiovascular disease. Isr Med Assoc J 2004;6(5):308–10.

51. Asleh R, Marsh S, Shilkrut M, et al. Genetically determined heterogeneity in hemoglobin scavenging and susceptibility to diabetic cardiovascular disease. Circ Res 2003;92(11):1193–200.

52. Asleh R, Guetta J, Kalet-Litman S, et al. Haptoglobin genotype- and diabetes-dependent differences in iron-mediated oxidative stress in vitro and in vivo. Circ Res 2005;96(4):435–41.

53. Levy AP, Roguin A, Hochberg I, et al. Haptoglobin phenotype and vascular complications in patients with diabetes. N Engl J Med 2000;343(13):969–70.

54. Levy AP, Hochberg I, Jablonski K, et al. Haptoglobin phenotype is an independent risk factor for cardiovascular disease in individuals with diabetes: The Strong Heart Study. J Am Coll Cardiol 2002;40(11):1984–90.

55. Roguin A, Koch W, Kastrati A, et al. Haptoglobin genotype is predictive of major adverse cardiac events in the 1-year period after percutaneous transluminal coronary angioplasty in individuals with diabetes. Diabetes Care 2003;26(9):2628–31.

56. Suleiman M, Aronson D, Asleh R, et al. Haptoglobin polymorphism predicts 30-day mortality and heart failure in patients with diabetes and acute myocardial infarction. Diabetes 2005;54(9):2802–6.

57. Granada JF, Kaluza GL, Wilensky RL, et al. Porcine models of coronary atherosclerosis and vulnerable plaque for imaging and interventional research. EuroIntervention 2009;5(1):140–8.

58. Granada JF, Kaluza GL, Raizner AE, et al. Vulnerable plaque paradigm: prediction of future clinical events based on a morphological definition. Catheter Cardiovasc Interv 2004;62(3):364–74.

59. Fujii K, Mintz GS, Carlier SG, et al. Intravascular ultrasound profile analysis of ruptured coronary plaques. Am J Cardiol 2006;98(4):429–35.

60. DeMaria AN, Narula J, Mahmud E, et al. Imaging vulnerable plaque by ultrasound. J Am Coll Cardiol 2006;47(8 Suppl):C32–9.

61. Ge J, Chirillo F, Schwedtmann J, et al. Screening of ruptured plaques in patients with coronary artery disease by intravascular ultrasound. Heart 1999; 81(6):621–7.

62. Kim SH, Hong MK, Park DW, et al. Impact of plaque characteristics analyzed by intravascular ultrasound on long-term clinical outcomes. Am J Cardiol 2009;103(9):1221–6.

63. Peters RJ, Kok WE, Havenith MG, et al. Histopathologic validation of intracoronary ultrasound imaging. J Am Soc Echocardiogr 1994;7(3 Pt 1): 230–41.

64. Komiyama N, Berry GJ, Kolz ML, et al. Tissue characterization of atherosclerotic plaques by intravascular ultrasound radiofrequency signal analysis: an in vitro study of human coronary arteries. Am Heart J 2000; 140(4):565–74.

65. Sano K, Kawasaki M, Ishihara Y, et al. Assessment of vulnerable plaques causing acute coronary syndrome using integrated backscatter intravascular ultrasound. J Am Coll Cardiol 2006;47(4): 734–41.

66. Yamagishi M, Terashima M, Awano K, et al. Morphology of vulnerable coronary plaque: insights from follow-up of patients examined by intravascular ultrasound before an acute coronary syndrome. J Am Coll Cardiol 2000;35(1):106–11.

67. Bayturan O, Tuzcu EM, Nicholls SJ, et al. Attenuated plaque at nonculprit lesions in patients enrolled in intravascular ultrasound atherosclerosis progression trials. JACC Cardiovasc Interv 2009; 2(7):672–8.

68. Lee SY, Mintz GS, Kim SY, et al. Attenuated plaque detected by intravascular ultrasound: clinical, angiographic, and morphologic features and post-percutaneous coronary intervention complications in patients with acute coronary syndromes. JACC Cardiovasc Interv 2009;2(1):65–72.

69. Schoenhagen P, Nissen SE, Tuzcu EM. Coronary arterial remodeling: from bench to bedside. Curr Atheroscler Rep 2003;5(2):150–4.

70. Feinstein SB. Contrast ultrasound imaging of the carotid artery vasa vasorum and atherosclerotic plaque neovascularization. J Am Coll Cardiol 2006;48(2):236–43.

71. Goertz DE, Frijlink ME, Tempel D, et al. Contrast harmonic intravascular ultrasound: a feasibility study for vasa vasorum imaging. Invest Radiol 2006;41(8):631–8.

72. Nair A, Kuban BD, Obuchowski N, et al. Assessing spectral algorithms to predict atherosclerotic plaque composition with normalized and raw intravascular ultrasound data. Ultrasound Med Biol 2001; 27(10):1319–31.

73. Nair A, Kuban BD, Tuzcu EM, et al. Coronary plaque classification with intravascular ultrasound radiofrequency data analysis. Circulation 2002; 106(17):2200–6.

74. Eagle_Eye_Gold_catheter. Available at: http://www.volcanotherapeutics.com/files/pdf/EEgold_US.pdf.

75. Van Herck J, De Meyer G, Ennekens G, et al. Validation of in vivo plaque characterisation by virtual histology in a rabbit model of atherosclerosis. EuroIntervention 2009;5(1):149–56.

76. Hong MK, Park DW, Lee CW, et al. Effects of statin treatments on coronary plaques assessed by volumetric virtual histology intravascular ultrasound analysis. JACC Cardiovasc Interv 2009;2(7):679–88.

77. Rodriguez-Granillo GA, Garcia-Garcia HM, Mc Fadden EP, et al. In vivo intravascular ultrasound-derived thin-cap fibroatheroma detection using ultrasound radiofrequency data analysis. J Am Coll Cardiol 2005;46(11):2038–42.

78. Serruys PW. Fourth annual American College of Cardiology international lecture: a journey in the interventional field. J Am Coll Cardiol 2006;47(9): 1754–68.

79. Nasu K, Tsuchikane E, Katoh O, et al. Accuracy of in vivo coronary plaque morphology assessment: a validation study of in vivo virtual histology compared with in vitro histopathology. J Am Coll Cardiol 2006;47(12):2405–12.

80. Davies MJ. Pathophysiology of acute coronary syndromes. Indian Heart J 2000;52(4):473–9.

81. Surmely JF, Nasu K, Fujita H, et al. Coronary plaque composition of culprit/target lesions according to the clinical presentation: a virtual histology intravascular ultrasound analysis. Eur Heart J 2006;24:2933–44.

82. Rodriguez-Granillo GA, Garcia-Garcia HM, Valgimigli M, et al. Global characterization of coronary plaque rupture phenotype using three-vessel intravascular ultrasound radiofrequency data analysis. Eur Heart J 2006;27(16):1921–7.

83. Rodriguez-Granillo GA, McFadden EP, Valgimigli M, et al. Coronary plaque composition of nonculprit lesions, assessed by in vivo intracoronary ultrasound radio frequency data analysis, is related to clinical presentation. Am Heart J 2006;151(5):1020–4.

84. Surmely JF, Nasu K, Fujita H, et al. Association of coronary plaque composition and arterial remodeling: a virtual histology intravascular ultrasound analysis. Heart 2007;93:928–32.

85. Rodriguez-Granillo GA, Serruys PW, Garcia-Garcia HM, et al. Coronary artery remodelling is related to plaque composition. Heart 2006;92(3): 388–91.

86. Schaar JA, De Korte CL, Mastik F, et al. Characterizing vulnerable plaque features with intravascular elastography. Circulation 2003;108(21):2636–41.

87. Low AF, Tearney GJ, Bouma BE, et al. Technology Insight: optical coherence tomography–current status and future development. Nat Clin Pract Cardiovasc Med 2006;3(3):154–62 [quiz 172].

88. Tearney GJ, Waxman S, Shishkov M, et al. Three-dimensional coronary artery microscopy by intracoronary optical frequency domain imaging. JACC Cardiovasc Imaging 2008;1:752–61.

89. Jang IK, Tearney GJ, MacNeill B, et al. In vivo characterization of coronary atherosclerotic plaque by use of optical coherence tomography. Circulation 2005;111(12):1551–5.

90. Giattina SD, Courtney BK, Herz PR, et al. Assessment of coronary plaque collagen with polarization sensitive optical coherence tomography (PS-OCT). Int J Cardiol 2006;107(3):400–9.

91. Tearney GJ, Yabushita H, Houser SL, et al. Quantification of macrophage content in atherosclerotic plaques by optical coherence tomography. Circulation 2003;107(1):113–9.

92. MacNeill BD, Jang IK, Bouma BE, et al. Focal and multi-focal plaque macrophage distributions in patients with acute and stable presentations of coronary artery disease. J Am Coll Cardiol 2004; 44(5):972–9.

93. Fuster V, Fayad ZA, Moreno PR, et al. Atherothrombosis and high-risk plaque: Part II: approaches by noninvasive computed tomographic/magnetic resonance imaging. J Am Coll Cardiol 2005;46(7): 1209–18.

94. Fuster V, Corti R, Fayad ZA, et al. Integration of vascular biology and magnetic resonance imaging in the understanding of atherothrombosis and acute coronary syndromes. J Thromb Haemost 2003;1(7):1410–21.

95. Sirol M, Fuster V, Fayad ZA. Plaque imaging and characterization using magnetic resonance imaging: towards molecular assessment. Curr Mol Med 2006;6(5):541–8.

96. Schneiderman J, Wilensky RL, Weiss A, et al. Diagnosis of thin-cap fibroatheromas by a self-contained intravascular magnetic resonance imaging probe in ex vivo human aortas and in situ coronary arteries. J Am Coll Cardiol 2005; 45(12):1961–9.

97. Lipinski MJ, Frias JC, Fayad ZA. Advances in detection and characterization of atherosclerosis using contrast agents targeting the macrophage. J Nucl Cardiol 2006;13(5):699–709.

98. Jaffer FA, Libby P, Weissleder R. Molecular and cellular imaging of atherosclerosis: emerging applications. J Am Coll Cardiol 2006;47(7):1328–38.

99. Rudd JH, Warburton EA, Fryer TD, et al. Imaging atherosclerotic plaque inflammation with

[^{18}F]-fluorodeoxyglucose positron emission tomography. Circulation 2002;105(23):2708–11.

100. Davies JR, Rudd JH, Weissberg PL, et al. Radionuclide imaging for the detection of inflammation in vulnerable plaques. J Am Coll Cardiol 2006;47(8 Suppl):C57–68.

101. Lipinski MJ, Amirbekian V, Frias JC, et al. MRI to detect atherosclerosis with gadolinium-containing immunomicelles targeting the macrophage scavenger receptor. Magn Reson Med 2006;56(3):601–10.

102. Fayad ZA, Amirbekian V, Toussaint JF, et al. Identification of interleukin-2 for imaging atherosclerotic inflammation. Eur J Nucl Med Mol Imaging 2006;33(2):111–6.

103. Sosnovik DE, Schellenberger EA, Nahrendorf M, et al. Magnetic resonance imaging of cardiomyocyte apoptosis with a novel magneto-optical nanoparticle. Magn Reson Med 2005;54(3):718–24.

104. Purushothaman KR, Sanz J, Zias E, et al. Atherosclerosis neovascularization and imaging. Curr Mol Med 2006;6(5):549–56.

105. Winter PM, Morawski AM, Caruthers SD, et al. Molecular imaging of angiogenesis in early-stage atherosclerosis with alpha(v)beta3-integrin-targeted nanoparticles. Circulation 2003;108(18):2270–4.

106. Matter CM, Schuler PK, Alessi P, et al. Molecular imaging of atherosclerotic plaques using a human antibody against the extra-domain B of fibronectin. Circ Res 2004;95(12):1225–33.

107. Kelly KA, Allport JR, Tsourkas A, et al. Detection of vascular adhesion molecule-1 expression using a novel multimodal nanoparticle. Circ Res 2005;96(3):327–36.

108. Takaya N, Yuan C, Chu B, et al. Presence of intraplaque hemorrhage stimulates progression of carotid atherosclerotic plaques: a high-resolution magnetic resonance imaging study. Circulation 2005;111(21):2768–75.

109. Takaya N, Yuan C, Chu B, et al. Association between carotid plaque characteristics and subsequent ischemic cerebrovascular events: a prospective assessment with MRI–initial results. Stroke 2006;37(3):818–23.

110. Puppini G, Furlan F, Cirota N, et al. Characterisation of carotid atherosclerotic plaque: comparison between magnetic resonance imaging and histology. Radiol Med (Torino) 2006;111(7):921–30.

111. Uchida Y, Nakamura F, Tomaru T, et al. Prediction of acute coronary syndromes by percutaneous coronary angioscopy in patients with stable angina. Am Heart J 1995;130(2):195–203.

112. Asakura M, Ueda Y, Yamaguchi O, et al. Extensive development of vulnerable plaques as a pan-coronary process in patients with myocardial infarction: an angioscopic study. J Am Coll Cardiol 2001;37(5):1284–8.

113. Ohtani T, Ueda Y, Mizote I, et al. Number of yellow plaques detected in a coronary artery is associated with future risk of acute coronary syndrome: detection of vulnerable patients by angioscopy. J Am Coll Cardiol 2006;47(11):2194–200.

114. Moreno PR, Muller JE. Detection of high-risk atherosclerotic coronary plaques by intravascular spectroscopy. J Interv Cardiol 2003;16(3):243–52.

115. Gardner CM, Tan H, Hull EL, et al. Detection of lipid core coronary plaques in autopsy specimens with a novel catheter-based near-infrared spectroscopy system. JACC Imaging 2008;1(5):638–48.

116. van de Poll SW, Kastelijn K, Bakker Schut TC, et al. On-line detection of cholesterol and calcification by catheter based Raman spectroscopy in human atherosclerotic plaque ex vivo. Heart 2003;89(9):1078–82.

117. Moreno PR, Lodder RA, Purushothaman KR, et al. Detection of lipid pool, thin fibrous cap, and inflammatory cells in human aortic atherosclerotic plaques by near-infrared spectroscopy. Circulation 2002;105(8):923–7.

118. Waxman S, Dixon SR, L'Allier P, et al. In vivo validation of a catheter-based near-infrared spectroscopy system for detection of lipid core coronary plaques: initial results of the SPECTACL study. JACC Imaging 2009;2(7):858–68.

119. Caplan JD, Waxman S, Nesto RW, et al. Near-infrared spectroscopy for the detection of vulnerable coronary artery plaques. J Am Coll Cardiol 2006;47(8 Suppl):C92–6.

120. Madjid M, Willerson JT, Casscells SW. Intracoronary thermography for detection of high-risk vulnerable plaques. J Am Coll Cardiol 2006;47(8 Suppl):C80–5.

121. Kawasaki M, Bouma BE, Bressner J, et al. Diagnostic accuracy of optical coherence tomography and integrated backscatter intravascular ultrasound images for tissue characterization of human coronary plaques. J Am Coll Cardiol 2006;48(1):81–8.

122. Romer TJ, Brennan JF 3rd, Puppels GJ, et al. Intravascular ultrasound combined with Raman spectroscopy to localize and quantify cholesterol and calcium salts in atherosclerotic coronary arteries. Arterioscler Thromb Vasc Biol 2000;20(2):478–83.

123. Ambrose JA, D'Agate DJ. Classification of systemic therapies for potential stabilization of the vulnerable plaque to prevent acute myocardial infarction. Am J Cardiol 2005;95(3):379–82.

124. Cannon CP, Steinberg BA, Murphy SA, et al. Meta-analysis of cardiovascular outcomes trials comparing intensive versus moderate statin therapy. J Am Coll Cardiol 2006;48(3):438–45.

125. Scirica BM, Morrow DA, Cannon CP, et al. Intensive statin therapy and the risk of hospitalization for heart failure after an acute coronary syndrome in

the PROVE IT-TIMI 22 study. J Am Coll Cardiol 2006;47(11):2326–31.

126. Goldenberg I, Goldbourt U, Boyko V, et al. Relation between on-treatment increments in serum high-density lipoprotein cholesterol levels and cardiac mortality in patients with coronary heart disease (from the Bezafibrate Infarction Prevention trial). Am J Cardiol 2006;97(4):466–71.

127. Corti R, Osende J, Hutter R, et al. Fenofibrate induces plaque regression in hypercholesterolemic atherosclerotic rabbits: In vivo demonstration by high-resolution MRI. Atherosclerosis 2006.

128. Naik SU, Wang X, Da Silva JS, et al. Pharmacological activation of liver X receptors promotes reverse cholesterol transport in vivo. Circulation 2006; 113(1):90–7.

129. Tso C, Martinic G, Fan WH, et al. High-density lipoproteins enhance progenitor-mediated endothelium repair in mice. Arterioscler Thromb Vasc Biol 2006;26(5):1144–9.

130. Cannon CP, Braunwald E, McCabe CH, et al. Intensive versus moderate lipid lowering with statins after acute coronary syndromes. N Engl J Med 2004;350(15):1495–504.

131. Waksman R, Leitch IM, Roessler J, et al. Intracoronary photodynamic therapy reduces neointimal growth without suppressing re-endothelialisation in a porcine model. Heart 2006;92(8):1138–44.

132. Waksman R. Photodynamic therapy. New York and London: Taylor & Francis; 2004.

133. Waksman R. Photodynamic therapy. In: Waksman R, Serruys P, editors. Handbook of the vulnerable plaque. 2004. p. 283–96.

134. Dorval JF, Geoffroy P, Sirois MG, et al. Endovascular cryotherapy accentuates the accumulation of the fibrillar collagen types I and III after percutaneous transluminal angioplasty in pigs. J Endovasc Ther 2006;13(1):104–10.

135. Triesscheijn M, Baas P, Schellens JH, et al. Photodynamic therapy in oncology. Oncologist 2006; 11(9):1034–44.

136. Waksman R. Novel photopoint photodynamic therapy for the treatment of atherosclerotic plaques [Abstract]. J Am Coll Cardiol 2003;41:259A.

137. Davies MJ. Detecting vulnerable coronary plaques. Lancet 1996;347(9013):1422–3.

138. Lafont A, Libby P. The smooth muscle cell: sinner or saint in restenosis and the acute coronary syndromes? J Am Coll Cardiol 1998;32(1):283–5.

139. Echeverri D, Purushothaman KR, Moreno PR. Plaque healing after bare metal and drug-eluting stents in an experimental rabbit model of thin-cap fibroatheroma. Brazilian Journal of Interventional Cardiology 2008; 16:478–81.

140. Echeverri D, Purushothaman KR, Kilpatrick D, et al. Plaque stabilization by bare metal and drug-eluting stents in a rabbit model of thin-cap fibroatheroma. Brazilian Journal of Interventional Cardiology 2008; 16:160–77.

141. Feder B. In quest to improve heart therapies, plaque gets a fresh look. New York Times November 27, 2006;. Health: front page.

142. Serruys PW, Kukreja N. Late stent thrombosis in drug-eluting stents: return of the 'VB syndrome'. Nat Clin Pract Cardiovasc Med 2006;3(12):637.

143. Waksman R. Biodegradable stents: they do their job and disappear. J Invasive Cardiol 2006;18(2):70–4.

Physiologic Lesion Assessment During Percutaneous Coronary Intervention

Narbeh Melikian, BSc (Hons), MD, MRCP[a],*,
Francesca Del Furia, MD[b], Carlo Di Mario, MD, PhD, FRCP[c]

KEYWORDS

- Percutaneous coronary intervention
- Coronary angiography • Fractional flow reserve
- Coronary flow reserve

The temporal and spatial resolution of coronary angiography has meant that despite major advances in noninvasive cardiac imaging invasive angiography continues to remain the gold standard for the diagnosis and management of coronary artery disease (CAD). However, the 2-dimensional silhouette image provided by coronary angiography has well-recognized limitations.[1,2] Angiographic images do not accurately represent the true complexity of the luminal morphology in coronary disease, and give no indication of the functional influence of luminal changes on coronary blood flow. These limitations are more pronounced in angiographically intermediate stenoses (40 to 70% of the luminal diameter stenosis) and in patients in whom there is a clear discrepancy between the clinical picture and angiographic findings. In addition, it is well recognized that in such cases there is often poor concordance between the estimated percentage angiographic stenosis and the corresponding intravascular ultrasound (IVUS) image or noninvasive functional data.

The absence of a close correlation between morphologic information derived from coronary angiography and functional evidence for myocardial ischemia has important clinical implications for coronary revascularization. Multiple studies have now confirmed that cardiac prognosis in patients with confirmed CAD is primarily dependent on the presence of myocardial ischemia as opposed to the extent of epicardial vessel stenosis.[2–8] The ACIP (Asymptomatic Cardiac Ischemia Pilot) Trial was one of the initial studies to confirm the role of ischemia in cardiac prognosis by demonstrating that suppression of symptomatic or electrocardiographic episodes of ischemia by revascularization or oral antianginal medication improved prognosis in patients with stable CAD.[4] More recently, long-term follow-up results from the DEFER and FAME (Fractional Flow Reserve versus Angiography for Multivessel Evaluation) trials have further confirmed the importance and clinical utility of ischemia-driven revascularization in patients with CAD.[5–7] In both trials, patients randomized to the ischemia-driven revascularization arm of the study had significantly lower major adverse cardiovascular events (MACE) at follow-up.

However, despite a clear understanding of the limitations of coronary angiography, few patients with angiographic intermediate stenoses routinely undergo evidence-based, ischemia-driven, coronary revascularization. To derive functional information patients in this important group often need to undergo extra investigations such as stress echocardiography or myocardial perfusion scanning as an adjunct to coronary angiography.

[a] Cardiology Department, King's College London British Heart Foundation Centre of Excellence and King's College Hospital, Denmark Hill, London SE5 9RS, UK
[b] Cardiology Department, Cittadella General Hospital, Padua, Italy
[c] Cardiology Department, Royal Brompton Hospital, Sydney Street, London SW3 6NP, UK
* Corresponding author.
E-mail address: narbeh.melikian@kcl.ac.uk (N. Melikian).

Cardiol Clin 28 (2010) 31–54
doi:10.1016/j.ccl.2009.10.002

The extra procedures and the in-/outpatient admissions required are often an inconvenience to patients, can be unattractive in financial terms, may be perceived to be delaying delivery of a definitive treatment, and hence are frequently avoided, giving rise to a large number of inappropriate decisions regarding revascularization. To address some of the perceived problems in deriving functional data in patients with intermediate epicardial stenoses and to facilitate ischemia-driven coronary revascularization, there has been a concerted effort over the past 10 to 15 years to develop physiologic indices that can be used as an adjunct to coronary angiography in the cardiac catheterization laboratory.

Fractional flow reserve (FFR) is the current "gold standard" index for functional evaluation of intermediate epicardial stenoses in the cardiac catheterization laboratory. FFR has superseded earlier indices such as coronary flow reserve (CFR) and relative coronary flow reserve (rCFR), which have important conceptual and clinical limitations. Hyperemic stenosis resistance (HSR) is an alternative index, which has recently been validated. However, the clinical applicability of HSR remains unclear and its use is primarily confined to research protocols. As discussed in this article, the ability to simultaneously obtain accurate anatomic and clinically applicable functional/physiologic data in the cardiac catheterization laboratory is an important step in the provision of a true "all-in-one" approach to evidence-based coronary revascularization.

PRINCIPLES OF CORONARY PRESSURE AND FLOW

Our understanding of the principles that govern the association between pressure and flow in the coronary circulation form the basis from which all aforementioned clinically applicable coronary physiologic indices have developed.[2,3,9]

According to Ohm's law, flow within a circuit is proportional to the ratio of the pressure gradient to resistance across the circuit. Ohm's principle can also be applied to determine myocardial blood flow, whereby the gradient within the circuit is derived from the pressure difference between the distal epicardial vessel and the central venous system and resistance from the functional state of the microcirculation and, to a lesser extent, the epicardial vessel (Fig. 1). In a normal epicardial artery, distal coronary pressure is theoretically equal to and dependent on the end-diastolic pressure in the aortic root as there is a minimal resistance and hence pressure drop along a normal vessel, and central venous pressure is equal to or very near to zero. Under physiologic conditions the functional state of the microcirculation is primarily responsible for determining overall resistance in the coronary circulation, with the resistive contribution of the epicardial vessel being negligible. Changes in vascular tone in resistance vessels (vessels of <400 μm in diameter) in response to local factors (including both vasodilator and vasoconstrictor molecules), metabolites, or sympathetic nervous stimulation regulate the overall microvascular response. As a result, small changes in microvascular resistance and/or distal coronary pressure alter myocardial blood flow, with microvascular vasodilatation (to reduce vascular resistance), and/or an increase in distal coronary end-diastolic pressure augmenting myocardial perfusion and microvascular vasoconstriction (to increase vascular resistance), and/or a decrease in distal coronary end-diastolic pressure having the opposite effect. In the healthy myocardium blood flow is continuously regulated as an adaptive response to ensure a close match between myocardial perfusion and metabolic

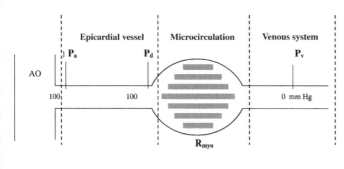

$$Q_{myo} = (P_d - P_v) / R_{myo}$$

Fig. 1. A coronary artery and its microvascular bed. According to Ohm's law, myocardial blood flow (Q_{myo}) is dependent on the ratio of the pressure gradient to resistance across the myocardium. The pressure gradient across the myocardium is determined by the difference between the distal coronary pressure (P_d) and central venous pressure (P_v). P_d in an unobstructed coronary artery is equal to the proximal coronary (P_a) pressure and P_v under physiologic conditions is often equal to or near to zero. The resistance across the myocardium (R_{myo}) is determined primarily by the functional state of the microcirculation, with the resistive contribution of an unobstructed/normal epicardial vessel being negligible. AO, aorta.

demands. Pathologic states that interfere with normal blood flow regulation adversely influence myocardial contraction.

In diseased states, impaired myocardial blood flow occurs in response to microvascular dysfunction, changes in epicardial vessel resistance, or a combination of both. Several conditions such as atherosclerosis, cardiomyopathies, and classic risk factors for vascular disease interfere with the normal vasodilator capacity of the microcirculation, thus blunting the potential for maximally increasing coronary blood flow. Atherosclerosis is also the main underlying cause of changes in epicardial vessel resistance. Diffuse atherosclerotic changes as well as more significant epicardial stenoses increase resistance through a combination of viscous friction, flow separation, turbulence, and micro-eddies in the epicardial vessel. This increase results in loss of energy, leading to a decrease in distal perfusion pressure and thus myocardial blood flow (**Fig. 2**). As depicted in **Figs. 2** and **3** there is a quadratic association between increases in velocity (caused by convective acceleration) and loss of pressure across a given epicardial stenosis.

CORONARY FLOW RESERVE

Gould and colleagues[10] introduced CFR as the fist clinically applicable functional index for assessment of epicardial vessel stenosis in the early 1990s. CFR is defined as *the ratio of steady-state hyperemic flow to baseline flow in a given artery.*

The concept of CFR is based on 2 important observations. First, myocardial oxygen extraction is maximal at rest, thus under physiologic conditions any increase in oxygen demand is met through an increase in myocardial blood flow.[11] In addition, as illustrated in **Fig. 4**, the percentage of epicardial stenosis required to cause a substantial decrease in coronary blood flow in a given vessel is significantly lower during maximal hyperemia (diameter stenosis of 45%) in comparison with flow at rest (diameter stenosis of 85%).[10] Therefore, the relative differences in flow during hyperemia and rest can theoretically provide an indication of the functional significance of an epicardial stenosis.

Validation and Cut-Off Threshold for CFR

The ischemic cut-off threshold for CFR is from less than 2.0 to 2.5.[2,3,9] This threshold is based on a series of studies comparing CFR values in vessels with differing levels of angiographic stenosis with evidence of reversible myocardial ischemia in the corresponding myocardial territory, as detected by standard noninvasive functional tests (**Table 1**).[11–26] Pooled results from multiple studies confirm that a CFR of less than 2.0 has a sensitivity of 86% to 92%, specificity of 89% to 100%, positive predictive value of 84% to 100%, negative predictive value of 77% to 95%, and predictive accuracy of 89% to 96% for detection of reversible myocardial ischemia.

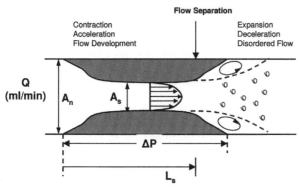

A_s = Area of stenosis

A_n = Area of normal segment

L_S = Effective length of stenosis (up to the point of flow separation)

Fig. 2. Pressure loss across a stenosis is derived from 2 sources: frictional losses along the entrance and throat of the stenosis, and inertial losses stemming from the sudden expansion immediately after the stenosis causing flow separation and eddies. Frictional losses are linearly related to flow (Q) (Law of Poiseuille) and exit losses increase with square of the flow caused by convective acceleration in the narrowed segment (Law of Bernoulli). The total pressure gradient (ΔP) is the sum of the 2 components: $\Delta P = (f_1 \times Q) + (f_2 \times Q^2)$. The loss coefficients f_1 and f_2 are a function of stenosis geometry and rheologic properties of blood (viscosity and density). The equation results in a quadratic relationship (**Fig. 3**), whereby the curvilinear shape demonstrates the presence of nonlinear exit losses. In the absence of stenosis, the second term is zero and the curve becomes straight, with a positive slope that depends on the diameter of the vessel (Law of Poiseuille). (*From* Kern MJ, Lerman A, Bech JW, et al. Physiological assessment of coronary artery disease in the cardiac catheterization laboratory. A scientific statement from the American Heart Association committee on diagnostic and interventional cardiac catheterization council on clinical cardiology. Circulation 2006;114:1321–41; with permission.)

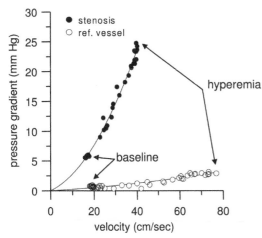

Fig. 3. The association between pressure drop (ΔP) and flow velocity (v) across a stenosis. In the presence of stenosis (*black circles*) there is a quadratic association between ΔP and velocity ($\Delta P = Av + Bv^2$), where A and B are the constants of viscous and separation losses that are determined by the geometry of the stenosis and fluid properties of blood, respectively. In an unobstructed vessel (*open circles*) there is a linear association between ΔP and v, which is dependent on the diameter the vessel (see **Fig. 2**). (*From* Kern MJ, Lerman A, Bech JW, et al. Physiological assessment of coronary artery disease in the cardiac catheterization laboratory. A scientific statement from the American Heart Association committee on diagnostic and interventional cardiac catheterization council on clinical cardiology. Circulation 2006;114:1321–41; with permission.)

Specific Features and Limitations of CFR

CFR is a measure of the capacity to achieve maximal myocardial blood flow in response to a hyperemic stimulus, which is directly dependent on the relative resistive influences of the epicardial vessel and its corresponding microvascular compartment. However, as an index it does not differentiate between the relative contributions of the epicardial or microvascular compartments toward changes in blood flow.[27] Therefore, the clinical applicability of CFR as a functional index of epicardial vessel stenosis is highly limited. There are currently only 2 frequently encountered clinical scenarios for which measurement of CFR may be of clinical value. (1) A normal CFR (>2.5), which implies low microvascular and epicardial resistance, and hence adequate myocardial perfusion. In such a case one can assume that there is no functionally significant epicardial stenosis and that microvascular function is normal. (2) Assessment of microvascular function in individuals who have an entirely normal epicardial vessel, whereby any abnormalities in flow and hence CFR are secondary to microvascular dysfunction.

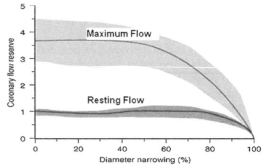

Fig. 4. Coronary flow reserve (CFR) (expressed as the ratio of maximum to resting blood flow) plotted as function of percentage epicardial vessel narrowing. At maximal hyperemia (maximal flow), CFR begins to be impaired at approximately 50% diameter narrowing. However, at rest similar changes occur at a much higher level of narrowing (approximately 80%). The *shaded area* represents the levels of variability about the mean. (*From* Gould KL, Lipscomb K, Hamilton GW. Physiologic basis for assessing critical coronary stenosis. Instantaneous flow response and regional distribution during coronary hyperaemia as measures of coronary flow reserve. Am J Cardiol 1974;33:87–94; with permission.)

Another important shortcoming of CFR is the observation that its value is altered by conditions that influence basal or hyperemic flow, thus limiting its applicability as index for serial measurements.[28,29] These conditions include changes in hemodynamic parameters (pulse rate, blood pressure, and contractility) and abnormal ventricular loading conditions (as seen in the context of advancing age, left ventricular hypertrophy, and fibrosis). The poor reproducibility of CFR is clearly illustrated by the inverse association between CFR and pulse rate, whereby for each 15-beat increase in heart rate there is a corresponding 10% decrease in CFR.

Clinical Applications of CFR

The inability of CFR to differentiate between the relative contributions of the epicardial and microvascular compartments toward myocardial ischemia, combined with clinical availability of alternative highly specific indices of epicardial stenoses such as FFR and HSR, has meant that CFR is now rarely used as a decision-making tool to either defer or recommend coronary revascularization in the catheterization laboratory.

However, despite its fundamental limitation, several studies have shown that deferral of revascularization based on a CFR of greater than 2.0 in patients with angiographically intermediate stenoses is associated with a low MACE rate

Table 1
Comparison of CFR, rCFR, FFR, and HSR to detect reversible myocardial ischemia with standard noninvasive functional tests

Study	n	Functional Test	BCV	Accuracy %
CFR				
Joyce[12]	30	SPECT	2.0	94
Miller[13]	33	SPECT	2.0	89
Deychak[14]	17	SPECT	1.8	96
Tron[15]	62	SPECT	2.0	84
Donohue[11]	50	SPECT	2.0	88
Heller[16]	55	SPECT	1.7	92
Schulman[17]	35	X-ECG	2.0	86
Danzi[18]	30	DSE	2.0	87
Verberne[19]	37	SPECT	1.9	85
Piek[20]	225	X-ECG	2.1	76
Abe[21]	46	SPECT	2.0	92
Chamuleau[23,a]	127	SPECT	1.7	76
Duffy[22]	28	DSE	2.0	88
El-Shafei[24]	48	SPECT	1.9	77
Meuwissen[25]	151	SPECT	1.7	75
Voudris[26]	48	SPECT	1.7	75
rCFR				
Verberne[19]	37	SPECT	0.65	85
Chamuleau[23,a]	127	SPECT	0.60	78
Duffy[22]	28	DSE	0.75	81
El-Shafei[24]	48	SPECT	0.75	75
Voudris[26]	48	SPECT	0.64	92
FFR				
Pijls[42,43]	60	X-ECG	0.74	97
De Bruyne[44]	60	X-ECG/SPECT	0.66	87
Pijls[42,43]	45	X-ECG/SPECT/DSE	0.75	93
Bartunek[45]	37	DSE	0.67	90
Abe[21]	46	SPECT	0.75	91
Chamuleau[23,a]	127	SPECT	0.74	77
Caymaz[46]	40	SPECT	0.75	95
Fearon[47]	10	SPECT	0.75	95
De Bruyne[49]	57	SPECT	0.78	85
Jimenez-Navarro[48]	21	DSE	0.75	90
Meuwissen[25]	151	SPECT	0.74	75
Usui[51]	167	SPECT	0.75	79
Yanagisawa[50]	165	SPECT	0.75	76
HSR				
Meuwissen[25]	151	SPECT	0.80	87

n indicates number of patients. BCV, best cut-off value (defined as the value with highest sum of sensitivity and specificity); X-ECG, exercise ECG test; DSE, dobutamine stress echocardiography.
[a] Multivessel disease.
Data from Kern MJ, Lerman A, Bech JW, et al. Physiologic assessment of coronary artery disease in the cardiac catheterization laboratory. A scientific statement from the American Heart Association committee on diagnostic and interventional cardiac catheterization council on clinical cardiology. Circulation 2006;114:1321–41.

(Table 2).[30–32] The clinical utility of CFR was best illustrated by the ILIAS (Intermediate Lesion: Intra-coronary flow ASsessment versus 99mTc-setamibi single-photon emission computed tomography [MIBI SPECT]) study wherein the role of CFR as an index of myocardial ischemia was compared with MIBI SPECT in angiographically intermediate stenosis in 191 patients with multivessel CAD.[32] Percutaneous coronary intervention (PCI) was performed when both CFR and MIBI SPECT were positive for ischemia, and deferred when both investigations were negative. In patients in whom there was a disparity between CFR and MIBI SPECT, revascularization was deferred (deferred patients n = 182). At 1-year follow-up 19 MACE had occurred in the deferred group, with CFR being a more accurate predictor of events than MIBI SPECT (relative risk: 3.9).

Assessment of CFR subsequent to balloon angioplasty or stent deployment has also played an important historical role in highlighting the importance of optimal lesion dilatation during PCI.[33] In the DEBATE (Doppler Endpoints Balloon Angioplasty Trial Europe) trial, Serruys and colleagues[33] demonstrated that in patients with single-vessel coronary disease a CFR of 2.5 or greater in association with angiographic stenosis of 35% or greater after balloon angioplasty was associated with a favorable medium-term clinical outcome (MACE rate of <20%). The DESTINI (Doppler Endpoint STenting International Investigation) study group further demonstrated that long-term clinical outcome in patients undergoing combined CFR and angiographic guided multivessel balloon angioplasty was comparable to elective stent deployment during PCI.[34] In addition, the DEBATE II study confirmed that coronary stent implantation subsequent to suboptimal balloon angioplasty, as detected by a CFR less than 2.5, improved clinical outcome by decreasing MACE rates from 26.7% to 10.7%.[35,36] Although CFR-guided balloon angioplasty is clinically valuable, this approach to PCI has been superseded by almost universal stent implantation, and has very limited value in modern "real world" interventional practice.

Clinical Techniques for Assessment of CFR

Estimation of coronary blood flow is essential for derivation of CFR. However, direct in vivo measurement of blood flow in the catheterization laboratory is not possible. Therefore, to derive CFR coronary blood flow is estimated through measurement of blood flow velocity or indirectly

Table 2
Outcomes after deferral of coronary intervention in intermediate coronary stenoses based on CFR and FFR values

Study	n	Defer Value	MACE	Follow-up Months
CFR				
Kern[30]	88	2.0	7%	9
Ferrari[31]	22	2.0	9%	15
Chamuleau[32b]	143	2.0	6%	12
FFR				
Bech[5,57,63]	100	0.75	8%	18
Bech[5,57,63]	150	0.75	8%	24
Hernández García[61]	43	0.75	12%	11
Bech[5,57,63a]	24	0.75	21%	29
Rieber[58,59]	47	0.75	13%	12
Chamuleau[60]	92	0.75	9%	12
Rieber[58,59]	24	0.75	8%	12
Leesar[62,65,73,c]	34	0.75	9%	12

n indicates number of patients. MACE, major adverse cardiovascular events (primarily recurrent rates of PCI as rates of death and myocardial infarction were not significant).
[a] Left main stem stenosis.
[b] Multivessel disease.
[c] Unstable angina.
Data from Kern MJ, Lerman A, Bech JW, et al. Physiologic assessment of coronary artery disease in the cardiac catheterization laboratory. A scientific statement from the American Heart Association committee on diagnostic and interventional cardiac catheterization council on clinical cardiology. Circulation 2006;114:1321–41.

by applying the principles of thermodilution to the coronary circulation.

Flow velocity and derivation of CFR

Volumetric coronary blood flow can be measured from the product of vessel surface area (cm^2) and blood flow velocity (cm/s) with separate measurements at baseline and during maximal hyperemia used to derive CFR. However, experimental data have shown that in a vessel with a constant surface area, volumetric flow is directly proportional to flow velocity, thus allowing CFR to simply be derived from the ratio of hyperemia to baseline coronary blood flow velocity (**Box 1**).

During cardiac catheterization, blood flow velocity is measured using a commercially available intracoronary Doppler angioplasty guidewire (FloWire; Volcano Inc, Rancho Cordova, CA). The Doppler guidewire has a microscopic ultrasound emitting and receiving crystal at its tip (Doppler crystal), which measures velocity through frequency shift (defined as the difference between the transmitted and returning frequency) as red blood cells go past the Doppler crystal [Velocity (v) = ($f_1 - f_0$) × $c/(2f_0)$ × cos θ, where v = velocity of blood flow, f_0 = transmitting transducer frequency, f_1 = returning frequency, c = constant for speed of sound in blood, and θ = angle of incidence]. The forward directed ultrasound beam diverges at 14° from the Doppler transducer to include as large a proportion of the flow velocity profile as possible.

Box 1
Derivation of $CFR_{Doppler}$

CFR is derived from the ratio of maximal hyperemic flow (Q_{max}) to baseline ($Q_{baseline}$) coronary blood flow:

$$CFR_{Doppler} = Q_{max}/Q_{baseline}$$

Volumetric blood flow in a given vessel can be derived from the product of the vessel surface area (SA) and blood flow velocity (v). As a result, Q can be substituted for the vessel surface area and velocity:

$$CFR_{Doppler} = (SA \times v_{max})/(SA \times v_{baseline})$$

Assuming a constant surface area (after administration of intracoronary isosorbide dinitrate [ISDN]), CFR can therefore simply be derived from the ratio of hyperemic (v_{max}) to baseline ($v_{baseline}$) blood flow velocity:

$$CFR_{Doppler} = v_{max}/v_{baseline}$$

where v_{max} = hyperemic blood flow velocity, $v_{baseline}$ = blood flow at baseline (rest).

The Doppler guidewire is introduced into the study artery under fluoroscopic guidance through a standard guiding catheter. Intracoronary nitrates (often 200 µg ISDN) are administered before any measurement to ensure vessel cross-sectional area remains constant over the measurement period (both hyperemic and baseline). In addition, intracoronary nitrates ensure maximal/near maximal dilatation of the epicardial vessel. The Doppler guidewire is connected to its dedicated interface (ComboMap), which uses on-line fast Fourier transformation to display real-time continuous gray-scale Doppler spectral traces (**Fig. 5**). The wire is advanced until the Doppler crystal at the tip of the wire is positioned the equivalent of 5 to 10 artery-diameter lengths (approximately >2.0 cm) beyond the stenosis and manipulated (through gentle rotation, advancement, or withdrawal) until optimal velocity traces are obtained. The position of the Doppler crystal approximately 2 cm beyond the stenosis will allow sampling of signals in an area of reestablished laminar flow. The software within the analyzer automatically tracks instantaneous peak velocity values from the Doppler traces and computes the average peak (blood flow) velocity (APV) over 2 to 5 heart beats. APV is measured at baseline and at peak steady-state hyperemia, and CFR computed from the ratio of the 2 values.

Thermodilution and derivation of CFR

Estimation of CFR using the thermodilution technique is based on the indicator dilution theory, which states that in a given vessel with a constant surface area flow is inversely proportional to the mean transit time (T_{mn}) of an injectate.[37] The indicator dilution theory has been validated in experimental and in vivo human studies demonstrating that the percentage decrease in T_{mn} of a hand-held intracoronary saline injectate correlates inversely with the percentage increase in true coronary flow (Coronary Flow $\propto 1/T_{mn}$).[37,38] Based on this association, CFR can be derived from the ratio of baseline to hyperemic T_{mn} (**Box 2**).

During cardiac catheterization T_{mn} is derived from the thermodilution profile of a hand-held injectate of room-temperature saline using a commercially available pressure/temperature sensor-tipped angioplasty guidewire (RadiWire; RadiMedical Systems Inc, Uppsala, Sweden). The thermodilution profile is generated from the specific properties of the RadiWire that detect changes in temperature (and pressure, see assessment of FFR) as the injectate passes along the wire. Temperature-dependent changes in electrical resistance in the shaft of the wire act as a proximal thermistor, allowing detection of the start of the

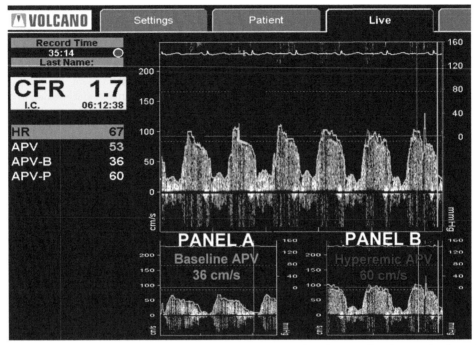

Fig. 5. Real-time continuous gray-scale Doppler spectral traces at baseline (*PANEL A*) and at maximal steady state hyperemia (*PANEL B*) as measured by an intracoronary Doppler wire (FloWire). CFR is derived from the ratio of the average peak velocity values over a prespecified number of heartbeats (2 beats in the example provided) at maximal hyperemia (APV_{max}) to baseline ($APV_{baseline}$) (CFR = $APV_{max}/APV_{baseline}$ = 60/36 = 1.7).

injection. A high-fidelity pressure/temperature sensor mounted at the tip of the wire detects distal passage of the injectate.[37,38] The wire is connected to its dedicated interface (Radi-Analyzer), which computes the thermodilution curve and its

---

Box 2
Derivation of CFR_{Thermo}

CFR is derived from the ratio of maximal hyperemic flow (Q_{max}) to baseline ($Q_{baseline}$) coronary blood flow:

$$CFR_{Thermo} = Q_{max}/Q_{baseline}$$

According to the indicator dilution theory, in a vessel with a constant surface area, flow is inversely proportional to the mean transit time (T_{mn}) of a hand-held injectate ($Q \propto 1/T_{mn}$). As a result Q can be represented as a change in T_{mn}:

$$CFR_{Thermo} = (1/\text{maximal } T_{mn})/$$
$$(1/\text{baseline } T_{mn})$$

Therefore, CFR can be derived from the ratio of baseline to maximal T_{mn}:

$$CFR_{Thermo} = \text{baseline } T_{mn}/\text{maximal } T_{mn}$$

---

corresponding T_{mn}. The RadiWire has an accuracy of 0.05°C within a temperature range of 15° to 42°C.

As for the Doppler guidewire, the RadiWire is introduced into the coronary artery through a standard angiography guiding catheter. Subsequent to calibration and equalization of pressure/temperature signals, the RadiWire is positioned in the distal third of the artery beyond the stenosis. Intracoronary nitrates are administered to ensure maximal dilatation and constant blood vessel surface area. Thermodilution curves are obtained (in triplicate) from a hand-held, 3- to 5-mL, brisk injection of room-temperature normal saline through the guiding catheter at baseline and at maximal steady state hyperemia (**Fig. 6**). Dedicated software within the Radi-Analyzer unit computes mean baseline and hyperemic T_{mn} values as well as CFR.

Both Doppler- and thermodilution-derived CFR ($CFR_{Doppler}$ and CFR_{Thermo}, respectively) are simple to perform as an adjunct to coronary angiography. However, CFR_{Thermo} has several advantages over $CFR_{Doppler}$. In 10% to 15% of cases the initial Doppler signal may be poor, requiring manipulation of the wire to change the orientation of the Doppler crystal and hence the sample volume. The Doppler signal is also highly sensitive to artifacts from cardiac or respiratory movement.

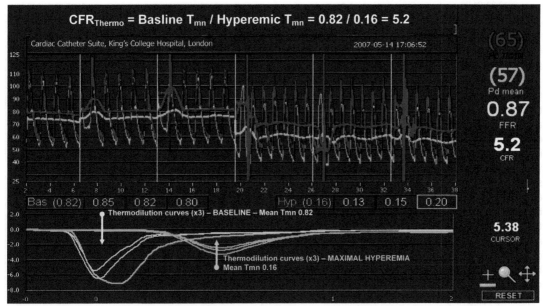

Fig. 6. Thermodilution curves and corresponding transit times (T_{mn}) (in triplicate) of a hand-held brisk intracoronary injection of 3 mL room-temperature saline as measured by an intracoronary temperature/pressure sensor-tipped angioplasty guidewire (RadiWire) and displayed by its dedicated interface (Radi-Analyzer Unit). CFR is computed on-line from the ratio of mean baseline to steady-state hyperemic T_{mn}. Continuous proximal (P_d; in red) and distal (P_a; in green) coronary pressures are also displayed at baseline and maximal hyperemia, allowing simultaneous computation of FFR.

In contrast, CFR_{Thermo} is not open to such artifacts, giving rise to a highly reproducible signal for measurement of CFR.[38,39] In addition, in comparison to measurement of true volumetric coronary blood flow (as measured in open chest in vivo experimental models), the thermodilution technique provides a more accurate estimate of flow whereas Doppler-derived estimates often underestimate volumetric flow and hence CFR.[40]

RELATIVE CORONARY FLOW RESERVE

As outlined, in daily practice CFR is rarely used as the sole indicator of epicardial lesion severity, as it simultaneously interrogates the epicardial and microvascular components of the coronary circulation. To overcome the 2-compartment limitation of CFR, the concept of relative CFR (rCFR) has been developed. rCFR attempts to reduce the influence of confounders on CFR by indexing flow reserve in the interrogated vessel to an adjacent reference "normal"/unobstructed vessel.[41] rCFR is defined *as the ratio of maximal flow in an artery with a stenosis to flow in an adjacent "normal"/unobstructed artery* (**Box 3**).

The proposed normal range for rCFR is 0.80 to 1.0, with an rCFR less than 0.80 indicating a functionally significant epicardial stenosis in the target

---

Box 3
Derivation of rCFR

rCFR attempts to index CFR in the stenosed vessel (CFR_S) to CFR in an adjacent vessel with no stenosis (CFR_N):

$$rCFR = CFR_S / CFR_N$$

Considering CFR can be derived from the ratio of maximal (Q_{max}) to baseline ($Q_{baseline}$) coronary flow, rCFR can be expressed as:

$$rCFR = \left(Q_S^{max} / Q_S^{baseline} \right) / \left(Q_N^{max} / Q_N^{baseline} \right)$$

Assuming uniform distribution of microvascular function, baseline flow in both the stenosed and reference vessel should be equal and thus cancel out. Therefore, rCFR can be expressed as:

$$rCFR = Q_S^{max} / Q_N^{baseline}$$

where S = stenosed artery, N = Normal (reference) artery, Q_S^{max} = Hyperemic blood flow in the stenosed artery, Q_N^{max} = Hyperemic blood flow in the normal (reference) artery.

vessel.[19,22–24,26] As for assessment of CFR, flow is derived from intracoronary Doppler velocity measurements or principles of thermodilution at maximal steady-state hyperemia in the target and reference vessels.

However, despite its conceptual advantages over CFR, rCFR also has several important limitations, which restrict its clinical applicability. To assess rCFR each patient must have at least one entirely normal epicardial vessel. Therefore, as an index of epicardial vessel stenosis, rCFR has very limited applicability in patients with multivessel CAD in whom there may be no suitable reference vessel. In addition, the concept of rCFR is based on the assumption that microvascular function is uniformly distributed throughout the myocardium. rCFR is consequently of no value in conditions with potentially heterogeneous distribution of microvascular function, such as previous myocardial infarction, asymmetric left ventricular hypertrophy, or myocardial fibrosis.

FRACTIONAL FLOW RESERVE

FFR is the current "gold standard" index for assessing functional severity of an epicardial vessel stenosis in catheterization laboratory. FFR has superseded other physiologic indices such as CFR and rCFR, which have important conceptual and clinical limitations. The concept of FFR was introduced by Pijls and colleagues[42,43] and is defined as *the ratio of maximal myocardial blood flow in the presence of an epicardial stenosis to the theoretical maximal flow in the absence of the same stenosis for a given epicardial coronary artery*. FFR can be derived simply from the ratio of distal (poststenotic) (P_d) to proximal (P_a) coronary pressures using an intracoronary pressure sensor-tipped angioplasty guidewire as an adjunct to coronary angiography (**Box 4**). Unlike CFR, which can be influenced by the epicardial vessel as well as the microcirculation, FFR is specific to the epicardial vessel and provides directly applicable clinical data.

Validation and Cut-Off Threshold for FFR

FFR has a well-defined cut-off threshold of less than 0.75 for myocardial ischemia, with a narrow gray zone of between 0.75 and 0.80. The cut-off threshold for FFR is derived from multiple clinical studies comparing FFR values across a range of epicardial vessel stenoses with noninvasive functional tests for reversible myocardial ischemia (see **Table 1**).[42–51] In a seminal study, Pijls and colleagues[43] compared FFR in patients with chest discomfort and angiographically moderate epicardial vessel stenoses with quantitative

---

Box 4
Derivation of FFR

FFR is defined as the ratio of maximal blood flow in the presence of an epicardial stenosis (Q_S^{max}) to the theoretical maximal flow in the absence of the stenosis (Q_N^{max}).

$$FFR = Q_S^{max}/Q_n^{max}$$

Considering flow (Q) can be derived from the pressure (P) gradient across the myocardium divided by the resistance across the myocardium, Q can also be represented according to the relationship between pressure gradient and resistance when deriving FFR:

$$FFR = \left[(P_d - P_v)/R_S^{max}\right]/\left[(P_a - P_v)/R_N^{max}\right]$$

Because all measurements are obtained under maximal hyperemia, resistances will be minimal and equal and thus cancel out:

$$FFR = (P_d - P_v)/(P_a - P_v)$$

In addition under physiologic conditions P_v is either 0 or negligible compared with P_d or P_a. Therefore, FFR can simply be derived from the ratio of distal to proximal coronary pressure at maximal hyperemia:

$$FFR = P_d/P_a$$

P_a = proximal coronary/aortic pressure, P_d = distal coronary pressure, P_v = central venous pressure, Q_S^{max} = hyperemic myocardial blood flow in the presence of a stenosis, Q_N^{max} = hyperemic myocardial blood flow in the absence of a stenosis, R_S^{max} = hyperemic myocardial resistance in the presence of a stenosis, R_N^{max} = hyperemic myocardial resistance in the absence of a stenosis.

---

coronary angiography (QCA) and 3 functional tests for myocardial ischemia (bicycle exercise test, thallium scintigraphy, and dobutamine stress echocardiography) (**Fig. 7**). In all patients with an FFR of less than 0.75, reversible myocardial ischemia was demonstrated unequivocally on at least one noninvasive functional test, and in 87% of patients with FFR greater than 0.75 all 3 noninvasive functional tests were also negative for ischemia. Based on this and other studies, it is now accepted that an FFR of less than 0.75 has a sensitivity of 88%, specificity of 100%, positive predictive value of 100%, negative predictive value of 88%, and overall accuracy of 93% for identification of reversible ischemia.

The theoretical normal value of FFR is 1.0 for every patient and every coronary artery where P_d/P_a is equal to or very close to unity. However, in clinical practice this is extremely rare, as most epicardial vessels, despite a normal angiographic appearance, will have some level of atherosclerosis that confers resistance to blood flow. The lowest FFR value identified in strictly normal angiographic vessels is 0.92, thus giving FFR a normal range of 0.92 to 1.00.[52] Another important feature of FFR is a narrow "gray zone" of 0.75 to 0.80, which spans less than 10% of the entire range of FFR values.

Specific Features and Limitations of FFR

In addition to being a highly sensitive and specific functional index of epicardial stenosis, FFR has several specific features, which contribute to its accuracy and clinical utility.

FFR is not influenced by hemodynamic parameters, and is reproducible

Unlike other physiologic indices, FFR is not influenced by changes in systemic hemodynamics (pulse rate, blood pressure, and contractility).[53] Therefore, the value of FFR for a given stenosis remains constant across a range of clinical conditions. In addition, FFR is highly reproducible (**Fig. 8**). This reproducibility is made possible in part due to the requirement to measure aortic and distal coronary pressures simultaneously in order to derive FFR, and in part due to the extraordinary ability of the microvasculature to vasodilate to exactly the same extent with an identical hyperemic stimulus.

FFR accounts for the influence of collateral vessels

The derivation of FFR requires measurement of P_d at maximal hyperemia. Therefore, the FFR value across a stenosis will account for the physiologic influence of collaterals in both: (1) the vessel that provides the collaterals to another more severely stenosed artery (retrograde flow) and (2) the vessel that receives collaterals from another less severely stenosed artery (anterograde flow).[54] Accounting for the functional influence of collaterals at maximal hyperemia has important implications for revascularization of intermediate stenoses in the "retrograde" vessel and the value of treating the more severe stenosis in the "antegrade" vessel (**Fig. 9**).

FFR has high spatial resolution

The exact position of the distal pressure sensor on the pressure sensor–tipped wire can easily be monitored during angiography and changed by

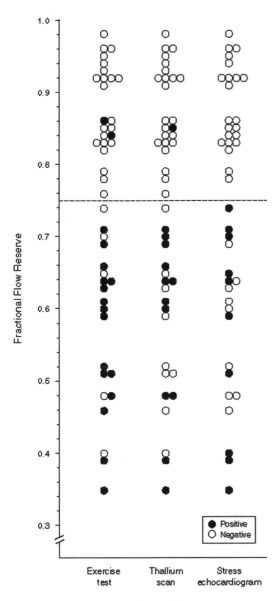

Fig. 7. Plots of FFR in 45 patients with an angiographically intermediate stenosis compared with 3 different noninvasive functional tests. *Black dots* indicate a positive result. A test was considered positive only if it was positive for ischemia before revascularization and negative for ischemia after revascularization. In the 21 patients with FFR less than 0.75 reversible myocardial ischemia was demonstrated unequivocally on at least one noninvasive functional test. In 4 patients with FFR less than 0.75 there was full concordance between all 3 functional tests and FFR. (*From* Pijls NH, De Bruyne B, Peels K, et al. Measurement of fractional flow reserve to assess the functional severity of coronary artery stenoses. N Engl J Med 1996;334:1703–08; with permission.)

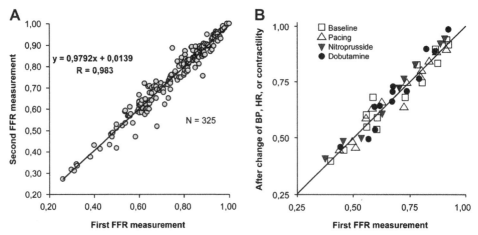

Fig. 8. FFR is highly reproducible. In 325 patients there was a close correlation between 2 serial FFR measurements in the same vessel within a 10-minute interval (*A*). FFR is not influenced by changes in hemodynamic parameters. There was no significant change in FFR before and after a 40% variation in heart rate (in response to temporary cardiac pacing), 35% variation in blood pressure (in response to systemic infusion of nitroprusside), and 50% change in contractility (in response to systemic infusion of dobutamine) across a given stenosis (*B*). (*Adapted from* Kern MJ, Lerman A, Bech JW, et al. Physiological assessment of coronary artery disease in the cardiac catheterization laboratory. A scientific statement from the American Heart Association committee on diagnostic and interventional cardiac catheterization council on clinical cardiology. Circulation 2006;114:1321–41; with permission.)

a few millimeters at a time to interrogate exact changes in FFR along a vessel. Although other functional tests reach a per-patient (for example, exercise electrocardiographic test) or per-vessel (for example, myocardial perfusion scan or dobutamine stress echocardiography) accuracy, FFR reaches a per-segment accuracy with a high spatial resolution of few millimeters. As outlined later, such a special resolution allows accurate identification of the exact anatomic position of a functionally significant stenoses, which is of particular clinical value in vessels with serial or ostial lesions.

FFR remains diagnostically accurate in patients with multivessel disease

The FFR value for a given coronary artery is unique to that vessel and is not influenced by stenoses or flow changes in remote vessels. Therefore, FFR is of particular diagnostic value in functional assessment of patients with multivessel CAD, for whom standard noninvasive functional tests are often negative for ischemia (normal test) or indicate only a single-vessel pattern of disease (**Fig. 10**).[55,56]

Clinical Applications of FFR

The 2 main clinical applications of FFR are functional evaluation of (1) angiographic intermediate (40%–70% luminal stenosis) epicardial vessel stenoses, and (2) epicardial stenoses wherein

there is discrepancy between clinical findings and observed percentage angiographic stenosis.

The clinical utility of FFR as a robust decision-making tool to defer or to perform revascularization has been validated in patients with both stable single- and multivessel CAD, as illustrated clearly by 2 landmark studies: DEFER and FAME.[5–7,57–62] The DEFER study examined the 12- and 24-month clinical outcome in 325 patients with single-vessel CAD who were referred for PCI (**Fig. 11**). All patients with FFR less than 0.75 underwent PCI as planned (Reference Group), and patients with FFR greater than 0.75 were randomly assigned to medical therapy (Deferral Group) or PCI (Performance Group). At 12- and 24-month follow-up, both event-free survival and recurrent angina were similar in the Deferral and Performance groups (**Fig. 12**).[5] Furthermore, the low event rate in the Deferral group was maintained at 5-year follow-up.[6] The FAME study evaluated the role of FFR as decision-making tool in patients with multivessel disease. On thousand and five patients with multivessel CAD, who were suited to undergo PCI, were randomized to FFR- or angiography-guided revascularization with drug-eluting stents (DES). At 1-year follow-up adverse events were lower (13.2% vs 18.3%; *P* = .02) and percentage of patients free of symptoms higher (81% vs 78%; *P* = .02) in the FFR-guided intervention group.[7] Based on the aforementioned, as well as other clinical studies, there is now clear evidence to

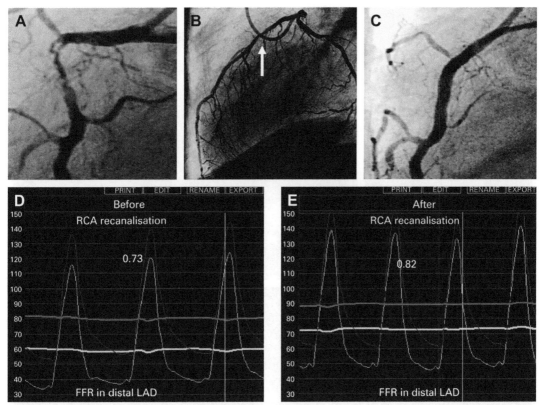

Fig. 9. An example of how FFR accounts for the influence of collateral vessels. A patient with angina underwent diagnostic coronary angiography, which demonstrated a critical stenosis in the right coronary artery (RCA) (*A*), collaterals from the left coronary system supplying the distal RCA (*B*), and an angiographically intermediate stenosis in the left anterior descending (LAD) artery (*white arrow, B*). FFR in the distal LAD was measured before (*A* and *D*) and after (*C* and *E*) treatment of the RCA. When antegrade flow was restored in the RCA, the LAD no longer supplied blood to the RCA territory. This situation resulted in a lower hyperemic flow in the LAD and hence an increase in FFR from 0.76 to 0.82. By taking into account the contribution of collateral vessels on flow, FFR in a given vessel provides clinically relevant functional information to guide the appropriateness of revascularization at the time of the measurement. This case also demonstrates clearly the relationship between FFR and the myocardial mass supplied by the artery: the larger the myocardial mass, the greater the hyperemic flow, and the lower the FFR for a given stenosis. (*From* De Bruyne B, Sarma J. Fractional flow reserve: a review. Heart 2008;94:949–59; with permission.)

confirm that FFR-guided PCI in the context of angiographically intermediate stenoses is associated with a superior short- and long-term clinical outcome in comparison with PCI decisions based on angiographic features alone.

The clinical utility of FFR also extends to management of left main stem (LMS) stenoses for which, as for patients with multivessel CAD, standard noninvasive functional tests have a high rate of false-negative results. Multiple clinical studies have demonstrated that a decision to defer LMS revascularization based on an FFR of greater than 0.75 is safe.[63–65] In 54 patients with LMS disease, Bech and colleagues[63] examined the value of FFR-guided LMS revascularization. Thirty patients had FFR of less than 0.75 and underwent

coronary artery bypass graft (CABG) surgery, and 24 patients with FFR of 0.75 or more were treated medically. At 3-year follow-up there was no difference in MACE or functional class between the 2 groups. In addition, none of the patients in the medical group had suffered a myocardial infarction or had died.

Emerging data indicate that hyperemic resistance in viable segments of myocardium within an infarcted area remains normal.[66] Therefore, standard FFR criteria, including the ischemic threshold of FFR less than 0.75, can be applied to functional evaluation of infarct-related arteries. However, it is important to note that for a given stenosis in an artery subtending an area of infarction, the FFR value pre- and post-infarct will often

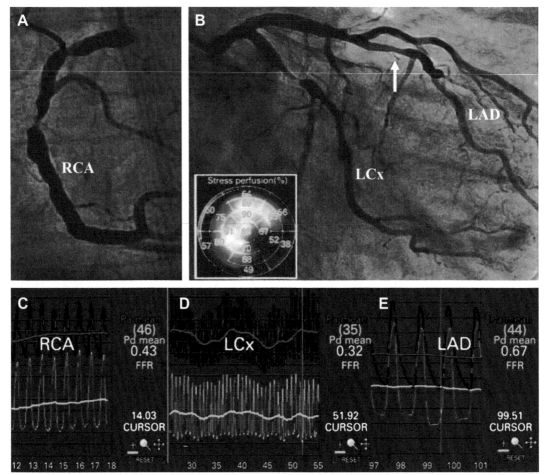

Fig. 10. Noninvasive functional tests, such as myocardial perfusion scans, use the principle of flow reserve by comparing hyperemic flow in the myocardial territory supplied by the stenotic artery with hyperemic flow in a myocardial territory subtended by a nonstenotic vessel to detect perfusion defects, which correspond to areas of myocardial ischemia.[76] The requirement of at least one "normal" vessel limits the diagnostic accuracy and application of perfusion scans in patients with multivessel disease. In contrast, derivation of FFR does not require comparison with a nonstenotic vessel. Therefore, FFR maintains its diagnostic accuracy in assessment of patients with multivessel disease. The superiority and accuracy of FFR in patients with multivessel CAD is illustrated in this case. Angiographic images from a patient with stable angina demonstrated critical stenoses in the right (RCA) (A) and circumflex (LCx) (B) coronary arteries, which clearly require revascularization without the requirement of functional information. However, there was also an angiographic mild stenosis in the left anterior descending (LAD) artery (*white arrow, B*). The functional significance of this stenosis has important clinical implications on prognosis as well as the mode of revascularization (PCI in 2-vessel disease versus coronary artery bypass grafting surgery in 3-vessel disease). A myocardial perfusion scan confirmed the presence of reversible defects in the inferolateral segments corresponding to the stenoses in the RCA and LCx arteries. In contrast, FFR was positive for ischemia in all 3 coronary vessels including the LAD artery (C–E). The LAD stenosis was undetected by the perfusion scan because the uptake of tracer is notably worse in the LCx/RCA territories where the ischemic burden is the greatest in comparison to the LAD territory. (*From* De Bruyne B, Sarma J. Fractional flow reserve: a review. Heart 2008;94:949–59; with permission.)

change, with the latter being higher, as the reduction in viable myocardium will result in lower hyperemic flow (**Fig. 13**). Furthermore, recent work indicates that hyperemic resistance in a myocardial territory remote to that of an acute infarction also remains normal.[67] Thus, FFR can be used to accurately evaluate a stenosis in a myocardial territory remote to that of an acute myocardial infarction.

FFR may also provide valuable medium- to long-term information subsequent to PCI. In a multi-center study, Pijls and colleagues[68] examined

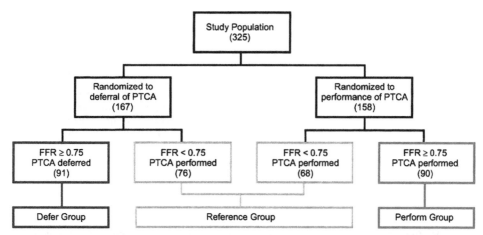

Fig. 11. An overview of the DEFER Study design, which examined the role of FFR in deferring or recommending PCI in 325 patients referred for PCI based on angiographic images. As outlined, all patients with an FFR less than 0.75 underwent PCI (Reference Group). Patients with FFR >0.75 were randomly assigned to medical therapy (Deferral Group) and PCI (Performance Group). (*From* Bech GJ, De Bruyne B, Bonnier HJ, et al. Long-term follow-up after deferral of percutaneous transluminal coronary angioplasty of intermediate stenosis on the basis of coronary pressure measurement. J Am Coll Cardiol 1998;31:841–7; with permission.)

FFR immediately after stent implantation in 705 patients after undergoing angiographically successful PCI. On multivariate analysis, FFR was an independent variable for all MACE, with an inverse association between immediate post-stent FFR values and adverse clinical events at 6-month follow-up. The lowest event rates (5%) were seen in patients with FFR immediately post-PCI in the normal range (FFR 0.96–1.00) and the highest event rates (30%) in patients with FFR in the gray zone (FFR 0.76–0.80). Potential causes for this association could be procedurally related problems (such as edge dissection) or untreated diffuse/discrete disease elsewhere in the vessel not detected by conventional angiographic images. Measurement of FFR after stent deployment is not routine, but can in selected cases provide important prognostic information. Nevertheless, it is important to appreciate that FFR does not provide anatomic information regarding the artery or the adequacy of stent deployment. Therefore, information from alternative imaging modalities such as IVUS or optical computed tomography (OCT) may be required to complement FFR-derived functional data post PCI.

Clinical Technique for Assessment of FFR

FFR can be derived from the ratio of P_a/P_d, with P_a measured from the tip of the angiography guiding

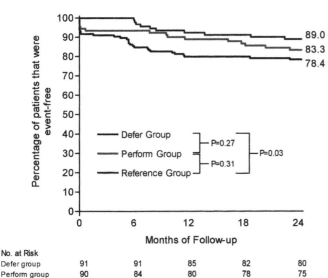

Fig. 12. Kaplan-Meier survival curves for freedom from adverse events during 24 months of follow-up in the DEFER Study. There were no significant differences in adverse events in the Deferral and Performance groups. (*From* Bech GJ, De Bruyne B, Bonnier HJ, et al. Long-term follow-up after deferral of percutaneous transluminal coronary angioplasty of intermediate stenosis on the basis of coronary pressure measurement. J Am Coll Cardiol 1998;31:841–7; with permission.)

No. at Risk					
Defer group	91	91	85	82	80
Perform group	90	84	80	78	75
Reference group	144	123	116	108	106

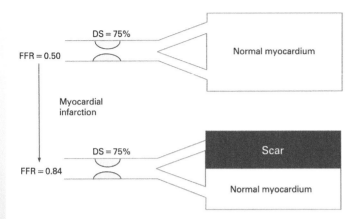

Fig. 13. The relationship between FFR and viable myocardial mass before and after a myocardial infarction. The reduction in viable myocardial mass subsequent to a myocardial infarction reduces coronary flow at maximal hyperemia and thus increases FFR for a given stenosis. (*From* De Bruyne B, Sarma J. Fractional flow reserve: a review. Heart 2008;94:949–59; with permission.)

catheter and P_d from an intracoronary pressure sensor–tipped angioplasty guidewire positioned distal to the stenosis within the epicardial vessel. At present, there are 3 commercially available guidewires in mainstream clinical use that can be used to derive FFR: Radi Pressure Wire (as outlined earlier, a combined pressure- and temperature-sensing guidewire), the Volcano (Volcano Inc, Rancho Cordova, CA) ComboWire (a combined Doppler and pressure-sensing guidewire), and PrimeWire (a single-modality pressure-sensing guidewire). All 3 wires have a solid-state pressure sensor mounted near the tip of a floppy angioplasty guide wire, which interfaces with a dedicated analyzer.

To assess the functional significance of an epicardial vessel stenosis, the guidewire is calibrated and introduced into the coronary vascular tree through a standard angioplasty guiding catheter, and the proximal and distal pressure readings are equalized (to ensure $P_a = P_d$). Under fluoroscopic guidance, the guidewire is placed in the distal vessel, ensuring the pressure sensor is distal to the stenosis being examined. As for assessment of CFR, intracoronary nitrates (200–400 μg ISDN) are always administered to ensure maximal epicardial vessel dilatation before any measurement. The dedicated interface (Radi-Analyzer for the Radi Pressure Wire and ComboMap or SmartMap for the Volcano wires) for the wire used provides simultaneous live pressure readouts from the tip of the guiding catheter (P_a) and the distal pressure sensor (P_d) to compute beat-to-beat FFR values. FFR is recorded at peak hyperemia, which is represented by the nadir or lowest P_d. At the end of the procedure the guidewire is often withdrawn with the distal sensor positioned at the tip of the guiding catheter to verify that proximal and distal pressure readings (Pa = Pd) remain equal, thus ensuring no error has occurred secondary to signal drift.

An important feature of having real-time continuous FFR readouts is the ability to confirm the

exact anatomic position of a functionally significant stenosis by demonstrating a step-up in FFR values during gentle manual pull-back of the pressure sensor–tipped guidewire (and thus the distal pressure sensor) under fluoroscopic guidance across a given stenosis (**Fig. 14**). In addition, the combination of the pull-back technique and the high spatial resolution of FFR also play an important role in functional interrogation of diffusely atheromatous epicardial vessels as well as angiographically intermediate serial and ostial stenoses.

FFR in diffuse epicardial disease
In diffusely diseased vessels or vessels with long segments of disease, pull-back of the pressure sensor under conditions of maximal steady-state hyperemia results in a gentle reduction in FFR as opposed to a clear step-up seen with a discrete stenosis (see **Fig. 14**). Vessels with a gradual pull-back pattern and a positive FFR are not suitable for treatment with PCI, and should be considered for either medical therapy or surgical revascularization.

FFR in serial epicardial stenoses
Serial discrete stenoses also pose a particular challenge where hyperemic flow and pressure gradient across the first stenosis is attenuated by the influences of the second stenosis, and vice versa.[9,56,69] The overall fluid dynamic interaction between 2 serial stenoses is dependent on the severity, distance, blood flow, and sequence of the lesions. In general, it is accepted that when the distance between 2 lesions is greater than 6 times the vessel diameter, the 2 stenoses behave independently, with the overall pressure gradient at maximal hyperemia equating to the sum of all individual pressure losses.[69] Although accurate calculation of FFR at each stenosis is possible, this requires estimation of the coronary wedge pressure (as derived from occlusion of the vessel using an angioplasty balloon) and thus is seldom

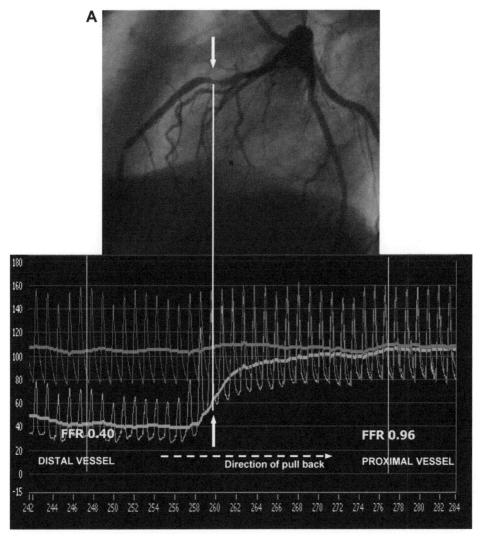

Fig. 14. Proximal (P_a, in red) and distal (P_d, in green) pressure traces as derived from an intracoronary pressure sensor-tipped wire (RadiWire) and displayed on the Radi-Analyzer. Changes in pressures traces and FFR with "pull-back" of the RadiWire along the length the left anterior descending (LAD) artery in 2 different patients with exertional angina are displayed. In *A* there is a clear step-up in P_d and hence the FFR value from 0.40 to 0.96 at the level of an angiographically intermediate mid-LAD (*white arrow*) stenosis, confirming the functional significance of the lesion that can be treated with PCI. In contrast, in *B* there is a gradual change in P_d and hence FFR in a diffusely diseased LAD.

performed. The current clinical recommendation for functional assessment of serial stenoses is to initially establish the pull-back FFR pattern across the length of the vessel. If there are discrete step-ups in FFR at the level of each stenosis, PCI is initially performed at the stenosis with the largest gradient, with repeat measurement of FFR to establish the functional significance of the remaining stenosis (**Fig. 15**). In the absence of discrete step-ups in FFR along a vessel with serial stenoses, the same principles used for diffusely diseased vessels apply.

FFR in ostial stenoses

Functional assessment of ostial stenoses (LMS or right coronary artery) using FFR also requires important technical considerations. In the context of an irregularly shaped or small ostium, the guiding catheter may obstruct the flow of blood during hyperemia, thus leading to an underestimation of FFR. Therefore, equalization of pressures at the start of the protocol and pressure measurements during maximal hyperemia should be performed with the guiding catheter disengaged from the ostium to prevent false negative results.[56]

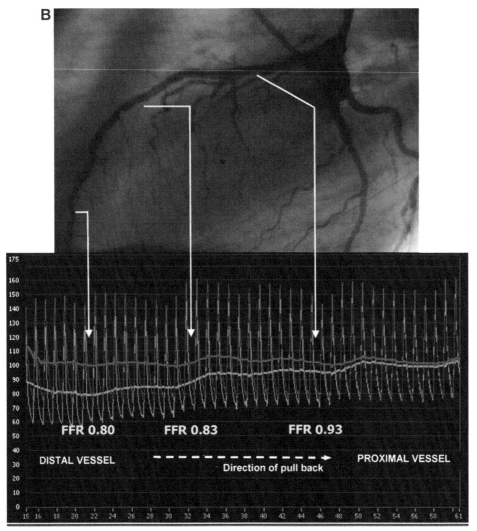

Fig. 14. (*continued*)

In addition, as for other nonostial stenoses, the pull-back technique can be used to accurately identify the exact anatomic location of the stenosis to guide the most suitable mode of revascularization.

HYPEREMIC STENOSIS RESISTANCE

HSR is an alternative emerging functional index of epicardial vessel stenosis that combines important diagnostic elements of CFR (distal blood flow velocity) and FFR (distal coronary pressure gradient). The concept of HSR was introduced by Meuwissen and colleagues,[25] and HSR is defined as the as *the ratio of distal coronary pressure gradient to distal coronary blood flow velocity at maximal hyperemia*. As for derivation of FFR, the distal coronary pressure gradient is derived from $P_a - P_d$.

It is reported that HSR provides a more refined physiologic measurement of epicardial vessel stenosis, as it quantifies the resistance to flow conferred by an epicardial stenosis. Meuwissen and colleagues[25] compared the ability of HSR, FFR, and CFR to accurately predict reversible ischemia as demonstrated by SPECT in 181 angiographic intermediate stenoses. HSR was the most powerful predictor of reversible ischemia. The level of agreement between HSR and SPECT (73%) was significantly higher than FFR (51%) and CFR (49%) in lesions where there were discordant results between FFR and CFR. A recent study has shown the prognostic value of HSR in deferring revascularization in angiographically intermediate stenoses.[70] In 186 intermediate lesions with a negative or nondiagnostic noninvasive stress test, HSR was a better predictor of medium-term adverse events than FFR and CFR.

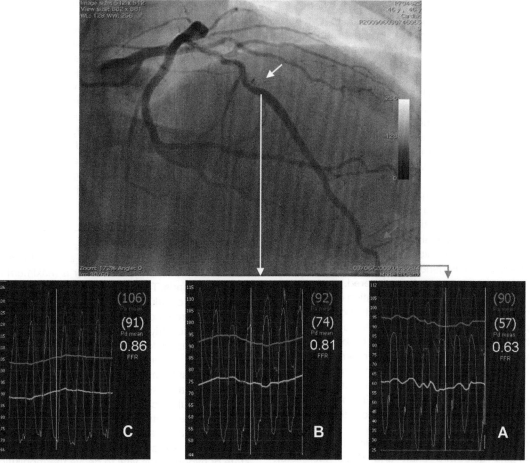

Fig. 15. Changes in FFR with "pull-back" of the RadiWire along the length of the left anterior descending artery (LAD) across 2 serial stenoses in the distal (*red arrow*) and proximal (*white arrow*) vessel. The step-up in FFR across the distal stenosis (*A*: from 0.63 to 0.81) was greater than the step-up across the proximal (*B*: from 0.81 to 0.0.88) stenosis. Therefore, the distal stenosis was treated with PCI. Post-PCI FFR in the distal vessel was negative (*C*: FFR 0.86), confirming that the angiographic intermediate proximal stenosis was not hemodynamically significant.

The cut-off ischemic threshold for HSR is greater than 0.8 mm Hg/cm/s, as derived from comparison with noninvasive standard functional tests.[25] In addition, HSR is independent of basal hemodynamic conditions, with high reproducibility and low variability. Although the exact clinical role of HSR needs to defined, it may potentially be important in the assessment of lesions with an FFR within the "gray zone" (FFR 0.75–0.80) or where there is a clear discrepancy between symptoms, CFR values, and FFR values.

As outlined later, the latest generation of physiologic guidewires allows accurate assessment of distal coronary pressure gradient and flow to be made using the same device during a single instrumentation of the target vessel. Therefore, HSR can be derived from: (1) a RadiWire measuring P_a, P_d (through the distal pressure sensor) and an estimate of flow by applying the principles of thermodilution; or (2) a ComboMap Wire to measure P_a, P_d (through the distal pressure sensor) and flow velocity (though the distal Doppler crystal).

FUNCTIONAL PROPERTIES OF PHYSIOLOGIC GUIDEWIRES

The current generations of both Doppler and pressure guidewires are 0.014 inch in diameter (0.356 mm) and have similar handling characteristics to standard angioplasty guidewires to facilitate passage across epicardial stenoses and tortuous vessels. In addition, the wires can be disconnected from their dedicated interface coupler to allow standard interventional devices to be advanced into the study artery (as for any standard PCI guidewire) and then reconnected for repeat physiologic measurements post PCI.

An important consideration remains whether the guidewire adds cross-sectional area to a stenosis that is being investigated. In most intermediate lesions this addition area is clinically not significant (cross-sectional area of a pressure sensor-tipped guide wire is approximately 0.099 mm^2, which equates to 1.4% of a 3-mm diameter vessel). However, if the guidewire does significantly reduce the cross-sectional area of stenosis (guidewire cross-sectional area of 0.099 mm^2 equates to 12% of a 1-mm diameter vessel), especially if it is also accompanied with a significant physiologic measure of stenosis (CFR <2.0 or FFR <0.75), it is highly likely that the index stenosis would have been severe enough to warrant revascularization regardless of functional assessment. In "real world" interventional practice the hemodynamic influences of the guidewire only arise in marginal cases where, in general, an overestimation of the lesion severity seems to be favored.

In addition, the current generation of physiologic guidewires has important multimodal functional properties that allow pressure measurements to be combined with estimates of blood flow or velocity in the target vessel. For example, the RadiWire has dual pressure- and temperature-sensing properties that allow measurement of pressure gradients (as for derivation of FFR) through a distal pressure sensor, and derivation of a thermodilution curve to estimate coronary flow (as for derivation of CFR) through the combined electrical properties of the guidewire shaft and distal thermistor. Indeed, experimental and in vivo human studies indicate that thermodilution-derived estimates of intracoronary blood flow using the RadiWire are better correlates of true flow than estimates derived from intracoronary Doppler velocity.[40] Another example is the ComboWire, which has dual distal pressure and Doppler transducers allowing measurement of both pressure gradients and blood flow velocity. The development of such multimodal wires has been an important step in encouraging detailed physiologic assessments in the catheterization laboratory.

INDUCTION OF MAXIMAL HYPEREMIA

Maximal hyperemia forms the cornerstone of the physiologic models used to assess epicardial vessel stenoses. Hyperemia is achieved by maximal vasodilatation of resistance vessels (vessels <400 μm diameter), which increase myocardial flow by reducing microvascular resistance. Although multiple agents have been shown to have a hyperemic influence, only adenosine and papaverine are commonly used in the clinical setting (**Table 3**).[71] Both agents cause vasodilatation of resistance vessels through relaxation of microvascular smooth muscle cells.

Adenosine

Adenosine has a short half-life ($t_{1/2}$) of less than 20 seconds, and when administered as an intracoronary bolus induces hyperemia for a maximum of 20 to 30 seconds. This route of administering adenosine is only of value when measuring FFR across a single discrete coronary stenosis, as it does not induce a sufficiently prolonged period of hyperemia to allow pull-back interrogation of the vessel/stenosis.[9,56,71] More complex FFR measurements (including assessment of LMS, ostial and serial stenoses, or a vessel with diffuse disease for which often FFR pull-back is required), Doppler-derived CFR measurements (whereby APV is derived from the mean of 3–5 heart beats), and thermodilution-derived CFR measurements (for which prolonged state of hyperemia is vital to derive thermodilution curves) all require a prolonged period of maximal steady-state hyperemia that is achieved through weight-adjusted central intravenous infusion of adenosine (140 μg/kg/min).[9,56,71]

Papaverine

Unlike adenosine, the $t_{1/2}$ of papaverine is longer (60–90 seconds). Therefore, an intracoronary bolus dose (10–15 mg) creates a sufficiently long enough period of maximal steady-state hyperemia to allow more complex FFR and CFR

Table 3		
Pharmacologic agents that can be used to induce hyperemia		
Agent	Route	Dose
Adenosine or ATP	IC	50 μg intracoronary bolus
Adenosine or ATP	IV	140 mg/kg/min infusion (for rapid response infused through a central vein, eg, femoral vein)
Papaverine	IC	8 mg in RCA and 12 mg LCA intracoronary bolus
Nitroprusside	IC	0.6 μg/kg intracoronary bolus

Abbreviations: RCA, right coronary artery; LCA, left coronary artery.

measurements to be made accurately. However, papaverine is rarely used routinely in the clinical setting as its can cause QT prolongation, resulting in ventricular arrhythmias.[71,72]

ECONOMIC CONSIDERATIONS AND PHYSIOLOGICALLY GUIDED REVASCULARIZATION

Several studies have shown that functional assessment of stenoses, as an adjunct to coronary angiography, is associated with a favorable medical economic outcome.[7,73–75] Fearon and colleagues[75] generated a decision model comparing long-term costs and benefits of 3 different strategies for management of patients with angiographic intermediate stenoses: (1) deferring the decision for PCI to obtain a nuclear perfusion scan (nuclear strategy), (2) measuring FFR at the time of angiography to guide PCI (FFR strategy), and (3) stent implantation for all intermediate stenoses (Stent strategy). The FFR strategy saved $1795 per patient in comparison with the nuclear strategy and $3830 per patient in comparison to the stent strategy. In addition, quality-adjusted life expectancy was similar amongst the 3 strategies. Preliminary health economic data from the FAME Trial, in which patients with multivessel CAD were randomized to FFR- and angiography-guided PCI, also indicate lower materials cost in the FFR group (angiography group: $6007 $\pm$ 2819; FFR group: $5332 $\pm$ 3261; $P<.01$).[7] Although the cost of obtaining the physiologic data may significantly increase the price of a diagnostic angiogram at the outset, the overall cost savings are more than offset by avoiding repeated in-/outpatient admissions, the requirement for alternative investigations, and lower complication rates in the short- as well as long-term.

SUMMARY

The validation and clinical availability of robust and accurate physiologic indices, which can be used as an adjunct to diagnostic angiography in the cardiac catheterization laboratory, have been pivotal in promoting ischemia-driven coronary revascularization. Deferral or revascularization based on such physiologic indices is associated with improved clinical outcome as well as more favorable health economic data. Although there are several clinical indices, FFR remains the "gold standard," with indications for physiologic assessment of angiographic intermediate stenoses, including LMS and ostial disease as well as serial lesions. The availability of such indices is an important step in streamlining

management of patients undergoing cardiac catheterization by allowing routine provision of an "all-in-one" ischemia-driven revascularization service.

REFERENCES

1. Topol EJ, Nissen SE. Our preoccupation with coronary luminology: the dissociation between clinical and angiographic findings in ischemic heart disease. Circulation 1995;92:2333–42.
2. Kern JM, De Bruyne B, Pijls NHJ. From research to clinical practice: current role of intracoronary physiologically based decision making in the cardiac catheterization laboratory. J Am Coll Cardiol 1997; 30:613–20.
3. Kern JM. Coronary physiology revisited. Practical insights from the cardiac catheterization laboratory. Circulation 2000;101:1344–51.
4. Bourassa MG, Pepine CJ, Forman SA, et al. Asymptomatic Cardiac Ischemia Pilot (ACIP) study: effects of coronary angioplasty and coronary artery bypass graft surgery on recurrent angina and ischemia: the ACIP investigators. J Am Coll Cardiol 1995;26: 606–14.
5. Bech GJ, De Bruyne B, Bonnier HJ, et al. Long-term follow-up after deferral of percutaneous transluminal coronary angioplasty of intermediate stenosis on the basis of coronary pressure measurement. J Am Coll Cardiol 1998;15(31):841–7.
6. Pijls NH, van Schaardenburgh P, Manoharan G, et al. Percutaneous coronary intervention of functionally non-significant stenosis: 5-year follow-up of the DEFER Study. J Am Coll Cardiol 2007;29:2105–7.
7. Tonino PAL, De Bruyne B, Pijls NHJ, et al. Fractional flow reserve versus angiography for guiding percutaneous coronary intervention. N Engl J Med 2009; 360:213–24.
8. Shaw LJ, Berman DS, Maron DJ, et al. Optimal medical therapy with or without percutaneous coronary intervention to reduce ischemic burden: results from the Clinical Outcomes Utilizing revascularization and aggressive drug evaluation (COURAGE) trial nuclear sub-study. Circulation 2008;117:1283–91.
9. Kern MJ, Lerman A, Bech JW, et al. Physiological assessment of coronary artery disease in the cardiac catheterization laboratory. A scientific statement from the American Heart Association committee on diagnostic and interventional cardiac catheterization council on clinical cardiology. Circulation 2006;114:1321–41.
10. Gould KL, Lipscomb K, Hamilton GW. Physiologic basis for assessing critical coronary stenosis. Instantaneous flow response and regional distribution during coronary hyperaemia as measures of coronary flow reserve. Am J Cardiol 1974;33:87–94.
11. Donohue TJ, Miller DD, Bach RG, et al. Correlation of poststenotic hyperemic coronary flow velocity

and pressure with abnormal stress myocardial perfusion imaging in coronary artery disease. Am J Cardiol 1996;77:948–54.

12. Joye JD, Schulman DS, Lasorda D, et al. Intracoronary Doppler guide wire versus stress single-photon emission computed tomographic thallium-201 imaging in assessment of intermediate coronary stenoses. J Am Coll Cardiol 1994;24:940–7.

13. Miller DD, Donohue TJ, Younis LT, et al. Correlation of pharmacological 99mTc-sestamibi myocardial perfusion imaging with poststenotic coronary flow reserve in patients with angiographically intermediate coronary artery stenoses. Circulation 1994;89:2150–60.

14. Deychak YA, Segal J, Reiner JS, et al. Doppler guide wire flow-velocity indexes measured distal to coronary stenoses associated with reversible thallium perfusion defects. Am Heart J 1995;129:219–27.

15. Tron C, Donohue TJ, Bach RG, et al. Comparison of pressure-derived fractional flow reserve with poststenotic coronary flow velocity reserve for prediction of stress myocardial perfusion imaging results. Am Heart J 1995;130:723–33.

16. Heller LI, Cates C, Popma J, et al. Intracoronary Doppler assessment of moderate coronary artery disease: comparison with 201Tl imaging and coronary angiography. FACTS Study Group. Circulation 1997;96:484–90.

17. Schulman DS, Lasorda D, Farah T, et al. Correlations between coronary flow reserve measured with a Doppler guide wire and treadmill exercise testing. Am Heart J 1997;134:99–104.

18. Danzi GB, Pirelli S, Mauri L, et al. Which variable of stenosis severity best describes the significance of an isolated left anterior descending coronary artery lesion? Correlation between quantitative coronary angiography, intracoronary Doppler measurements and high dose dipyridamole echocardiography. J Am Coll Cardiol 1998;31:526–33.

19. Verberne HJ, Piek JJ, van Liebergen RA, et al. Functional assessment of coronary artery stenosis by Doppler derived absolute and relative coronary blood flow velocity reserve in comparison with (99m)Tc MIBI SPECT. Heart 1999;82:509–14.

20. Piek JJ, Boersma E, di Mario C, et al. Angiographical and Doppler flow-derived parameters for assessment of coronary lesion severity and its relation to the result of exercise electrocardiography. DEBATE study group. Doppler Endpoints Balloon Angioplasty Trial Europe. Eur Heart J 2000;21:466–74.

21. Abe M, Tomiyama H, Yoshida H, et al. Diastolic fractional flow reserve to assess the functional severity of moderate coronary artery stenoses: comparison with fractional flow reserve and coronary flow velocity reserve. Circulation 2000;102(19):2365–70.

22. Duffy SJ, Gelman JS, Peverill RE, et al. Agreement between coronary flow velocity reserve and stress echocardiography in intermediate-severity coronary stenoses. Catheter Cardiovasc Interv 2001;53:29–38.

23. Chamuleau SA, Meuwissen M, van Eck-Smit BL, et al. Fractional flow reserve, absolute and relative coronary blood flow velocity in relation to the results of technetium-99m sestamibi single-photon emission computed tomography in patients with two-vessel coronary artery disease. J Am Coll Cardiol 2001;37:1316–22.

24. El-Shafei A, Chiravuri R, Stikovac MM, et al. Comparison of relative coronary Doppler flow velocity reserve to stress myocardial perfusion imaging in patients with coronary artery disease. Catheter Cardiovasc Interv 2001;53:193–201.

25. Meuwissen M, Siebes M, Chamuleau SA, et al. Hyperemic stenosis resistance index for evaluation of functional coronary lesion severity. Circulation 2002;106:441–6.

26. Voudris V, Avramides D, Koutelou M, et al. Relative coronary flow velocity reserve improves correlation with stress myocardial perfusion imaging in assessment of coronary artery stenoses. Chest 2003;124:1266–74.

27. Melikian N, Kearney MT, Thomas MR, et al. A simple thermodilution technique to assess coronary endothelium-dependent microvascular function in humans: validation and comparison with coronary flow reserve. Eur Heart J 2007;28:2188–94.

28. McGinn AI, White CW, Wilson RF. Inter-study variability of coronary flow reserve: influence of heart rate, arterial pressure and ventricular preload. Circulation 1990;81:1319–30.

29. Hoffma JI. Problems of coronary flow reserve. Ann Biomed Eng 2000;28:884–96.

30. Kern MJ, Donohue TJ, Aguirre FV, et al. Clinical outcome of deferring angioplasty in patients with normal translesional pressure-flow velocity measurements. J Am Coll Cardiol 1995;25:178–87.

31. Ferrari M, Schnell B, Werner GS, et al. Safety of deferring angioplasty in patients with normal coronary flow velocity reserve. J Am Coll Cardiol 1999;33:83–7.

32. Chamuleau SA, Tio RA, de Cock CC, et al. Prognostic value of coronary blood flow velocity and myocardial perfusion in intermediate coronary narrowings and multivessel disease. J Am Coll Cardiol 2002;39:852–8.

33. Serruys PW, di Mario C, Piek J, et al. Prognostic value of intracoronary flow velocity and diameter stenosis in assessing the short- and long-term outcomes of coronary balloon angioplasty: the DEBATE Study (Doppler Endpoints Balloon Angioplasty Trial Europe). Circulation 1997;96:3369–77.

34. Di Mario C, Moses JW, Anderson TJ, et al. Randomized comparison of elective stent implantation and coronary balloon angioplasty guided by online quantitative angiography and intracoronary Doppler. DESTINI Study Group (Doppler Endpoint Stenting

International Investigation). Circulation 2000;102: 2910–4.

35. Serruys PW, de Bruyne B, Carlier S, et al. Randomized comparison of primary stenting and provisional balloon angioplasty guided by flow velocity measurement. Doppler Endpoints Balloon Angioplasty Trial Europe (DEBATE) II Study Group. Circulation 2000;102:2930–7.

36. Voskuil M, van Liebergen RA, Albertal M, et al. Coronary hemodynamics of stent implantation after suboptimal and optimal balloon angioplasty. J Am Coll Cardiol 2002;39:1513–7.

37. De Bruyne B, Pijls NH, Smith L, et al. Coronary thermodilution to assess coronary flow reserve: experimental validation. Circulation 2001;104:2003–6.

38. Pijls NH, De Bruyne B, Smith L, et al. Coronary thermodilution to assess flow reserve: validation in humans. Circulation 2002;105:2482–6.

39. Barbato E, Aarnoudse W, Aengevaeren WR, et al. Validation of coronary flow reserve measurements by thermodilution in clinical practice. Eur Heart J 2004;25:219–23.

40. Fearon WF, Farouque HM, Balsam LB, et al. Comparison of coronary thermodilution and Doppler velocity for assessing coronary flow reserve. Circulation 2003;108:2198–200.

41. Gould KL, Kirkeeide RL, Buchi M. Coronary flow reserve as a physiologic measure of stenosis severity. J Am Coll Cardiol 1990;15:459–74.

42. Pijls NH, Van Gelder B, Van der Voort P, et al. Fractional flow reserve. A useful index to evaluate the influence of an epicardial coronary stenosis on myocardial blood flow. Circulation 1995;92: 3183–93.

43. Pijls NH, De Bruyne B, Peels K, et al. Measurement of fractional flow reserve to assess the functional severity of coronary-artery stenoses. N Engl J Med 1996;334:1703–8.

44. De Bruyne B, Bartunek J, Sys SU, et al. Relation between myocardial fractional flow reserve calculated from coronary pressure measurements and exercise-induced myocardial ischemia. Circulation 1995;92:39–46.

45. Bartunek J, Van Schuerbeeck E, de Bruyne B. Comparison of exercise electrocardiography and dobutamine echocardiography with invasively assessed myocardial fractional flow reserve in evaluation of severity of coronary arterial narrowing. Am J Cardiol 1997;79:478–81.

46. Caymaz O, Fak AS, Tezcan H, et al. Correlation of myocardial fractional flow reserve with thallium-201 SPECT imaging in intermediate-severity coronary artery lesions. J Invasive Cardiol 2000;12:345–50.

47. Fearon WF, Takagi A, Jeremias A, et al. Use of fractional myocardial flow reserve to assess the functional significance of intermediate coronary stenoses. Am J Cardiol 2000;86:1013–4.

48. Jiménez-Navarro M, Alonso-Briales JH, Hernández García MJ. Measurement of fractional flow reserve to assess moderately severe coronary lesions: correlation with dobutamine stress echocardiography. J Interv Cardiol 2001;14:499–504.

49. De Bruyne B, Pijls NHJ, Bartunek J, et al. Fractional flow reserve in patients with prior myocardial infarction. Circulation 2001;104:157–62.

50. Yanagisawa H, Chikamori T, Tanaka N, et al. Correlation between thallium-201 myocardial perfusion defects and the functional severity of coronary artery stenosis as assessed by pressure-derived myocardial fractional flow reserve. Circ J 2002;66:1105–9.

51. Usui Y, Chikamori T, Yanagisawa H, et al. Reliability of pressure-derived myocardial fractional flow reserve in assessing coronary artery stenosis in patients with previous myocardial infarction. Am J Cardiol 2003;92:699–702.

52. De Bruyne B, Hersbach F, Pijls NH, et al. Abnormal epicardial coronary resistance in patients with diffuse atherosclerosis but "normal" coronary angiography. Circulation 2001;104:2401–6.

53. De Bruyne B, Bartunek J, Sys SU, et al. Simultaneous coronary pressure and flow velocity measurements in humans: feasibility, reproducibility, and hemodynamic dependence of coronary flow velocity reserve, hyperemic flow versus slope index, and fractional flow reserve. Circulation 1996;94:1842–9.

54. Melikian N, Cuisset T, Hamilos M, et al. Fractional flow reserve—the influence of the collateral circulation. Int J Cardiol 2009;132:109–10.

55. Botman M, Pijls NH, Bech JW, et al. Percutaneous coronary intervention or bypass surgery in multivessel disease? A tailored approach based on coronary pressure measurement. Catheter Cardiovasc Interv 2004;63:184–91.

56. De Bruyne B, Sarma J. Fractional flow reserve: a review. Heart 2008;94:949–59.

57. Bech GJ, Pijls NH, De Bruyne B, et al. Usefulness of fractional flow reserve to predict clinical outcome after balloon angioplasty. Circulation 1999;99:883–8.

58. Rieber J, Schiele TM, Koenig A, et al. Long-term safety of therapy stratification in patients with intermediate coronary lesions based on intracoronary pressure measurements. Am J Cardiol 2002;90: 1160–4.

59. Rieber J, Jung P, Schiele TM, et al. Safety of FFR-based treatment strategies: the Munich experience. Z Kardiol 2002;91(Suppl 3):115–9.

60. Chamuleau SA, Meuwissen M, Koch KT, et al. Usefulness of fractional flow reserve for risk stratification of patients with multivessel coronary disease and an intermediate stenosis. Am J Cardiol 2002;89: 377–80.

61. Hernández García MJ, Alonso-Briales JH, Jiménez-Navarro M, et al. Clinical management of patients with coronary syndromes and negative fractional

flow reserve findings. J Interv Cardiol 2001;14: 505–9.

62. Leesar MA, Abdul-Baki T, Yalamanchili V, et al. Conflicting functional assessment of stenoses in patients with previous myocardial infraction. Catheter Cardiovasc Interv 2003;59:489–95.

63. Bech GJ, Droste H, Pijls NH, et al. Value of fractional flow reserve in making decisions about bypass surgery for equivocal left main coronary artery disease. Heart 2001;86(5):547–52.

64. Jasti V, Ivan E, Yalamanchili V, et al. Correlations between fractional flow reserve and intravascular ultrasound in patients with an ambiguous left main coronary artery stenosis. Circulation 2004;110:2831–6.

65. Leesar MA, Mintz GS. Hemodynamic and intravascular ultrasound assessment of an ambiguous left main coronary artery stenosis. Catheter Cardiovasc Interv 2007;70:721–30.

66. Marques KM, Knaapen P, Boellaard R, et al. Microvascular function in viable myocardium after chronic infarction does not influence fractional flow reserve measurements. J Nucl Med 2007;48:1987–99.

67. Marques KM, Knaapen P, Boellaard R, et al. Hyperaemic microvascular resistance is not increased in viable myocardium after chronic myocardial infarction. Eur Heart J 2007;28:2320–5.

68. Pijls NH, Klauss V, Siebert U, et al. Coronary pressure measurement after stenting predicts adverse events at follow-up: a multicenter registry. Circulation 2002;105:2950–4.

69. Pijls NH, De Bruyne B, Bech GJ, et al. Coronary pressure measurement to assess hemodynamic significance of serial stenoses within one coronary artery: validation in humans. Circulation 2000;102:2371–7.

70. Meuwissen M, Chamuleau SA, Siebes M, et al. The prognostic value of combined intracoronary pressure and blood flow velocity measurements after deferral of percutaneous coronary intervention. Catheter Cardiovasc Interv 2008;71:291–7.

71. De Bruyne B, Pijls NH, Barbato E, et al. Intracoronary and intravenous adenosine 5′-triphosphate, adenosine, papaverine, and contrast medium to assess fractional flow reserve in humans. Circulation 2003;107:1877–83.

72. Wilson RF, White CW. Serious ventricular dysrhythmia after intracoronary papaverine. Am J Cardiol 1988;62:1301–5.

73. Leesar MA, Abdul-Baki T, Akkus NI, et al. Use of fractional flow reserve versus stress perfusion scintigraphy after unstable angina: effect on duration of hospitalization, cost, procedural characteristics, and clinical outcome. J Am Coll Cardiol 2003;41: 1115–21.

74. Joye LD, Cates C, Farah T, et al. Cost analysis of intracoronary Doppler determination of lesion significance: preliminary results of the PEACH study. J Invasive Cardiol 1994;7:22A.

75. Fearon WF, Yeung AC, Lee DP, et al. Cost-effectiveness of measuring fractional flow reserve to guide coronary interventions. Am Heart J 2003; 145(5):882.

76. Ragosta M, Bishop AH, Lipson LC, et al. Comparison between angiography and fractional flow reserve versus single-photon emission computed tomographic myocardial perfusion imaging for determining lesion significance in patients with multi-vessel coronary disease. Am J Cardiol 2007;99: 896–902.

Coronary Bifurcation Lesions: A Current Update

Samin K. Sharma, MD, FACC*, Joseph Sweeny, MD,
Annapoorna S. Kini, MD, MRCP, FACC

KEYWORDS

- Coronary bifurcation • Simultaneous kissing stent
- Kissing balloon inflation

Coronary bifurcations are prone to develop atherosclerotic plaque because of turbulent blood flow and high shear stress, and these lesions account for 15% to 20% of the total number of percutaneous coronary interventions (PCIs) performed. A true coronary bifurcation lesion consists of more than 50% diameter obstruction of the main vessel (MV) and the side branch (SB) vessel in an inverted "Y" fashion.

When compared with nonbifurcation coronary interventions, bifurcation interventions have historically reported a lower rate of procedural success, higher procedural costs, longer hospitalization, and higher clinical and angiographic restenosis.[1–5] Consequently, the treatment of coronary bifurcation lesions represents a challenging area in interventional cardiology. However, recent advances in stent design, selective use of a 2-stent technique, acceptance of a suboptimal SB result, and various percutaneous techniques (high-pressure postdilatation, kissing balloon inflation, and intravascular ultrasound) have led to a dramatic increase in the number of patients with bifurcation lesions who are being successfully treated with excellent long-term outcome.

ANATOMIC CLASSIFICATION

Bifurcation lesions are variable not only in their anatomy (eg, location of plaque, plaque burden, angle between branches, site of bifurcation, size of branches) but also in the dynamic changes in anatomy during treatment (dissections and carina shift). As a result, there are no 2 identical bifurcations, and hence, there is no single strategy to be used on every bifurcation.[1]

Coronary bifurcations have been previously classified according to both the angulation between the MV and the SB and the location of the plaque burden. Depending on the degree of SB angulation, a bifurcation lesion can be classified as (1) "Y-angulation" (when the angulation is <70°; access to the SB is usually less difficult but plaque shifting is more pronounced, and precise stent placement in the ostium is more difficult) and (2) "T-angulation" (when the SB angulation is more than 70°; access to the SB is usually more difficult but plaque shifting is often minimal, and precise stent placement in ostium is more straightforward). There are 2 classification patterns commonly used to describe bifurcation plaque distribution: the Duke classification (**Fig. 1**) and the Medina classification (**Fig. 2**).[1] Both of these classifications underestimate plaque distribution and plaque burden when compared with intravascular ultrasound and do not take into account the fate of the SB on dilatation of the MV. A new, simple, practical, and prognostic classification of bifurcation lesions has been suggested by Movahed[6] that takes into account the

There is no conflict of interest or financial support to be disclosed by the authors.
Cardiac Catheterization Laboratory of the Cardiovascular Institute, Mount Sinai Hospital, Box 1030, One Gustave L. Levy Place, New York, NY 10029-6754, USA
* Corresponding author.
E-mail address: samin.sharma@mountsinai.org (S.K. Sharma).

Cardiol Clin 28 (2010) 55–70
doi:10.1016/j.ccl.2009.10.001

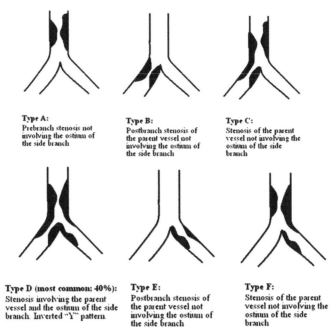

Fig. 1. Duke classification of bifurcation lesions based on the location of the obstructive plaque. (*From* Sharma SK, Kini AS. Coronary bifurcation lesions. Cardiol Clin 2006;24:233–46; with permission.)

size of proximal MV (**Fig. 3**), which is very important while considering 1- or 2-stent techniques.

BIFURCATION STENT TECHNIQUES

The introduction of drug-eluting stents (DESs) has specifically resulted in a lower event rate and reduction of MV restenosis in comparison with previous studies using balloon angiography (percutaneous transluminal coronary angioplasty) and/or bare metal stent placement. Nonetheless, ostial SB stenosis and long-term restenosis remain a problem. Although stenting the MV with provisional SB stenting seems to be the prevailing

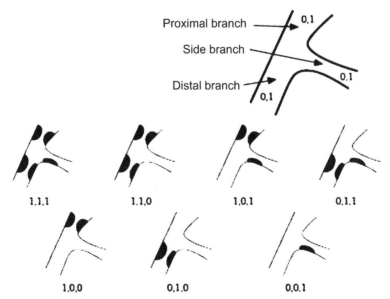

Fig. 2. Medina classification of bifurcation lesions based on the location of the obstructive plaque. Number 1 is assigned to the location of plaque. (*From* Louvard Y, Thomas M, Dzavik V, et al. Classification of coronary artery bifurcation lesions and treatments: time for a consensus! Catheter Cardiovasc Interv 2008;71:175–83; with permission.)

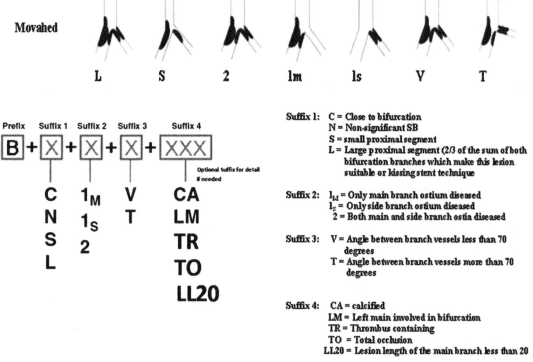

Movahed L S 2 lm ls V T

Prefix Suffix 1 Suffix 2 Suffix 3 Suffix 4

B + X + X + X + XXX

Optional Suffix for detail if needed

C 1$_M$ V CA
N 1$_S$ T LM
S 2   TR
L   TO
            LL20

Suffix 1: C = Close to bifurcation
N = Non-significant SB
S = small proximal segment
L = Large proximal segment (2/3 of the sum of both bifurcation branches which make this lesion suitable or kissing stent technique

Suffix 2: 1$_M$ = Only main branch ostium diseased
1$_S$ = Only side branch ostium diseased
2 = Both main and side branch ostia diseased

Suffix 3: V = Angle between branch vessels less than 70 degrees
T = Angle between branch vessels more than 70 degrees

Suffix 4: CA = calcified
LM = Left main involved in bifurcation
TR = Thrombus containing
TO = Total occlusion
LL20 = Lesion length of the main branch less than 20

Fig. 3. Mohaved classification incorporating location of the obstructive plaque, vessel size, and angulation, with optional suffix for further details. (*Adapted from* Movahed MR, Stinis CT. A new proposed simplified classification of coronary artery bifurcation lesions and bifurcation interventional techniques. J Invas Cardiol 2006;18:199–204; with permission.)

approach, various 2-stent techniques have emerged in the DES era to present a systematic approach to stenting of large SB vessels **(Fig. 4)**.[7–11]

The most important issue in bifurcation PCI is selecting the most appropriate strategy for an individual bifurcation and optimizing the performance of this technique. In 2007, an accurate

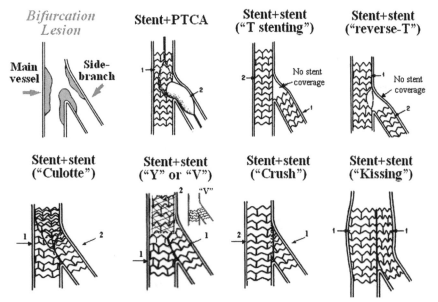

Bifurcation Lesion Stent+PTCA Stent+stent ("T stenting") Stent+stent ("reverse-T")

Main vessel Side-branch

No stent coverage No stent coverage

Stent+stent ("Culotte") Stent+stent ("Y" or "V") Stent+stent ("Crush") Stent+stent ("Kissing")

Fig. 4. Various stenting techniques used for bifurcation lesions. (*From* Sharma SK, Kini AS. Coronary bifurcation lesions. Cardiol Clin 2006;24:233–46; with permission.)

definition of each of the various techniques used, combined with a precise classification to facilitate their description, was proposed by Louvard and colleagues.[1] This classification of the techniques (MADS, or *main, across, distal, side*) was based on the manner in which the first stent was implanted, which often corresponds to a technical strategy related to the importance of the vessel treated first, ie, beginning the procedure (**Fig. 5**).[12]

The strategies to use 1 stent (in MV) or 2 stents (1 in the MV and 1 in the SB) for the treatment of bifurcation lesions have been debated for a long time. There are currently 7 randomized trials and 3 large registries designed to compare a provisional stenting strategy (1-stent) with a 2-stent strategy in patients with bifurcation lesions. Zhang and colleagues[13] recently published a meta-analysis of 5 randomized studies using DES, with a simple stenting strategy (provisional approach) versus a more complex 2-stent strategy to treat 1553 patients with coronary bifurcation lesions; the risk of early myocardial infarction at 30-day or at 6- to 9-months' follow-up was markedly lower (approximately half) in patients treated with a simple stenting strategy. Some earlier studies showed a trend toward higher stent thrombosis (ST) with 2-stent strategy, but recent randomized studies have shown no difference in ST incidence between the 2 techniques (**Fig. 6**).[14] The target lesion revascularization (TLR) rates of 1-stent strategy are comparable with those of the 2-stent strategy (**Fig. 7**), with a trend toward lower angiographic restenosis rates in the 2-stent approach (**Table 1**).[15–24]

Despite the overall momentum of treating bifurcation lesions with a provisional 1-stent approach, this strategy still has several limitations (maintaining access to the SB, jailing the SB ostium, or difficulty rewiring the SB), and therefore, an in-depth understanding of the 2-stent strategy is necessary for any operator who wishes to successfully treat coronary bifurcations. The most important initial question when deciding on a 2-stent versus 1-stent approach is whether the SB is large enough (>2.75 mm) with a sufficient territory of distribution to justify stent implantation. If the SB is small (<1.5 mm) and supplies a small area of myocardium, it should be ignored, and a stent can be placed in the MV, across the SB ostium. In the medium size SB (2–2.75 mm), a strategy of keep-it-open by predilatation using a cutting balloon (or a noncompliant balloon) and leaving the jailed wire is appropriate with stent placement only if SB ostium is severely compromised. In large-size SB (>2.75 mm), 2-stent strategy may be preferred, especially if SB is angulated (>50°), has long lesions beyond the ostium, and if there is significant dissection after predilatation.

Treatment of coronary bifurcations frequently requires simultaneous insertion of 2 balloons or 2 stents; therefore, an appropriately sized guiding catheter should be selected.[25] With the currently available low-profile balloons, it is possible to

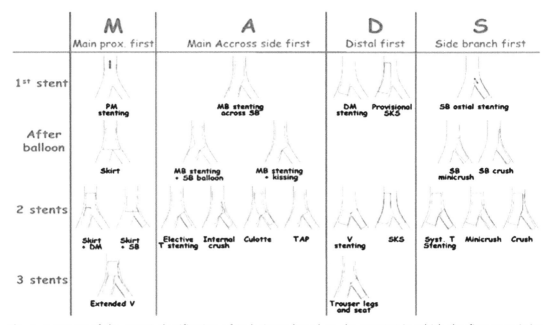

Fig. 5. Summary of the MADS classification of techniques based on the manner in which the first stent is implanted with multiple final stent strategies.

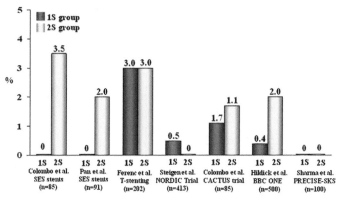

Fig. 6. Stent thrombosis incidence in clinical trials comparing 1-stent (1S) with 2-stent (2S) strategies in treating coronary bifurcations.

insert 2 balloons inside a large-lumen 6F guiding catheter with an internal lumen diameter of more than 0.070 in (1.75 mm). If 2 stents are needed, they can only be inserted one after the other, not simultaneously, in a large-lumen 6F guiding catheter. The crush or simultaneous kissing stents (SKS) technique require a minimum 7F or 8F guiding catheter, with an internal lumen diameter of 0.081 in (2.06 mm). Therefore, unless limited by peripheral arterial disease or ostial lesions, a routine use of a 7F guiding catheter is recommended.

Stenting Techniques

Conventional stent technique with provisional SB stent approach

The most common approach in the treatment of bifurcations is stenting only the MV and provisional stenting of the SB if needed for suboptimal angiographic results before or after stent deployment in the MV.[26-28] This technique

usually requires wiring of the SB (first) and the MV, followed by predilatation of the MV and then the SB (preferably with atherotomy by cutting balloon or noncompliant balloon). The predilatation is then followed by stenting of the MV. In more heavily calcified lesions, rotational atherectomy may be required in the MV or SB using a single burr with a burr-to-artery ratio of 0.4:0.5. The stent should be deployed while leaving the SB wire in place to prevent plaque shift, closure, or dissections in the SB ostium. Rarely, postdilatation with a high-pressure balloon may be needed at the area of maximal plaque burden for full stent expansion. If angiographic results in the MV and SB are satisfactory, the procedure is completed and the trapped guidewire in the SB behind the stent struts can be removed gently. If the SB ostium remains narrow or dissected, the next step is to place a wire into the SB across the MV stent strut and perform kissing balloon dilatations after dilatation of the SB ostium; this procedure

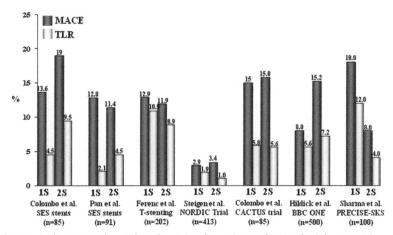

Fig. 7. Major adverse cardiac event (MACE) and TLR incidence in randomized trials comparing 1-stent (1S) with 2-stent (2S) strategies.

Table 1
Recent randomized trials of coronary bifurcation lesion management using DES; intention-to-treat analysis

Study	Technique Used	Number	Mean Follow-up Months	Procedural Success (%)	Follow-up MACE (%)	TLR (%)	Angiographic Restenosis MV (%)	Angiographic Restenosis SB (%)	ST (%)
BBK	T stent vs provisional stent	202	9	98 vs 98	11.9 vs 12.9	8.9 vs 10.9	3.1 vs 7.3	98.2 vs 19	3 vs 3
NORDIC	MV+SB stent vs MV stent	413	6	94 vs 97	3.4 vs 3.9	1 vs 1.9	2.5 vs 2.6	10.2 vs 19.2	0 vs 0.5
CACTUS	Crush vs provisional stent	350	6	90.4 vs 91.3	18.6 vs 17.6	5.6 vs 5.8	4.6% vs 6.7	13.2 vs 14.7	1.7 vs 1.1
BBC ONE	Crush/culotte vs provisional stent	500	9	98 vs 98	15.2 vs 8	5.6 vs 7.2	NR	NR	2.0 vs 0.4
PRECISE-SKS	SKS vs provisional stent	100	9	100 vs 92	8 vs 18	4 vs 12	2.4 vs 4.9	7.1 vs 24.4	0 vs 0
NORDIC II	Crush vs culotte stent	424	8	98 vs 98	4.3 vs 3.7	2.4 vs 2.8	4.7 vs 2	9.2 vs 4.5	1.4 vs 1.9

Abbreviations: MACE, major adverse cardiac event; NR, not reported; TLR, target lesion revascularization.

can be performed with the wire trapped behind the stent serving as a marker. Regarding the wire of choice for reentering the SB, a hydrophilic wire, such as Fielder or Whisper wires (Abbott Vascular Devices, Redwood City, CA, USA) or Luge Guidewire (Boston Scientific Corporation, Natick, MA, USA) is recommended. In this case, first, dilatation of the SB and then kissing balloon inflation in the MV and the SB are performed. If the SB result is satisfactory (even with a 50%–70% residual obstruction but no dissection), the stenting procedure is complete. If the SB result is suboptimal, stenting of the SB is performed in a "reverse T" approach, advancing the stent via the MV stent struts with final kissing balloon inflation.

There are some circumstances in which, due to the location of the plaque in the MV and/or the angulation of the SB, the wire cannot be advanced into the SB. Although this is a rare occurrence, after attempting different types of wires with all types of curves and techniques, it may still be difficult to advance a wire in the SB. At this point, few options are available: (1) stop the procedure, because the risk of losing the SB will be too high, considering also the size and distribution of the branch (typically an angulated circumflex artery when stenting the distal bifurcation of an unprotected left main); (2) use the Venture wire control catheter (St Jude Medical, Minnetonka, MN, USA) to direct the guidewire entry in the SB; and (3) dilate the MV with a balloon after advancing the intended SB wire into the MV distally, with the rationale that the plaque modification with a favorable plaque shift will facilitate access toward the SB. After balloon dilatations, the SB wire is withdrawn gently from the MV and directed into the SB ostium. In the past, plaque removal by directional coronary atherectomy has been suggested to facilitate the wire passage into the SB ostium.

SKS and "V" stenting techniques

The V technique consists of the delivery and implantation of 2 stents together. One stent is advanced in the SB, the other in the MV, and the 2 stents touch each other, forming a small proximal stent carina (<2 mm). When new stent carina extends a considerable length (3 mm or more) into the MV, this technique is called SKS (**Fig. 8**A), with its modified alternative ("trouser SKS," see **Fig. 8**B) for the long proximal lesions (to avoid new long carina).[24,28,29] The type of lesion the authors consider most suitable for this technique is a very proximal lesion, such as a bifurcation lesion of distal left main vessel and other bifurcation with moderate to large SB (>2.75

mm), with the vessel portion proximal to the bifurcation free of significant disease (see **Fig. 8**C).

SKS technique SKS technique involves using 2 appropriately sized stents (1:1 stent-to-artery ratio), 1 for the MV and 1 for the SB, with an overlap of the 2 stents in the proximal segment of the MV (stent sized 1:1 to the MV after the bifurcation). The proximal part of the MV should be able to accommodate the 2 stents, and its size should be approximately two-thirds of the aggregate diameter of the 2 stents (eg, for two 3.0-mm stents in left anterior descending artery and the diagonal branch, the proximal MV size should be approximately 4 mm). Stent lengths are selected visually to cover the entire length from the distal end of the SB and MV lesions to the proximal end in the MV. Debulking of the MV and/or SB using a cutting balloon or Rotablator (Boston Scientific Corporation, Natick, MA, USA), with or without balloon angioplasty, is performed as clinically indicated. Both MV and SB are wired, and lesions with more than 80% stenosis are dilated by appropriate sized balloons. Two stents are then advanced one by one, initially to the SB followed by 1 to the MV. After this step, both stents are pulled simultaneously back to the bifurcation, making a "V" and then into the proximal part of the MV to configure a "Y," with the stem of the Y in the MV (allowing for complete coverage of the proximal end of the lesion), with 1 arm of the Y in distal MV (covering the distal end of the MV lesion), and another arm in the SB (covering the distal end of SB lesions). The proximal overlapping part of the stents is kept as short as possible but long enough to cover the proximal end of the MV lesion. Once the position of the stents is confirmed and proximal stent markers are aligned, stents are deployed with simultaneous inflation at 10 to 12 atm for 10 to 20 seconds and then deflated. This is followed by a second dilatation of the MV stent at 16 to 20 atm for 10 to 20 seconds to fully expand the MV stent struts while the other SB stent balloon remains deflated in the SB stent. Then a third dilatation of the SB stent at 14 to 20 atm for 10 to 20 seconds is performed to allow full expansion of the SB stent struts while the other MV stent balloon remains deflated in the MV stent. This is then followed by a fourth and final simultaneous inflation and deflation at 10 to 12 atm for 10 to 20 seconds to form the uniform carina of the fully expanded kissing stents. Deflated stent balloons are withdrawn simultaneously. In cases of stent under expansion, 2 high-pressure balloons of similar length (may be different sizes) are advanced for the simultaneous kissing balloon dilatations. In cases of distal dissection, prolonged

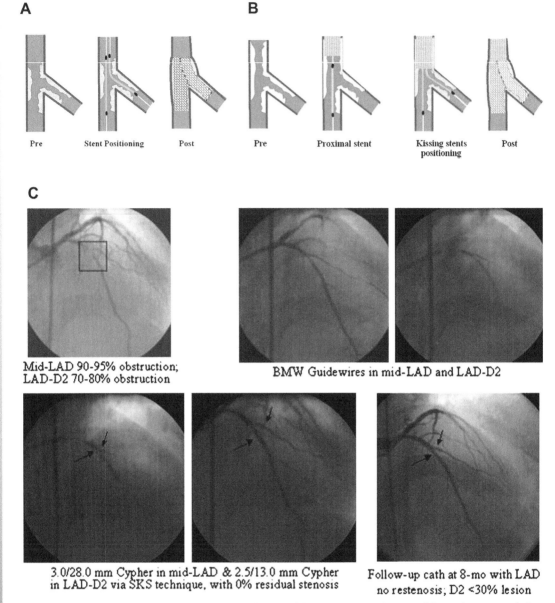

Fig. 8. (*A*) "Simultaneous kissing stents" (SKSs) technique. (*B*) Trouser SKS technique. (*C*) SKS for LAD-D2 bifurcation with 8-month angiographic follow-up. (*Adapted from* Sharma SK, Kini AS. Coronary bifurcation lesions. Cardiol Clin 2006;24:233–46; with permission.)

balloon dilatation is performed to avoid the need for stenting. In cases of proximal dissection, 2-balloon (1 in each stent) dilatation or a perfusion balloon dilatation at low pressure in the MV is done. If there is a need to place a stent at the proximal segment of a vessel treated with SKS stenting, there are 2 options: (1) a stent is placed proximally, leaving a small gap between the kissing stents and the proximal stent and (2) the kissing stent technique is converted into a crush technique, with the stent in the MV compressing

the other stent (1 arm of the V) in the SB. A wire will then cross the struts into the SB, and a balloon will be inflated toward the SB. After wire removal from the SB, the proximal stent will be advanced toward the MV.

Trouser SKS technique In cases that involve a long lesion in the proximal part of MV, before the bifurcation, a large stent is first deployed proximally over the guidewire in the MV. This is followed by wiring the SB via the proximal stent and then

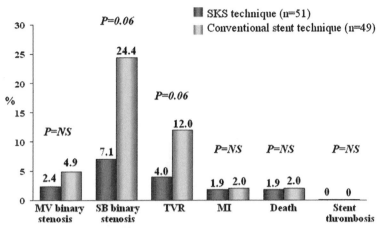

Fig. 9. PRECISE-SKS trial comparing simultaneous kissing stent technique with conventional technique: 9- to 12-months follow-up results.

advancing the 2 stents through the MV stent to the distal MV and the SB and deploying the stent as described earlier (in "trouser-and-seat" pattern) (see **Fig. 8**B).

The SKS technique obviates the need for recrossing a stent strut and reducing stent deformation and has been shown to provide excellent short- and long-term results when compared with the conventional stenting strategy for medium-to-large coronary bifurcation lesions.

Precise-SKS pilot study (**Fig. 9**) of 100 large bifurcation lesions showed a trend toward lower SB restenosis by SKS technique as compared with conventional technique (with 28% provisional stent use), with higher acute procedural success of SB (90% vs 92% in conventional group).

There was no ST in this study, with no difference in major adverse cardiac event (MACE) rates between the 2 techniques.

Crush technique

In the crush technique, 2 stents are placed in the MV and the SB, with the former more proximal than the latter.[17,30–32] The stent of the SB is deployed, and its balloon and wire are removed. The stent subsequently deployed in the MV flattens the protruding cells of the SB stent, hence the name crushing or crush technique. Wire recrossing and dilatation of the SB with a balloon of a diameter at least equal to that of the stent followed by final kissing balloon inflation is recommended. The implementation of final kissing balloon inflation is done to allow better strut contact against the ostium of the SB and therefore better drug delivery in the case of DES. The crush technique, therefore, became a sort of simplified culotte technique. The positive aspect is that whenever restenosis occurs, this narrowing is

very focal (<5 mm in length) and most of the time it is not associated with symptoms or ischemia.

The CACTUS (Coronary Bifurcations: Application of the Crushing Technique Using Sirolimus-Eluting Stents) trial of 350 cases, comparing crush with provisional stent technique, showed similar acute clinical and procedural success. At 6 months, angiographic restenosis rates were not different between the crush group (4.6% and 13.2% in the main branch and SB, respectively) and the provisional stenting group (6.7% and 14.7% in the main branch and SB, respectively; P = not significant). Additional stenting of the SB in the provisional stenting group was required in 31% of the lesions. Rates of MACEs and ST were also similar in the 2 groups (**Fig. 10**).

When using the crush stenting technique, use of kissing balloon after dilatation is mandatory to reduce the restenosis rate of SB and the need for TLR. The main disadvantage is that the performance of the final kissing balloon inflation makes the procedure more laborious because of the need to recross multiple struts with a wire and a balloon.

Reverse crush technique

The main indication for performing the reverse crush is to allow an opportunity for provisional SB stenting. A stent is deployed in the MV, and balloon dilatation with final kissing inflation toward the SB is performed. The result at the ostium or at the proximal segment of the SB is suboptimal for deploying a stent at this site. A second stent is advanced into the SB and is left in position without being deployed. Then a balloon sized according to the diameter of the MV is positioned at the level of the bifurcation, with the operator making sure to keep the stent inside the stent previously deployed in the MV. The stent in the SB is retracted to about

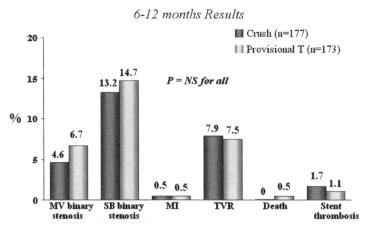

Fig. 10. CACTUS study: 6- to 12-month restenosis, myocardial infarction (MI), target vessel revascularization (TVR), death, and stent thrombosis rates in the crush stenting (crush) and provisional T-stenting (provisional) groups. (*Data from* Colombo A, Bramucci E, Saccà S, Violini R, Lettieri C, Zanini R, et al. Randomized study of the crush technique versus provisional side-branch stenting in true coronary bifurcations: the CACTUS (Coronary bifurcations: application of the crushing technique using sirolimus-eluting stents) study. Circulation 2009;119:71–8.)

2 to 3 mm into the MV and deployed, the deploying balloon is removed, and an angiogram is obtained to verify that a good result is present at the SB (no further distal stent in the SB is needed). If this is the case, the wire from the SB is removed, and the balloon in the MV is inflated at high pressure (12 atm or more). The other steps are similar to the ones described for the crush technique and involve recrossing into the SB and performing SB dilatation and final kissing balloon inflation.

The main advantages of the reverse crush technique are that the immediate patency of both branches is assured and that the technique can be performed using a 6F guiding catheter. This technique has the same disadvantages as the standard crush technique and is even more laborious.

Double-kissing crush technique

The classic crush technique consists of 3 steps: SB stenting, crushing, and final kissing balloon inflations, and it is limited by residual stenosis of the SB ostium. The double-kissing (DK) crush technique consists of 5 steps: SB stenting, balloon crush, first kissing, MV stenting and crushing, and final kissing.[33] In the DK crush technique, first, a balloon is used in the MV, and a stent is loaded into the SB. The SB stent is inflated, and after removing the guidewire and the SB-stented balloon, the balloon in the MV is inflated, and the protruding SB stent is crushed against the MV wall. Then, the first kissing balloon inflation is done after successfully rewiring the SB. Another stent in the MV is inflated to further crush the SB stent after removing the SB guidewire and balloon. Final kissing balloon inflations are performed after

successfully rewiring the SB. DK crush technique has shown improved SB results compared with classical crush technique.

T-stenting and modified T-stenting techniques

The classic T-stenting technique consists of positioning a stent first at the ostium of the SB, being careful to avoid stent protrusion into the MV (see **Fig. 10**).[34] Some operators leave a balloon in the MV to help to further locate the MV. After deployment of the stent and removal of the balloon and the wire from the SB, a second stent is advanced in the MV. A wire is then readvanced into the SB, and final kissing balloon inflation is performed. Modified T-stenting is a variation performed by simultaneous positioning of stents at the SB and the MV. The SB stent is deployed first, and then after wire and balloon removal from the SB, the MV stent is deployed. A final kissing balloon dilatation is required to complete the procedure.

Culotte technique

The culotte technique uses 2 stents and leads to full coverage of the bifurcation at the expense of an excess of metal covering of the proximal end. Both branches are predilated.[35] First, a stent is deployed across the most angulated branch, usually the SB. The nonstented branch is then rewired through the struts of the stent and dilated. A second stent is advanced and expanded into the nonstented branch, usually the MV. Finally, kissing balloon inflation is performed.

The culotte technique is suitable for all angles of bifurcations and provides near-perfect coverage of the SB ostium. Similar to the crush technique, it leads to a high concentration of metal with a double-stent layer at the carina and at the proximal part of the bifurcation. The main disadvantage of the technique is that rewiring both branches through the stent struts can be difficult and time consuming.

Y-stent technique

This technique involves an initial predilatation, followed by stent deployment in each branch. If the results are not adequate, a third stent may also be deployed in the MV. This technique is not commonly used at the present time and is a last resort for treating very demanding bifurcations in which there is a need to maintain wire access to both branches. The modification of this Y-stent technique could be deployment of the stent proximal to bifurcation and then advance 1 or 2 stents distally into each branch. This technique has gained favor with a new, self-expanding, dedicated bifurcation stent.[36]

Technique for isolated ostial lesions involving the MV or the SB

With isolated ostial lesions, it is important to accurately place a stent to cover the lesion entirely without having the stent protrude into the other branch. Some operators use intravascular ultrasound to facilitate appropriate stent placement. The following techniques are suggested based on the lesion location.

Isolated ostial lesions of MV There are 2 approaches for treating these lesions: (1) placement of a stent at the ostium of the MV with a balloon protecting the SB, and with inflation of the SB balloon and kissing balloon only if plaque shift occurs, and (2) placement of a stent in the MV covering the origin of the SB and then wiring the SB and performing kissing balloon inflation in case the ostium of the SB deteriorates.

Isolated ostial lesions of SB The most common approach in treating these lesions is to place a stent at the ostium of the SB, frequently with a low-pressure balloon inflated in the MV (stent pull-back technique). If after stent placement there is deterioration of the MV at the site of the bifurcation, the balloon in the MV is inflated, protecting the stent by a simultaneous inflation of the stent delivery balloon. In cases of suboptimal angiographic results in MV, a stent can be deployed with final kissing balloon dilatation.[37]

Dedicated Bifurcation Stents

Based on the results from randomized trials, the provisional stent approach to bifurcation lesions seems to be the prevailing approach. Despite the simplified 1-stent approach, this technique does have disadvantages as previously described.

Dedicated bifurcation stents have been designed to specifically overcome some of the disadvantages of the provisional approach to bifurcations lesions; that is, they enable the treatment of the SB ostium simultaneously with the main branch, thereby preserving a permanent access to SB during the procedure. There are currently several devices available (**Fig. 11**) that are undergoing or have undergone clinical trials, but larger controlled studies are needed before these stents are routinely used in everyday clinical practice.[34]

Frontier (Abbott Vascular Devices, Redwood City, CA, USA/Guidant Corporation, Santa Clara, CA, USA). The Frontier coronary stent system is a balloon-expandable stainless steel stent mounted on a delivery system with 2 balloons (a monorail for the MV and an over-the-wire inner lumen for the SB) and 2 guidewire lumens. The stent system is advanced into the MV over a coronary wire and the joining mandrel is retracted, releasing the over-the-wire SB tip. A 300-cm wire is inserted into the SB balloon lumen and into the SB. The system is then advanced to the carina, and a single indeflator provides simultaneous kissing inflation of the 2 balloons to expand the stent on the MV and the SB.[38]

Petal (Boston Scientific, Natick, MA, USA). The Petal stent has a side aperture located at the middle of the stent with deployable struts and is designed to prevent SB occlusion after MV stenting. The Petal stent is crimped over 2 balloons such that an elliptical balloon is under the side aperture and petal elements. On inflation, the main balloon deploys the stent into the MV, whereas the elliptical balloon deploys the petal elements into the SB ostium.

Stentys (Stentys S.A.S., Clichy, France). The Stentys-bifurcated DES is the first of the second-generation bifurcation stents. The Stentys is a self-expanding, paclitaxel-coated nitinol stent made of Z-shaped mesh linked by small interconnections. A unique advantage of this stent is its ability to disconnect the stent struts with an angioplasty balloon, thereby allowing an opening for the SB to be created anywhere in the stent after it is implanted in the vessel.

Tryton (Tryton Medical, Inc, Durham, NC, USA). The Tryton SB stent is a slotted tube, cobalt-chromium balloon-expandable stent designed for the SB implantation. Treatment with the Tryton stent generally allows the operator to implant 2 stents in the bifurcation in a technique that is identical when performing the culotte technique.

Antares SAS (TriReme Medical, Inc, Pleasanton, CA, USA). The TriReme Antares Side Branch Adaptive System (SAS) is made of a single balloon-expandable, stainless steel stent. Stent

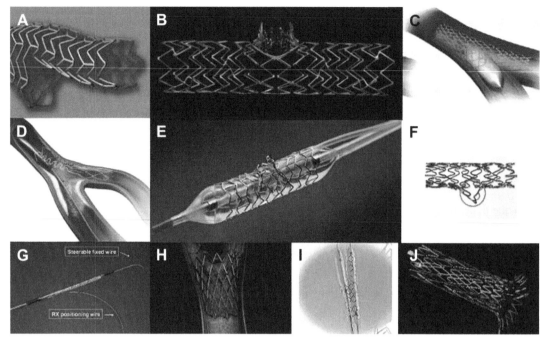

Fig. 11. Dedicated bifurcation stents. (*A*) Frontier coronary stent system (Abbott Vascular Devices, Redwood City, CA, USA/Guidant Corporation, Santa Clara, CA, USA). (*B*) Petal (Boston Scientific Corporation, Natick, MA, USA). (*C*) Stentys (Stentys S.A.S., Clichy, France). (*D*) Tryton (Tryton Medical, Inc, Durham, NC, USA). (*E*) Antares SAS (TriReme Medical, Inc, Pleasanton, CA, USA). (*F*) Twin-Rail (Invatec S.r.l., Brescia, Italy). (*G*) Y-Med Sidekick (Ymed, Inc, San Diego, CA, USA). (*H*) Devax AXXESS PLUS (Devax, Inc, Irvine, CA, USA). (*I*) Nile Croco (Minvasys, Genevilliers, France). (*J*) Cappella Sideguard (Cappella, Inc, Galway, Ireland).

deployment is achieved by using a single rapid-exchange balloon catheter. On expansion of the main stent body, the ostial crown is automatically deployed with elements protruding approximately 2 mm into the SB to scaffold the ostium.

Twin-Rail (Invatec S.r.l., Brescia, Italy). This is a slotted tube, stainless steel stent premounted on double balloons in its proximal portion and on the MV balloon in its distal portion. The stent has a closed-cell type design with variable stent geometry. The stent is deployed by simultaneous kissing inflation with a single indeflator.

Y-Med Sidekick (Ymed, Inc, San Diego, CA, USA). The Y-Med Sidekick is a low-profile stent delivery system that integrates an MV fixed-wire platform with a rapid-exchange, steerable SB guidewire that is designed to preserve SB access during bifurcation stenting. When the device is close to the carina, a guidewire is passed through the SB exit port and the MV stent struts into the SB, thus avoiding recrossing into the SB.

Devax AXXESS PLUS (Devax, Inc, Irvine, CA, USA). The Devax AXXESS PLUS stent is a self-expanding, nickel-titanium stent that delivers biolimus-A9, a sirolimus derivative via polymer carrier and must be precisely placed at the carina of the bifurcation to be effective. However, in most cases, it requires another stent to fully treat the bifurcation lesions.

Nile Croco (Minvasys, Genevilliers, France). This is a double-balloon cobalt stent delivery system with 2 independent, yet joined, catheters that require independent manipulation and pressure monitoring. After the stent is deployed into the MV, the SB balloon is advanced into the SB and final kissing balloon inflation is performed.

Sideguard (Cappella, Inc, Galway, Ireland). The Cappella Sideguard ostium protection device is a self-expanding, trumpet-shaped nitinol stent that is deployed using a special balloon-release sheath system. The stent is deployed using a nominal-pressure balloon, which helps tear a protective sheath that keeps the Cappella Sideguard in place until deployment. A conventional stent is placed in the MV. The SB is reaccessed with a conventional guidewire, and the procedure is completed after final kissing balloon inflation.

Lesion Preparation and Adjunct Pharmacotherapy

Plaque removal before stent implantation, using directional atherectomy in noncalcified lesions and rotational atherectomy in calcified lesions,

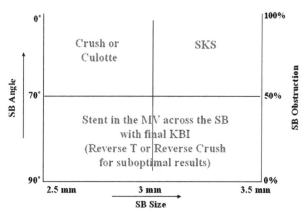

Fig. 12. Suggested approach for large bifurcation lesions based on the SB size, angulation, and obstruction. KBI, kissing balloon inflation.

has been attractive. However, some encouraging results of many single-center experiences have not been reproduced in the randomized trials. Rotational atherectomy for heavy calcification is essential for lesion dilatation and, hence, facilitates stent delivery and expansion. In most catheterization laboratories, the use of this procedure is less than 5% of all interventions. Most of the time, rotational ablation is performed only on the MV, but occasionally also or only on the SB because of heavily calcified lesion. Therefore, lesion preparation with compliance change for a calcified lesion can substantially facilitate stent delivery and symmetric stent expansion with more homogeneous drug delivery after DES implantation.[39]

Techniques using plaque modification by cutting balloon (Boston Scientific Corporation, Inc, MA) or AngioSculpt balloon (AngioScore, Inc,

Fremont, CA) have reported the beneficial combination of stenting preceded by atherotomy. In bifurcation lesions, in which there is a large fibrotic plaque at the ostium of the SB, the use of the cutting balloon as a sole device or as a predilatation strategy before stenting seems reasonable. Currently, the authors suggest the use of the cutting balloon in moderately calcific and fibrotic lesions. Symmetric stent expansion, avoidance of SB recoil, and stent compression are all attractive hypotheses for the use of these devices.

Unfractionated heparin to keep activated clotting time (ACT) of approximately 250 seconds or bivalirudin to keep ACT of more than 300 seconds are usual antithrombotic therapy. Use of glycoprotein IIb/IIIa inhibitors is reserved for thrombus-containing lesions, when multiple stents or overlapping stents are implanted on both branches. These

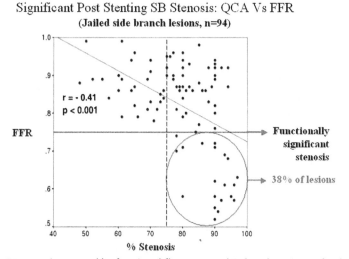

Fig. 13. Poststenting SB stenosis assessed by fractional flow reserve (FFR) and angiography. (*Adapted from* Koo B, Kang H, Youn T, et al. Physiologic assessment of jailed side branch lesions using fractional flow reserve. J Am Coll Cardiol 2005;46:633–37; with permission.)

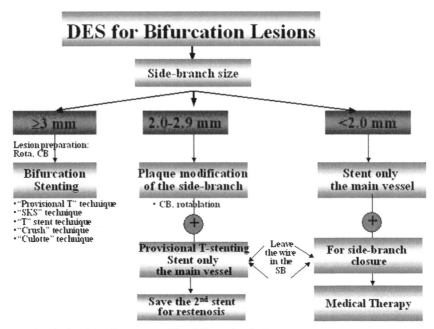

Fig. 14. Interventional algorithm for approaching bifurcation lesions.

agents are sometimes administered when the final result at the SB seems suboptimal and for other procedural complications, such as dissection or slow flow. A 162- to 325-mg loading dose or 81- to 162-mg maintenance dose of aspirin is recommended, and a 600-mg loading dose of clopidogrel is routinely used in most catheterization laboratories, with 75 mg daily for 1 to 3 years after DES implantation.[40] The duration of combined thienopyridine and aspirin treatment after stent implantation varies according to the length of the stent implanted, the type of stent used, and the clinical conditions of the patient (acute coronary syndrome or diabetes mellitus).

SUMMARY AND FUTURE DIRECTIONS

Treating bifurcation lesions is challenging, but a simple algorithm based on the SB size, stenosis, and angulation can be used (**Fig. 12**). When treating bifurcation lesions, close attention must be paid in choosing the right guiding catheter size. It should be large enough to accommodate 2 balloons or 2 stents when needed a priori or when there is a high likelihood of being used. A wire should be placed in the SB, especially if there is disease at the ostium or if a problematic take off. The general consensus is to try to keep the procedure safe and simple. When the SB is not severely diseased, implantation of a stent in the MV and provisional stenting in the SB are the preferred strategies. Implantation of 2 stents as the initial approach is appropriate when both branches are large

(>2.75 mm) and significantly diseased (>50% diameter stenosis) and suitable for stenting.

Although dedicated stents are being developed, their clinical use in the format of DES is very limited. However, these devices may have potentially important applications in proximal large bifurcations and in the left main trunk.

Despite all of the unanswered questions and some persisting problems, 2 major achievements cannot be overlooked in bifurcational stenting since the introduction of DES: (1) single-digit restenosis rates on the MV and (2) focal restenosis at the SB that is very frequently clinically silent. Also, many ostially narrow-jailed SBs are not functionally significant as assessed by fractional flow reserve (>0.75), and the operator should resist temptation to improve the angiographic appearance (**Fig. 13**).[41] The ongoing development of novel DES devices designed specifically for coronary bifurcations and the large randomized clinical trials being conducted to address their utility will add to the already present literature regarding treatment of coronary bifurcation lesions.

In conclusion, an algorithm for bifurcation lesions treatment based on SB size has been proposed (**Fig. 14**).

REFERENCES

1. Louvard Y, Thomas M, Dzavik V, et al. Classification of coronary artery bifurcation lesions and

treatments: time for a consensus!. Catheter Cardio-vasc Interv 2008;71:175–83.

2. Dauerman H, Higgins P, Sparano A, et al. Mechanical debulking versus balloon angioplasty for the treatment of true bifurcation lesions. J Am Coll Cardiol 1998;32:1845–52.

3. Al Suwaidi J, Berger P, Rihal C, et al. Immediate and long-term outcome of intracoronary stent implantation for true bifurcation lesions. J Am Coll Cardiol 2000;35:929–36.

4. Yamashita T, Nishida T, Adamian M, et al. Bifurcation lesions: two stents versus one stent—immediate and follow-up results. J Am Coll Cardiol 2000;35: 1145–51.

5. Pan M, Suarez de Lezo J, Medina A, et al. Simple and complex stent strategies for bifurcated coronary arterial stenosis involving the side branch origin. Am J Cardiol 1999;83:1320–5.

6. Movahed MR. Coronary artery bifurcation lesion classifications, interventional techniques and clinical outcome. Expert Rev Cardiovasc Ther 2008;6: 261–74.

7. Kobayashi Y, Colombo A, Akiyama T, et al. Modified "T" stenting: a technique for kissing stents in bifurcational coronary lesions. Cathet Cardiovasc Diagn 1998;43:323–6.

8. Chevalier B, Glatt B, Royer T, et al. Placement of coronary stents in bifurcation lesions by the "culotte" technique. Am J Cardiol 1998;82:943–9.

9. Brueck M, Scheinert D, Flachskampf F, et al. Sequential vs. kissing balloon angioplasty for stenting of bifurcation coronary lesions. Catheter Cardiovasc Interv 2002;55:461–6.

10. Cervinka P, Foley D, Sabaté M, et al. Coronary bifurcation stenting using dedicated bifurcation stents. Catheter Cardiovasc Interv 2000;49:105–11.

11. Colombo A, Stankovic G, Orlic D, et al. Modified T-stenting technique with crushing for bifurcation lesions: immediate results and 30-day outcome. Catheter Cardiovasc Interv 2003;60:145–51.

12. Stankovic G, Darremont O, Ferenc M, et al. Percutaneous coronary intervention for bifurcation lesions: 2008 consensus document from the fourth meeting of the European Bifurcation Club. EuroIntervention 2009;5:39–49.

13. Zhang F, Dong L, Ge J. Simple versus complex stenting strategy for coronary artery bifurcation lesions in the drug-eluting stent era: a meta-analysis of randomised trials. Heart 2009;95:1676–81.

14. Iakovou I, Schmidt T, Bonizzoni E, et al. Incidence, prediction and outcome of thrombosis after successful implantation of drug-eluting stents. JAMA 2005;293:2126–30.

15. Colombo A, Moses J, Morice M, et al. Randomized study to evaluate sirolimus-eluting stents implanted at coronary bifurcation lesions. Circulation 2004; 109:1244–9.

16. Pan M, de Lezo SJ, Medina A, et al. Rapamycin-eluting stents for the treatment of bifurcated coronary lesions; a randomized comparison of a simple versus complex strategy. Am Heart J 2004;148:857–64.

17. Colombo A, Bramucci E, Saccà S, et al. Randomized study of the crush technique versus provisional side-branch stenting in true coronary bifurcations: the CACTUS (coronary bifurcations: application of the crushing technique using sirolimus-eluting stents) study. Circulation 2009;119:71–8.

18. Ferenc M, Gick M, Kienzle R, et al. Randomized trial on routine vs. provisional T-stenting in the treatment of de novo coronary bifurcation lesions. Eur Heart J 2008;29:2859–67.

19. Collins N, Seidelin P, Daly P, et al. Long-term outcomes after percutaneous coronary intervention of bifurcation narrowings. Am J Cardiol 2008;102: 404–10.

20. Tsuchida K, Colombo A, Lefèvre T, et al. The clinical outcome of percutaneous treatment of bifurcation lesions in multivessel coronary artery disease with the sirolimus-eluting stent: insights from the Arterial Revascularization Therapies Study part II (ARTS II). Eur Heart J 2007;28:433–42.

21. Steigen T, Maeng M, Wiseth R, et al. Randomized study on simple versus complex stenting of coronary artery bifurcation lesions. The Nordic Bifurcation Study. Circulation 2006;114:1955–61.

22. Hildick-Smith D. BBC-ONE (British Bifurcation Coronary Study: Old, New, and Evolving Strategies) trial. Paper presented at Transcatheter Cardiovascular Therapeutics (TCT), October 17, 2008, Washington, DC.

23. Erglis A, Kumsars I, Niemela M, et al. Randomized comparison of coronary bifurcation stenting with the crush versus the culotte technique using sirolimus eluting stents. (Nordic bifurcation II study). Circ Cardiovasc Interv 2009;2:27–34.

24. Sharma S, Labana S, Krishnan P, et al. A randomized pilot trial for treatment of large bifurcation lesions with simultaneous kissing stents: PRECISE-SKS trial [abstract]. Circulation 2008;118: II-S901.

25. Latib A, Colombo A. Bifurcation disease. What do we know, what should we do? JACC Cardiovasc Interv 2008;1:218–26.

26. Routledge H, Morice MC, Lefevre T, et al. 2-year outcome of patients treated for bifurcation coronary disease with provisional side branch T-stenting using drug-eluting stents. JACC Cardiovasc Interv 2008;1:358–65.

27. Ormiston JA, Webster MW, El Jack S, et al. Drug-eluting stents for coronary bifurcations: bench testing of provisional side-branch strategies. Catheter Cardiovasc Interv 2006;67:49–55.

28. Sharma S, Ahsan C, Lee J, et al. Simultaneous kissing stents (SKS) technique for treating bifurcation lesions in medium-to-large size coronary arteries. Am J Cardiol 2004;94:913–7.

29. Sharma SK. Simultaneous kissing drug-eluting stent technique for percutaneous treatment of bifurcation lesions in large-size vessels. Catheter Cardiovasc Interv 2005;65:10–6.

30. Ge L, Airoldi F, Iakovou I, et al. Clinical and angiographic outcome after implantation of drug-eluting stents in bifurcation lesions with the crush stent technique: importance of final kissing balloon post-dilatation. J Am Coll Cardiol 2005;46:613–20.

31. Hoye A, Iakovou I, Ge L, et al. Long-term outcomes after stenting of bifurcation lesions with the "crush" technique: predictors of an adverse outcome. J Am Coll Cardiol 2006;47:1949–58.

32. Costa RA, Mintz GS, Carlier SG, et al. Bifurcation coronary lesions treated with the "crush" technique: an intravascular ultrasound analysis. J Am Coll Cardiol 2005;46:599–605.

33. Chen S, Zhang J, Chen Y, et al. Study comparing the double kissing (DK) crush with classical crush for the treatment of coronary bifurcation lesions: the DKCRUSH-1. Bifurcation study with drug-eluting stents. Eur J Clin Invest 2008;38:361–71.

34. Latib A, Colombo A, Sangiorgi GM. Bifurcation stenting: current strategies and new devices. Heart 2009;95:495–504.

35. Adriaenssens T, Byrne R, Dibra A, et al. Culotte stenting technique in coronary bifurcation disease: angiographic follow-up using dedicated quantitative coronary angiographic analysis and 12-month clinical outcome. Eur Heart J 2008;29:2868–76.

36. Verheye S, Agostoni P, Dubois C, et al. 9-month clinical, angiographic and intravascular ultrasound results of a prospective evaluation of the Axxess self-expanding biolimus A9-eluting stent in coronary bifurcation lesions. The DIVERGE (Drug-Eluting Stent Intervention for Treating Side Branches Effectively) study. J Am Coll Cardiol 2009;53:1031–9.

37. Kini A, Moreno P, Steinheimer A, et al. Effectiveness of the stent pull-back technique for non-aorto ostial coronary narrowings. Am J Cardiol 2005;96:1123–8.

38. Lefèvre T, Ormiston J, Guagliumi G, et al. The Frontier stent registry: safety and feasibility of a novel dedicated stent for the treatment of bifurcation coronary artery lesions. J Am Coll Cardiol 2005;46:592–8.

39. Dahm J, Dorr M, Scholz E, et al. Cutting-balloon angioplasty effectively facilitates the interventional procedure and leads to a low rate of recurrent stenosis in ostial bifurcation coronary lesions: a subgroup analysis of the NICECUT multicenter registry. Int J Cardiol 2008;124:345–50.

40. Pan M, Suárez de Lezo J, Medina A, et al. Drug-eluting stents for the treatment of bifurcation lesions: a randomized comparison between paclitaxel and sirolimus stents. Am Heart J 2007;153:15–7.

41. Koo B, Kang H, Youn T, et al. Physiologic assessment of jailed side branch lesions using fractional flow reserve. J Am Coll Cardiol 2005;46:633–7.

Coronary Chronic Total Occlusion

John M. Galla, MD, Patrick L. Whitlow, MD*

KEYWORDS

- Coronary artery disease • Coronary intervention
- Chronic total occlusion

Chronic total coronary occlusions (CTOs) are a frequent finding in patients with coronary disease and when clinically indicated, remain one of the most challenging target lesion subsets for intervention. Comprised of a combination of fibrocalcific and thrombotic elements, CTOs have been reported in approximately one-third of patients undergoing diagnostic coronary angiography.[1] By nature of their complexity, CTO percutaneous interventions (PCI) are associated with lower rates of procedural success, higher complication rates, greater radiation exposure, and longer procedure times compared with interventions in non-CTO stenoses. Despite these obstacles, reported benefits of successful CTO PCI include a reduction in symptoms and improvement in both ventricular function and survival.[2–5]

Defined angiographically as a complete occlusion—thrombolysis in myocardial infarction (TIMI) grade 0 or 1 antegrade flow—the chronicity to qualify as lesion as a CTO has ranged from 1 to 3 months. A universal CTO classification system has recently been proposed that grades lesions on both the technical challenges of and risk associated with attempted recanalization.[6] Factors associated with higher success of recanalization include a stem of patent vessel longer than 10 mm, no branches within 5 mm of the occlusion, a tapering configuration or visible track through the lesion, and no evidence of calcification on fluoroscopy. A CTO occurring at the coronary ostium, at a bifurcation point, with significant calcification, or a long lesion evidenced by retrograde filling of the distal vessel all portend a high level of difficulty with a reduced likelihood of success. The risk of adverse outcomes during attempted percutaneous revascularization is highest for patients with bridging collateral vessels and aneurysmal appearance at the point of occlusion. Consideration of the technical challenges of recanalization and the risk associated with attempted reopening are valuable when planning CTO PCI.

APPROACH TO PERCUTANEOUS CORONARY INTERVENTION OF CHRONIC TOTAL OCCLUSIONS

Given the technical challenges, most operators who specialize in CTO revascularization recognize the importance of planning prior to any attempted PCI. Although an experienced interventionalist may elect to pursue a straightforward occlusion, strong consideration should be given to deferring ad hoc CTO PCI to allow for patient discussion and determination of the appropriate strategy and equipment. Novel imaging techniques such as 3-dimensional cineangiography or computed tomographic angiogram offer the opportunity to more completely analyze a candidate lesion, and may significantly benefit CTO PCI outcomes.[7,8] In addition, imaging studies to determine distal myocardial viability might be needed to estimate the benefit versus risk of CTO PCI. Once the CTO anatomy has been delineated, additional considerations include choice of devices and approach whereby development of new devices and technical variations has given the CTO operator a list of highly functional choices when planning a CTO PCI. The ultimate decision to offer CTO PCI to patients may be based on several factors including technical difficulty, chances for successful outcome, and the amount of viable myocardium supplied by the CTO vessel. Appropriate patients should have the possibility of significant benefit in limiting chest discomfort or have

Division of Interventional Cardiology, Heart and Vascular Institute, Cleveland Clinic J2-3, 9500 Euclid Avenue, Cleveland, OH 44195, USA
* Corresponding author.
E-mail address: whitlop@ccf.org (P.L. Whitlow).

Cardiol Clin 28 (2010) 71–79
doi:10.1016/j.ccl.2009.10.003

a significant amount of viable myocardium at risk, and proceed only after a thoughtful consideration of either continued aggressive medical therapy or surgical revascularization.

Choosing an approach is an appropriate first step in CTO PCI. Broadly characterized as either antegrade or retrograde, several successfully employed variations have been described on both techniques. The antegrade approach may be performed in a similar way to standard PCI whereby the lesion is wired, dilated, and stented with standard equipment. As with any PCI, proper guide selection is critical to ensure a successful outcome. Guide support is paramount in CTO PCI whereby the ability to push wires and equipment through long tortuous or occluded segments is essential for success. Larger guides, 7F or 8F lumen, are frequently employed for their increased stiffness and ability to handle adjunctive equipment (ie, intravascular ultrasound). Guide shapes for CTOs arising from the left coronary tree are typically the Amplatz or Extra Backup, and either traditional or modified Amplatz for those in the right system. The Amplatz guides are particularly useful in that they provide excellent support even when seated in the coronary sinus noncoaxial with the proximal vessel, thus lowering the chances of dissection. For particularly challenging lesions, additional guide support can be achieved through the use of an anchor balloon, typically a small over-the-wire (OTW) balloon placed in a small side branch and inflated to low pressure to provide counterforce for firm engagement of the guide catheter.[9]

Advances in guidewire design have played a significant role in the improved success in CTO PCI. It is reasonable to attempt CTO PCI with standard workhorse wires and select progressively stiffer wires as necessary to reenter the distal true lumen. Several wire families are particularly useful in attempting CTO PCI, and offer choices in hydrophilicity and varying tip stiffness. Hydrophobic wires (Miracle Bros/Confianza, Abbott Vascular Inc, Abbott Park, IL) offer better tactile response when attempting to penetrate the CTO and are favored when blunt dissecting through a fibrocalcific cap or organized thrombotic core. Hydrophilic wires (Fielder/Whisper, Abbott Vascular Inc) are preferred when navigating microchannels or tortuous segments where increased tip lubricity is helpful in overcoming frictional forces.

The addition of an OTW balloon or support catheter offers reinforcement when attempting to penetrate demanding lesions. By providing a fulcrum for the wire, these devices, when advanced close to the lesion, increase the buckling load on the wire tip, thus allowing for maximum penetrating force. The authors generally prefer

microcatheters to angioplasty balloons for this purpose because of reduced wire bias and optimal wire torque response. In addition, these devices improve maneuverability by reducing friction along the length of the wire and permitting guidewire exchanges without loss of progress through the lesion. Catheters currently approved for use and with widespread popularity in the CTO community are primarily marketed as neurovascular devices, and include the Transit (Cordis Corp, Warren, NJ), Tracker (Boston Scientific, Natick, MA), and the Finecross (Terumo Medical Corp, Somerset, NJ) catheters. An adaptation of the standard support catheter, the Tornus (Abbott Vascular Inc) is a braided stainless steel catheter with a tapered threaded tip that allows the catheter to be advanced through a lesion while twisting to provide additional penetrating force. Commonly used guidewires and devices for CTO PCI are listed in **Table 1**.

A novel modification of the support catheter concept by BridgePoint Medical Systems (Minneapolis, MN) has produced a complete CTO PCI crossing system particularly applicable to an antegrade approach. The system is comprised of 3 elements: the CrossBoss CTO catheter, the Stingray CTO orienting balloon catheter, and the Stingray reentry guidewire with a tapered tip. The CTO catheter has a highly torqueable coiled-wire shaft and an atraumatic 1-mm rounded tip that tracks in advance of a guidewire via the facilitated antegrade steering spin technique (see Video 1, available in the online version of this article at http://www.cardiology.theclinics.com). Depending on whether the crossing catheter remains within the true lumen during penetration of the lesion, the CrossBoss may be removed, leaving a guidewire in place to allow either balloon angioplasty and stenting or implementation of the second element, the Stingray reentry balloon catheter. To facilitate reentry into the true lumen, the Stingray balloon is advanced within the subintimal space adjacent to or just past the distal cap and inflated, which provides a fulcrum with orthogonal orientation of 2 exit holes within the balloon (see Video 2, courtesy of Dr Etsuo Tsuchikane, available in the online version of this article at http://www.cardiology.theclinics.com). Then, using a proprietary reentry guidewire, the distal true lumen is entered via the adluminal exit hole. In its first-in-man all-comers registry, this system was used to place a guidewire in the distal true lumen in 87.5% of patients, with no in-hospital major adverse cardiac events (Whitlow, personal communication, 2009).

A compilation of these antegrade techniques can be seen in the case of a 61-year-old man with refractory angina and a known left anterior descending artery (LAD) CTO (**Fig. 1**). The patient

Table 1
Commonly used equipment for CTO PCI

Guidewires	Tip Load (g)	Utility
Fielder, FC, XT	1	Excellent for antegrade microchannel and retrograde collateral tracking
Miracle Bros	3, 4.5, 6, 9, 12	Variable penetrating power with excellent tactile feedback
Confianza	9, 12	Excellent penetrating force with great tip steering against resistance
Confianza Pro	9, 12	Improved torqueability associated with hydrophilic coating
Pilot 50, 150, 200	1, 5, 3, 4.5	Hydrophilic with a nitinol shaping wire
Choice PT, PT Graphix	3.2, 3.0	Hydrophilic and good support for device tracking
Runthrough	1	Soft tip with nitinol core and hydrophilic coating
Persuader	3, 6, 9	Variable power for penetration
Whisper LS, MS	1, 3	Excellent tracking in tortuous vessels
Support Catheters	**Crossing Profile (F)**	**Length (cm)**
Finecross	Tapered 1.8–2.6	130, 150
Progreat	Tapered 2.4–2.9	110, 130
Tracker	Tapered 1.9–2.4	150
Transit	Tapered 2.5–2.8	100–170
Tornus	2.1, 2.6	135
Corsair	Tapered 1.3–2.8	135–150

was brought to the catheter laboratory and 8F catheter access obtained. Using an XB 3.5 guide, a diagnostic angiogram confirmed the presence of a long occluded segment of the mid LAD with left-to-left collateralization (**Fig. 1**A). With the assistance of a Finecross microcatheter, attempts were made to advance coronary wires with increasing stiffness through the occluded segment. Ultimately, the lesion was crossed with the wire subintimal adjacent to the distal true lumen (**Fig. 1**B). The subintimal location of the guidewire was confirmed by intravascular ultrasound (**Fig. 1**C). A Stingray balloon catheter was advanced to the segment adjacent to the true lumen past the distal cap and inflated. The reentry wire was used to gain access to the distal true lumen and placement confirmed (**Fig. 1**D). The length of the occluded segment was treated with 3 overlapping drug-eluting stents with an excellent mid-vessel result (**Fig. 1**E).

Guidewire entry into the subintimal space is a common occurrence during attempted penetration CTO PCI. Several techniques have been developed to deal with wire excursions from the true lumen. The use of the subintimal guidewire left behind as a marker to help guide penetration of a second guidewire into the true lumen has been termed the parallel wire method.[10]

When present, contralateral collateral vessels offer several benefits to the conduct of CTO PCI. During an antegrade attempt, contrast injection through collateral vessels (via an additional diagnostic catheter if necessary) assists with visualization of the distal true lumen and provides a visible target for guidewire manipulation. An adaptation of the technique first described by Kahn and Hartzler,[11] the retrograde approach to CTO, uses collateral vessels in an attempt to cross the occluded segment through an initial penetration of the distal cap. Given its technical complexity and requirement of specialized equipment, retrograde attempts at CTO PCI performed following detailed planning and are commonly considered following a failed antegrade attempt. Due to the possibility of long intravascular distances to reach the occluded segment, short guides (80–90 cm) and long wires are employed. Through this approach, an appropriate collateral vessel is wired to allow for passage of a guidewire and equipment to engage the CTO via the distal cap.

Collateral channels exist both as epicardial and endomyocardial (septal perforator) vessels. The latter are preferred in retrograde CTO PCI as they are generally less tortuous and more elastic, thus facilitating guidewire passage and reducing

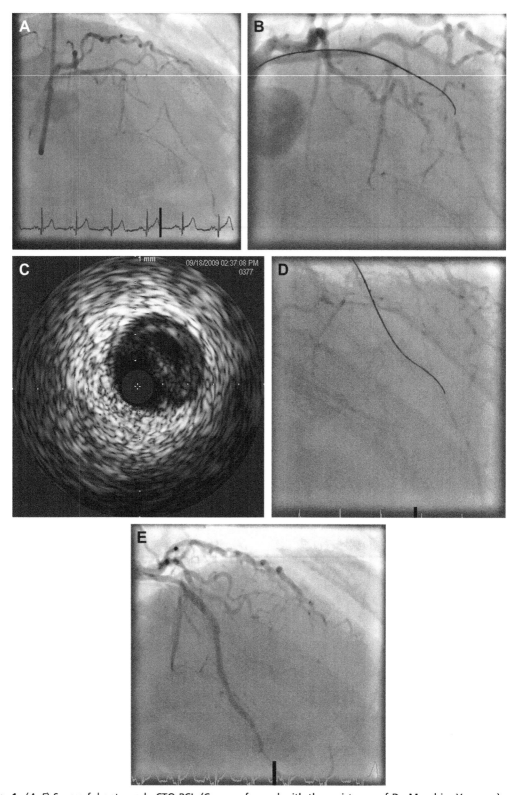

Fig. 1. (*A–E*) Successful antegrade CTO PCI. (Case performed with the assistance of Dr. Masahisa Yamane.)

the risk of perforation during wire transit. Septal collaterals can also be dilated to allow easy passage of balloons and even stents if necessary. Epicardial collaterals are less ideal given they are generally very fragile, thin-walled vessels that can be perforated by balloon dilation or aggressive wire manipulation. Navigation of collateral vessels is typically approached with the assistance of one of the many commercially available end-hole, microsupport catheters like the Finecross. In addition to their previously mentioned benefits in CTO PCI, they allow for selective injections of candidate collateral vessels with significantly less contrast. Recently approved for use in the United States, the Corsair microcatheter (Asahi Intecc Co Ltd, Aichi, Japan) is specially designed for retrograde collateral navigation and acts as a septal channel dilator with a flexible, gradually tapering tip. Constructed with a braided tungsten core, the Corsair has an outer diameter of 2.6F and has a 20-cm screw-head tip comprised of a tungsten wire helix that enables progress through septal or epicardial channels by rotating the catheter. Designed to maximize flexibility, the tip is made from a polyamide and tungsten powder mixture, while the hydrophilic coating minimizes friction.

Passage of the guidewire through the distal cap and into the proximal true lumen is accomplished in a similar way to antegrade techniques. An additional method for traversing the occluded segment that may be applied to either approach is controlled antegrade and retrograde tracking (CART).[12] This mode is conducted by creating a dissection plane with a gentle inflation of a small-diameter retrograde balloon, which is advanced over a wire that has entered the occluded segment. After creating the short-distance, controlled dissection with the balloon, an antegrade wire is advanced from the proximal true lumen toward the dissection plane and with a short sharp curve an attempt is made to reenter the distal true lumen. Intravascular ultrasound may be used to help guide the reentry if necessary. The CART technique may also be employed in a "reverse" variation whereby a balloon over an antegrade wire from the proximal true lumen is inflated in the subintimal plaque, creating a space for the retrograde wire to enter. The retrograde wire is then used to engage the proximal true lumen.

In the case of a 59 year-old woman with type 1 diabetes and the recurrence of lifestyle-limiting angina 2 months following coronary artery bypass grafting at an outside facility, a retrograde approach was chosen in an attempt to revascularize the previously grafted left circumflex system, which received rich collaterals from a patent saphenous vein graft to the right coronary. An antegrade approach was also considered, but the origin of the left circumflex could not be visualized clearly from left coronary injections. A 6F multipurpose guide catheter was engaged in the saphenous vein graft to the right coronary artery and a 7F XB 3.5 guide in the left main coronary artery (**Fig. 2**A). With the assistance of a short OTW balloon, a Fielder FC coronary wire was advanced through the vein graft and distal right coronary. Due to difficulty penetrating the proximal cap, the Fielder wire was exchanged for a Miracle Bros 6, which allowed the wire to cross through into the true lumen and ultimately the ascending aorta (**Fig. 2**B). With the guidewire in the ascending aorta, the occluded segment was ballooned and an antegrade wire placed in the distal circumflex (**Fig. 2**C). In addition, on antegrade injection, separate ostia of the LAD and circumflex arteries were identified. The occluded segment was treated with a single long drug-eluting stent, with an excellent result (**Fig. 2**D).

Experiences with several new devices specifically designed for CTO PCI have been recently reported. The RVT CTO Guidewire Device (ReVascular Therapeutics, Sunnyvale, CA) is a 0.014-inch guidewire system that offers a rotating wire tip housed within a hollow outer shaft that can be engaged to facilitate passage through difficult to cross lesions. The rotating tip is combined with video and audio feedback of the load condition on the wire tip. A first-in-man study of the device in a consecutive cohort of patients undergoing CTO PCI reported an overall success rate of 62.5%, with no major adverse events through 30 days of follow-up.[13] The CROSSER (FlowCardia, Sunnyvale, CA) is a 6F-compatible monorail catheter with irrigation outlets housed within a vibrating stainless steel tip. When activated at the site of occlusion, the device is advanced in front of the guidewire while the blunt tip vibrates at 20 kHz and delivers saline irrigation for cooling. The high-frequency motion of the catheter tip is designed to fragment the fibrous tissue along the length of the CTO with potentially lower risk of perforation. In a safety and feasibility trial, the device was used in 125 consecutive patients who had a failed CTO attempt using conventional techniques. The device successfully crossed the lesion in 60.8% of cases with an average fluoroscopy time of 12.4 minutes.[14] The results of this study led to the Food and Drug Administration's approval of the CROSSER in 2008.

PROCEDURAL COMPLICATIONS AND ADVERSE EVENTS FOLLOWING CTO PCI

Given their complexity, CTO lesions occasionally require power and force to achieve successful

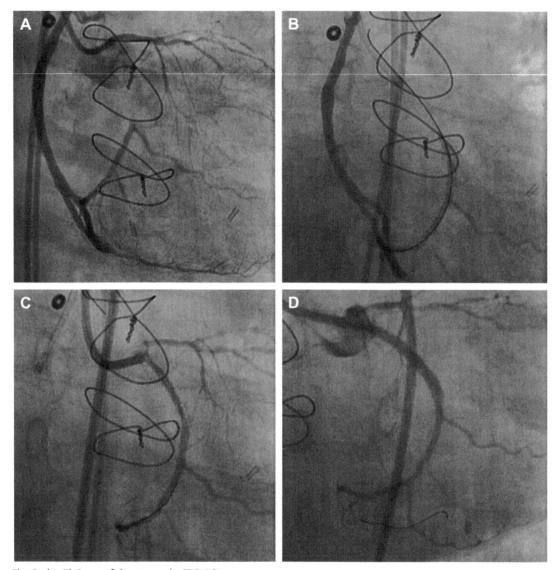

Fig. 2. (A–D) Successful retrograde CTO PCI.

revascularization. In this setting, it is not unexpected that complications can and do occur. Adverse intraprocedural events during attempted CTO PCI include coronary perforation, dissection, thrombosis, and collateral vessel occlusion. Due to increased procedure duration, contrast-induced nephropathy and radiation injury are also concerns of CTO PCI.

Coronary perforation is likely the most feared acute complication of CTO PCI. Categorized as ranging from the appearance of an angiographic crater outside the lumen to contrast spilling directly into an extravascular space, successful management of coronary perforations requires rapid action.[15] Type I and II perforations may be treated with serial angiographic observation to

evaluate for signs of progression with or without reversal of anticoagulation. Heparin is the preferred anticoagulant for CTO PCI because of its ability to rapidly reverse its effects with protamine. More serious perforations should be initially managed with balloon occlusion of the coronary artery proximal to the perforations and subsequent gentle balloon dilation at the site of perforation for several minutes. Because the perforated artery is occluded before the PCI attempt, prolonged inflations are usually well tolerated. Patients with more than a type 1 perforation should be monitored in an intensive care unit for at least 6 hours. Serial echocardiograms should be performed to evaluate for signs of pericardial effusion, and patients should be monitored closely for the development of tamponade physiology. Urgent pericardiocentesis accompanied by aggressive volume resuscitation and intravenous vasopressors may be required in more severe cases. If the anatomic location of the perforation permits, a covered stent may be placed to seal the perforation, and should be followed by subsequent angiographic confirmation of hemostasis. Urgent surgical consultation for open repair is an alternative for patients who fail the more conservative approaches described.

Coronary dissection in the setting of CTO PCI typically occurs at the coronary ostium due to aggressive guide manipulation, or in the body of the vessel due to subintimal tracking of the guidewire. Dissections within the coronary ostium can be avoided by careful attention to guide positioning, but when present may be treated with prolonged balloon inflations or stenting as necessary. Within the body of the artery, dissection may be helpful in allowing the guidewire to bypass the occluded segment in the subintimal space and potentially allow for stenting, as previously mentioned. Body dissections associated with CTO PCI should be managed in the typical fashion with either balloon angioplasty or stenting to prevent propagation or vessel closure. Dissection involving the coronary ostium and ascending aorta is a rare complication of CTO PCI, but given the occasional need for strong guide support and use of additional techniques to augment force generation for device delivery, aortic dissection can rarely occur during CTO intervention. Ascending aortic dissections have been reported to occur most commonly during PCI of the right coronary artery.[16] Dissections limited to the aortic sinus may be reasonably managed by stenting of the coronary artery dissection entry point; however, surgical intervention should be considered in cases where the dissection extends extensively up the aorta.[17]

Loss of collateral flow to the vessel distal to a CTO may be considered a complication of the procedure in the event that it is due to dissection or embolization of ipsilateral collaterals during an antegrade attempt, or disruption of collaterals while using a retrograde approach. Preservation of collateral circulation may be a consideration in the choice of initial approach when planning subintimal tracking near or cannulation of a prominent collateral vessel.

Periprocedural myocardial infarction, as diagnosed by significant elevations of biomarkers of myocardial necrosis, has been associated with worse long-term outcomes, and is a potential complication of CTO PCI.[18,19] Potential mechanisms for infarction during CTO PCI include side-branch closure, coronary dissection, atheroembolism, and prolonged balloon inflation.

Several single-center analyses have reported an incidence of 6% to 13% of biomarker defined myocardial infarction following CTO PCI, and have highlighted the strong association with side-branch closure.[20,21] Care should be taken to preserve any major vessels distal to the occluded segment and consideration given for adjunctive antiplatelet therapy in patients with significant disruption in coronary flow during CTO PCI.

OUTCOMES FOLLOWING REVASCULARIZATION OF CHRONIC TOTAL CORONARY OCCLUSIONS

Chronically occluded coronary arteries are a relatively common finding among patients with coronary disease, and remain a common indication for referral for coronary artery bypass grafting. When offering CTO PCI as a strategy for complete revascularization, careful consideration of both adverse outcomes and potential benefits is necessary to allow patients realistic informed consent. PCI has been reported to benefit patients with CTO by reducing ischemic symptoms and mortality while improving myocardial function.[2–5] A recent temporal analysis of CTO PCI trends from the Mayo Clinic documented improved procedural success for attempted revascularization following the introduction of coronary stents, but no significant improvement above the 70% mark in the subsequent 15 years.[3]

Unrevascularized CTO has been reported to increase mortality in the setting of incomplete revascularization with multivessel coronary artery disease. Successful CTO PCI also seems to provide a survival advantage over those patients who undergo an unsuccessful CTO PCI attempt. Definitive data on a possible survival advantage following successful CTO PCI are lacking due to the absence of any prospective randomized comparisons. Compared with patients with non-CTO lesions who undergo incomplete revascularization, the presence of a CTO is associated with increased mortality in both the stable and acute settings.[22,23] Numerous single-center registries have reported improved mortality for patients undergoing a successful CTO PCI compared with those who undergo an unsuccessful attempt. The largest and most comprehensive study was by the Mid America Heart Institute and included 2066 patients with 10-year follow-up, wherein successfully revascularized patients demonstrated a 7.6% absolute reduction in mortality.[4] In an updated publication from this institution, investigators reported a variable benefit of successful CTO PCI by target vessel. When evaluating 5-year survival, patients who underwent successful revascularization of a LAD

CTO demonstrated a significant improvement over patients with a failed PCI, 88.9% versus 80.2% (P<.001).[24] Multivariable analysis including numerous coronary disease risk factors confirmed mortality reduction, with a relative 39% decrease (hazard ratio 0.61, 95% confidence interval 0.42–0.89) in favor of subjects who underwent a successful PCI of a LAD CTO. Whereas the previous reports were largely limited to patients prior to the advent of drug-eluting stents (DES), Valenti and colleagues[25] corroborated the survival advantage in an updated cohort of more than 300 patients in whom those with successful CTO PCI including DES had a significant improvement in 2-year cardiac survival: 91.6% compared with 87.4% for those whose attempt was unsuccessful.

In patients with ischemic coronary disease, there is a well-documented correlation between survival and left ventricular function. The hypothesis that improved left ventricular function is in part responsible for the survival advantage seen in patients who achieve long-term vessel patency following CTO PCI is supported by several reports. Global improvements in left ventricular function have been documented by qualitative cineangiography in patients following successful CTO PCI.[26] Of note, patients without prior myocardial infarction (MI) in the revascularized territory demonstrated significant improvements when compared with those with either historical or electrocardiographic evidence of previous MI. Magnetic resonance imaging (MRI) has also confirmed the benefits of successful CTO PCI on measures of left ventricular function. As compared with non-CTO lesions, successful CTO PCI has shown improvements in myocardial blood flow, and improvements in the magnitude and temporal aspects of contractility within the affected myocardium.[27] Using more sensitive measures including segmental wall thickening and volumes assessed by MRI, improvement in left ventricular remodeling and function was seen for up to 3 years following successful CTO PCI.[5] The extent of transmural infarction prior to revascularization was shown to predict early and late improvements in regional left ventricular function.

FUTURE DIRECTIONS FOR CTO PCI

Exciting developments within the area of coronary CTO modeling and stem cell application offer insight into the future of the field. Efforts to develop a suitable environment for developing novel devices for CTO have been imperfect. In a recent report, Suzuki and colleagues[28] detail the development of a large animal model for CTO. Created by the injection of bone chips and gelatin foam, the resulting occlusion within a porcine coronary artery demonstrated histologic characteristics similar to human CTO, including neointimal proliferation, abundant microchannels, and rich collateralization. The availability of this model will allow a realistic platform for the preclinical evaluation of CTO technology.

There has been significant interest in the ability of progenitor cells to improve cardiac function in territories of myocardial ischemia and infarction. Kendziorra and colleagues[29] randomized 26 patients to receive autologous circulating progenitor cells or placebo following successful CTO PCI. Using nuclear techniques to measure relative changes in myocardial perfusion and metabolism, the investigators were able to show modest benefits in this investigatory cohort, and concluded that the use of these imaging techniques is satisfactory for monitoring outcomes following treatment with stem cell therapy. These improvements also provide support for further investigations of the benefit of progenitor cell therapy in the treatment of chronic ischemic coronary disease.

SUMMARY

Throughout the evolution of both specific equipment and techniques, percutaneous revascularization of coronary CTO remains a formidable endeavor. Ongoing observations of the benefits of CTO PCI, hopefully enhanced by data from randomized comparisons and embracing novel validated measures, promise continued interest in improving this technique. Collaborative efforts to share successful procedural methodology and overcome challenges through device improvement are vital to continue the advance of this exciting and important area of research.

REFERENCES

1. Christofferson RD, Lehmann KG, Martin GV, et al. Effect of chronic total coronary occlusion on treatment strategy. Am J Cardiol 2005;95(9):1088–91.
2. Olivari Z, Rubartelli P, Piscione F, et al. Immediate results and one-year clinical outcome after percutaneous coronary interventions in chronic total occlusions: data from a multicenter, prospective, observational study (TOAST-GISE). J Am Coll Cardiol 2003;41(10):1672–8.
3. Prasad A, Rihal CS, Lennon RJ, et al. Trends in outcomes after percutaneous coronary intervention for chronic total occlusions: a 25-year experience from the Mayo Clinic. J Am Coll Cardiol 2007; 49(15):1611–8.
4. Suero JA, Marso SP, Jones PG, et al. Procedural outcomes and long-term survival among patients undergoing percutaneous coronary intervention of

a chronic total occlusion in native coronary arteries: a 20-year experience. J Am Coll Cardiol 2001;38(2): 409–14.

5. Kirschbaum SW, Baks T, van den Ent M, et al. Evaluation of left ventricular function three years after percutaneous recanalization of chronic total coronary occlusions. Am J Cardiol 2008;101(2):179–85.

6. Jayasinghe R, Paul V, Rajendran S. A universal classification system for chronic total occlusions. J Invasive Cardiol 2008;20(6):302–4.

7. Dvir D, Assali A, Kornowski R. Percutaneous coronary intervention for chronic total occlusion: novel 3-dimensional imaging and quantitative analysis. official journal of the Society for Cardiac Angiography & Interventions. Catheter Cardiovasc Interv 2008;71(6):784–9.

8. Garcia-Garcia HM, van Mieghem CA, Gonzalo N, et al. Computed tomography in total coronary occlusions (CTTO registry): radiation exposure and predictors of successful percutaneous intervention. EuroIntervention 2009;4(5):607–16.

9. Fujita S, Tamai H, Kyo E, et al. New technique for superior guiding catheter support during advancement of a balloon in coronary angioplasty: the anchor technique. Catheter Cardiovasc Interv 2003;59(4):482–8.

10. Ochiai M, Ashida K, Araki H, et al. The latest wire technique for chronic total occlusion. Ital Heart J 2005;6(6):489–93.

11. Kahn JK, Hartzler GO. Retrograde coronary angioplasty of isolated arterial segments through saphenous vein bypass grafts. Cathet Cardiovasc Diagn 1990;20(2):88–93.

12. Surmely JF, Tsuchikane E, Katoh O, et al. New concept for CTO recanalization using controlled antegrade and retrograde subintimal tracking: the CART technique. J Invasive Cardiol 2006;18(7):334–8.

13. Chamié D, Abizaid A, Costa JR, et al. The revascular active percutaneous interventional device for coronary total occlusions study. official journal of the Society for Cardiac Angiography & Interventions. Catheter Cardiovasc Interv 2008;72(2):156–63.

14. Tiroch K, Cannon L, Reisman M, et al. High-frequency vibration for the recanalization of guidewire refractory chronic total coronary occlusions. official journal of the Society for Cardiac Angiography & Interventions. Catheter Cardiovasc Interv 2008;72(6):771–80.

15. Ellis SG, Ajluni S, Arnold AZ, et al. Increased coronary perforation in the new device era. Incidence, classification, management, and outcome. Circulation 1994;90(6):2725–30.

16. Dunning DW, Kahn JK, Hawkins ET, et al. Iatrogenic coronary artery dissections extending into and involving the aortic root. Catheter Cardiovasc Interv 2000;51(4):387–93.

17. Gomez-Moreno S, Sabate M, Jiminez-Quevedo P, et al. Iatrogenic dissection of the ascending aorta following heart catheterisation: incidence, management and outcome. EuroIntervention 2006;2:197–202.

18. Cavallini C, Savonitto S, Violini R, et al. Impact of the elevation of biochemical markers of myocardial damage on long-term mortality after percutaneous coronary intervention: results of the CK-MB and PCI study. Eur Heart J 2005;26(15):1494–8.

19. Prasad A, Singh M, Lerman A, et al. Isolated elevation in troponin T after percutaneous coronary intervention is associated with higher long-term mortality. J Am Coll Cardiol 2006;48(9):1765–70.

20. Bahrmann P, Ferrari M, Figulla HR, et al. Low incidence of cardiac biomarker elevation following PCI of chronic total coronary occlusions. EuroIntervention 2006;2:231–7.

21. Paizis I, Manginas A, Voudris V, et al. Percutaneous coronary intervention for chronic total occlusions: the role of side-branch obstruction. EuroIntervention 2009;4:600–6.

22. Hannan EL, Racz M, Holmes DR, et al. Impact of completeness of percutaneous coronary intervention revascularization on long-term outcomes in the stent era. Circulation 2006;113(20):2406–12.

23. van der Schaaf RJ, Vis MM, Sjauw KD, et al. Impact of multivessel coronary disease on long-term mortality in patients with ST-elevation myocardial infarction is due to the presence of a chronic total occlusion. Am J Cardiol 2006;98(9):1165–9.

24. Safley DM, House JA, Marso SP, et al. Improvement in survival following successful percutaneous coronary intervention of coronary chronic total occlusions: variability by target vessel. JACC Cardiovasc Interv 2008;1(3):295–302.

25. Valenti R, Migliorini A, Signorini U, et al. Impact of complete revascularization with percutaneous coronary intervention on survival in patients with at least one chronic total occlusion. Eur Heart J 2008;29(19): 2336–42.

26. Chung CM, Nakamura S, Tanaka K, et al. Effect of recanalization of chronic total occlusions on global and regional left ventricular function in patients with or without previous myocardial infarction. Catheter Cardiovasc Interv 2003;60(3):368–74.

27. Cheng AS, Selvanayagam JB, Jerosch-Herold M, et al. Percutaneous treatment of chronic total coronary occlusions improves regional hyperemic myocardial blood flow and contractility: insights from quantitative cardiovascular magnetic resonance imaging. JACC Cardiovasc Interv 2008;1(1):44–53.

28. Suzuki K, Saito N, Zhang G, et al. Development of a novel calcified total occlusion model in porcine coronary arteries. J Invasive Cardiol 2008;20(6):296–301.

29. Kendziorra K, Barthel H, Erbs S, et al. Effect of progenitor cells on myocardial perfusion and metabolism in patients after recanalization of a chronically occluded coronary artery. J Nucl Med 2008;49(4): 557–63.

Percutaneous Coronary Intervention for Unprotected Left Main Coronary Artery Stenosis

Seung-Jung Park, MD, PhD*, Young-Hak Kim, MD, PhD

KEYWORDS
- Stent • Left main • Restenosis
- Prognosis • Bypass surgery

Because of the long-term benefit of coronary artery bypass graft (CABG) surgery in medical therapy, CABG has been the standard treatment of unprotected left main coronary artery (LMCA) stenosis.[1–3] However, with the advancement of techniques and equipment the percutaneous interventional approach for implantation of coronary stents has been shown to be feasible for patients with unprotected LMCA stenosis.[3] The recent introduction of drug-eluting stents (DESs), together with advances in periprocedural and postprocedural adjunctive pharmacotherapies, has improved outcomes of percutaneous coronary interventions (PCIs) for these complex coronary lesions.[4–29] PCI for unprotected LMCA stenosis has still been indicated for patients at a high surgical risk or in emergent clinical situations, such as bailout procedures or acute myocardial infarction (MI), as an alternative therapy to CABG, because the recent registry or randomized study failed to prove superiority, or at least noninferiority, of DES placement for unprotected LMCA stenosis, compared with CABG.[21,30,31] In contrast, there is concern about the long-term safety of DES. The incidence of late stent thrombosis has been reported to be higher with DES than with bare-metal stent (BMS) implantation.[32–36] The US Food and Drug Administration has warned that the risk of stent thrombosis may outweigh the benefits of DES in off-label use, such as for unprotected LMCA stenosis.[37]

Patients with LMCA stenosis have traditionally been classified into 2 subgroups: protected (a previous patent CABG surgery graft to 1 or more major branches of the left coronary artery), and unprotected LMCA diseases (without such bypasses). This review evaluates the current outcomes of PCI with DES in research conducted in several countries.

DEFINITION OF SIGNIFICANT LMCA STENOSIS

Coronary angiography has been the standard tool to determine the severity of coronary artery disease. Although a traditional cutoff of significant coronary stenosis has been diameter stenosis of 70% in non-LMCA lesions, its cutoff in LMCA has been diameter stenosis of 50%. However, because the conventional coronary angiogram is only a lumenogram, providing information about lumen diameter but yielding little insight into lesion and plaque characteristics themselves, it has several limitations due to peculiar anatomic and hemodynamic factors. In addition, the LMCA segment is the least reproducible of any coronary segment, with the largest reported intraobserver and interobserver variabilities.[38–40] Therefore, intravascular ultrasound (IVUS) is often used to assess the severity of LMCA stenosis.

A decision of significant stenosis at LMCA necessitating revascularization should be

Cardiac Center, Asan Medical Center, University of Ulsan College of Medicine, 388-1 Pungnap-dong, Songpa-gu, Seoul, 138–736, Korea
* Corresponding author.
E-mail address: sjpark@amc.seoul.kr (S.-J. Park).

Cardiol Clin 28 (2010) 81–95
doi:10.1016/j.ccl.2009.09.001
0733-8651/09/$ – see front matter © 2010 Published by Elsevier Inc.

cardiology.theclinics.com

determined by the absolute luminal area, not by the degree of plaque burden or area of stenosis. Because of remodeling, a larger plaque burden can exist in the absence of lumen compromise.[41] Abizaid and colleagues[42] reported 1-year follow-up in 122 patients with LMCA. The minimal lumen diameter by IVUS was the most important predictor of cardiac events with a 1-year event rate of 14% in patients with a minimal luminal diameter less than 3.0 mm.[42] Fassa and colleagues[43] reported that the long-term outcomes of patients having LMCA with a minimal lumen area less than 7.5 mm^2 without revascularization were considerably worse than those of patients who were revascularized. Jasti and colleagues[44] compared fractional flow reserve (FFR) and IVUS in patients with an angiographically ambiguous LMCA stenosis. However, accurate assessment for ostial LMCA is not always possible. It is important to keep the IVUS catheter coaxial with the LMCA and to disengage the guiding catheter from the ostium so that the guiding catheter is not mistaken for a calcific lesion with a lumen dimension equal to the inner lumen of the guiding catheter. When assessing distal LMCA disease, it is important to begin imaging in the most coaxial branch vessel. Nevertheless, distribution of plaque in the distal LMCA is not always uniform; and it may be necessary to image from more than 1 branch back into the LMCA.

FFR may play an adjunctive role in determining significant stenosis at LMCA. FFR is the ratio of the maximal blood flow achievable in a stenotic vessel to the normal maximal flow in the same vessel.[45] An FFR value of less than 0.75 is considered a reliable indicator of significant stenosis producing inducible ischemia.[46] In patients with an angiographically equivocal LMCA stenosis, a strategy of revascularization versus medical therapy based on an FFR cut-point of 0.75 was associated with excellent survival and freedom from events for up to 3 years of follow-up.[44]

OUTCOMES OF DES
Safety in Terms of the Risk of Death, MI, or Stent Thrombosis

Although there are disputes regarding the long-term safety of DES, the possibility of late or very late thrombosis has still been the major factor limiting global use of DES, especially for unprotected LMCA stenosis. **Table 1** shows the results of recent studies demonstrating the outcomes of DES implantation for unprotected LMCA stenosis. None of the clinical studies showed a significant increase in the cumulative rates of death or MI in DES implantation for unprotected LMCA,

compared with BMS. In the 3 early pilot studies comparing the outcomes of DES with those of BMS, the incidences of death, MI, or stent thrombosis were comparable in the 2 stent types during the procedure and at follow-up.[4–6] In the study by Valgimigli and colleagues,[6] DES was associated with significant reduction in the rate of MI (hazard ratio 0.22, $P = .006$) and the composite of death or MI (hazard ratio 0.26, $P = .004$) compared with BMS. Considering that restenosis can lead to an acute MI in 3.5% to 19.4%, a significant reduction of restenosis achieved by DES might contribute to the better outcome of DES. In fact, a previous study was concerned that the episode of restenosis with BMS in the LMCA could present as late mortality.[48] In addition, more frequent repeat revascularization to treat BMS restenosis, in which CABG is the standard of care for unprotected LMCA, may also be related to the increase in hazardous accidents compared with DES. A recent meta-analysis supported the safety of DES, in that DES did not increase the risk of death, MI, or stent thrombosis compared with BMS.[18] In this meta-analysis of 1278 patients with unprotected LMCA stenosis, for a median of 10 months, mortality rate in DES-based PCI was only 5.5% (3.4%–7.7%) and was not higher than BMS-based PCI.

Recently, 3 registry studies assessed the safety risk outcomes for the use of DES compared with BMS over 2 years, as shown in **Fig. 1**.[25–27] After rigorous adjustment using the propensity score or inverse probability of treatment weighting (IPTW) methods to avoid selection bias, which is an inherent limitation of registry studies, DES was at least not associated with long-term increase of death or MI. The report by Palmerini and colleagues[26] showed the survival benefit of DES over 2 years. These studies agreed with the previous pilot studies that elective PCI with DES for unprotected LMCA stenosis seems to be a safe alternative to CABG.

In the series of LMCA DES studies, the incidence of stent thrombosis at 1 year ranged from 0% to 4% and was not statistically different from that of BMS.[4–6] Recently, a multicenter study confirmed the finding that the incidence of definite stent thrombosis at 2 years was only 0.5% in 731 patients treated with DES.[19] In addition, the DELFT (Drug Eluting stent for LeFT main) multicenter registry, which included 358 patients undergoing LMCA stenting with DES, reported the incidence of definite, probable, and possible stent thrombosis as 0.6%, 1.1%, and 4.4% at 3 years.[29] In recent large, multicenter studies for the ISAR-LEFT-MAIN (Intracoronary Stenting and Angiographic Results: Drug-Eluting Stents for Unprotected Coronary Left Main Lesions) study or MAIN-COMPARE (COMparison of Percutaneous Coronary Angioplasty Versus Surgical REvascularization) study, the incidence of definite or probable stent thrombosis was less than 1%.[21,47] However, because these studies were underpowered to completely exclude the possibility of increased risk of stent thrombosis over a long period, further research is needed on this topic. The previous studies assessing the long-term outcomes of DES for complex lesions produced inhomogeneous results. For example, recent large registries evaluating the safety of DES for complex lesions showed comparable risks of death or MI for the 2 stent types.[49,50] The recent large National Heart, Lung, and Blood Institute (NHLBI) registry in the United States reported that the off-label use of DES, compared with BMS, for similar indications was associated with a comparable 1-year risk of death and a lower 1-year risk of MI after adjustment.[49] A large registry of 13,353 patients in Ontario found that the 3-year mortality rate in a propensity-matched population was significantly higher with BMS than with DES.[50] The comparable, or lower, incidence of death or MI with the use of DES, compared with BMS, may be due, at least in part, to the offsetting risks of restenosis versus stent thrombosis.

Prognostic Factors

Several attempts have been made to predict long-term outcomes of complex LMCA intervention. Predictably, periprocedural and long-term mortality depend strongly on patient clinical presentation. In the ULTIMA (Unprotected Left Main Trunk Investigation Multicenter Assessment) multicenter registry, which included 279 patients treated with BMS, 46% of whom were inoperable or high surgical risk, the in-hospital mortality was 13.7%, and the 1-year incidence of all-cause mortality was 24.2%.[51] However, in the 32% of patients with low surgical risk (age <65 years and ejection fraction >30%), there were no periprocedural deaths and a 1-year mortality of 3.4%. Similarly, in the DES implantation, high surgical risk represented by high EuroSCORE or Parsonnet score, was the independent predictor of death or MI.[13,52] Therefore, it is recommended that attention should continue to be paid to the procedure for patients at high surgical risk. More recently, the SYNTAX (Synergy between PCI with Taxus and Cardiac Surgery) score, which was an angiographic risk stratification model, has been created to predict long-term outcomes after coronary revascularization with PCI or CABG.[30] In the recent SYNTAX study comparing PCI with paclitaxel-eluting stent versus CABG for multivessel or LMCA disease, the long-term mortality was significantly associated

with the SYNTAX score.[30] Therefore, for patients with high clinical risk profiles or complex lesion morphologies, who are defined using these risk stratification models, the PCI procedures need to be performed by experienced interventionalists with the aid of IVUS, mechanical hemodynamic support, and optimal adjunctive pharmacotherapies, after the judicious selection of patients.

Recurrent Revascularization

Compared with BMS, DES reduced the incidence of angiographic restenosis and subsequently the need of repeat revascularization in unprotected LMCA stenosis. In early pilot studies, the 1-year incidence of repeat revascularization in DES implantation was 2% to 19%, compared with 12% to 31% in BMS (see **Table 1**).[4–6] In the long-term (3 year) study, the incidence of repeat revascularization remained steady with no significant "late catch-up" phenomenon of late restenosis noted after coronary brachytherapy.[21] Recently, 2 larger registries confirmed the efficacy of DES.[25,27] The risk of target lesion revascularization (TLR) over 3 years was reduced by 60% with the use of DES (see **Fig. 1**).[27]

The risk of restenosis was significantly influenced by lesion location. DES treatment of the ostial and shaft LMCA lesions had a low incidence of angiographic or clinical restenosis.[14] In a study including 144 patients with ostial or shaft stenosis in the 3 cardiac centers, angiographic restenosis and target vessel revascularization at 1 year occurred in only 1 (1%) and 2 (1%) patients, respectively. Although the lack of DES sizes bigger than 3.5 mm required an overdilation strategy to match the LMCA reference diameter, there was no incidence of cardiac death, MI or stent thrombosis in this study.

PCI for LMCA bifurcation has been more challenging, although the prevalence was more than 60% across the previous studies.[4–6,10,21] However, repeat revascularization was exclusively performed in patients with PCI for bifurcation stenosis.[4–6] A recent study assessing the outcomes of LMCA DES showed that the risk of target vessel revascularization was sixfold (95% CI, 1.2–29) in bifurcation stenosis compared with nonbifurcation stenosis (13% vs 3%).[13] The risk of bifurcation stenosis was highlighted in a recent study by Price and colleagues,[11] which showed that the TLR rate after sirolimus-eluting stent implantation was 44%. In this study, 94% (47/50) of patients had lesions at the bifurcation, and 98% underwent serial angiographic follow-up at 3 or 9 months. This discouraging result questioned the efficacy of DES and highlighted the need for

Table 1
Outcomes of DESs for unprotected LMCA stenosis

	Chieffo et al[4]		Valgimigli et al[6]		Park et al[5]		De Lezo et al[28]	Price et al[11]	Kim et al[20]	Meliga et al[29]	Mehilli et al[47]	
Stent type	SES, PES	BMS	SES, PES	BMS	SES	BMS	SES	SES	SES, PES	SES, PES	PES	SES
Design	Single center registry		Single center registry		Single center registry		Single center registry	Single center registry	Single center registry	Multicenter DELFT registry	Multicenter randomized study	
No. of patients	85	64	95	86	102	121	52	50	63	358	302	305
Age, y	63	66	64	66	60	58	63	69	67	66	69	69
Ejection fraction (%)	51[a]	57	41	42	60	62	57	NA	50	49	53	54
Acute MI (%)	NA	NA	17	20[a]	9.8	6.6	NA	NA	5	8.4	NA	NA
Bifurcation involvement (%)	81[a]	58	65	66	71[a]	43	42	94	54	74	63	63
Two-stent technique (%)	74	NA	40[a]	15	41[a]	18	18	89	17	43	51	49
Initial clinical outcomes	In-hospital		30 d		In-hospital		In-hospital	In-hospital	In-hospital	In-hospital	30 d	
Death (%)	0	0	11	7	0	0	0	0	0	3	1	2

MI (%)	6	8	4	9	7	8	4	8	10	7	4	4
Stent thrombosis (%)	0	0	0	0	0	0	0	4	0	NA	0.3	0.7
TVR (%)	0	2	0	2	0	0	0	6	0	0.8	0.3 (TLR)	0.7 (TLR)
Any events (%)	NA	NA	15	19	7	8	4	10	10	11	5.0	4.6
Long-term outcomes (%)	Cumulative	Cumulative	Cumulative	Cumulative	Cumulative	Cumulative	Cumulative	After discharge	Cumulative	Cumulative 3 y	2 y	
Mean follow-up, months	6	6	17	12	12	12	12	9	11	NA	NA	NA
Death (%)	4	14	14	16	0	0	0	10	5	9	10	9
MI (%)	NA	NA	4a	12	7	8	4	2	11	9	5	5
Stent thrombosis (%)	0.1	0	NA	NA	0	0	0	0	0.2	0.6	0.3	0.7
TVR (%)	19	31	6a	12	2a	17	2	38	19	14	9 (TLR)	11 (TLR)
Any MACE (%)	NA	NA	24a	45	8a	26	NA	44	29	32	21	21

Abbreviations: BMS, bare-metal stent; MACE, major adverse cardiac events including death, MI, and TVR; NA, not available; PES, paclitaxel-eluting stent; SES, sirolimus-eluting stent; TVR, target vessel revascularization.

a $P<.05$ for DES (SES or PES) versus BMS.

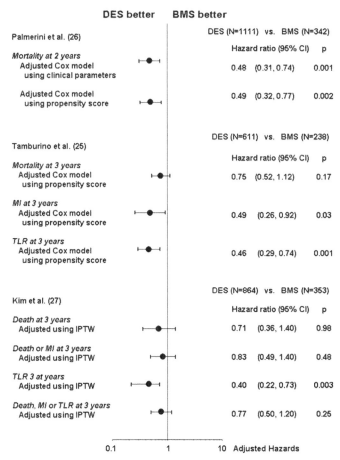

Fig. 1. Adjusted hazard ratios for clinical outcomes after stenting. DES compared with BMS. Hazard ratios were measured using propensity score or IPTW methods for adverse outcomes including death, MI, or target lesion revascularization (TLR) from registries performed by Palmerini and colleagues,[26] Tamburino and colleagues,[25] and Kim and colleagues.[27]

meticulous surveillance of angiographic follow-up in PCI for LMCA bifurcation stenosis. However, this study was limited by the exclusive use of a complex stenting strategy (2 stents in both branches) in 84% of patients, which may increase the need for repeat revascularization. Although there was some debate,[53] a current report proposes a probability that the complex stenting technique might be associated with high occurrence of restenosis compared with the simple stenting technique.[8] A subgroup analysis of the large Italian registry supported the hypothesis that the single-stenting strategy for bifurcation LMCA lesions had long-term outcomes comparable to those of nonbifurcation lesions.[24] Taken together, before the novel treatment strategy is settled, the simple stenting approach (LMCA to left anterior descending artery with optional treatment in the circumflex artery) is primarily recommended in patients with patent or diminutive circumflex arteries. Furthermore, future stent

platforms specifically designed for LMCA bifurcation lesions may provide better scaffolding, and more uniform drug delivery, to the bifurcation LMCA stenosis.

Regarding the differential benefit of the DES type for prevention of restenosis, the 2 most widely applicable DESs, sirolimus- and paclitzel-eluting stents, were evaluated in the previous studies. An early study comparing the 2 DESs from a RESEARCH registry showed a comparable incidence of major adverse cardiac events with 25% in sirolimus-eluting stents (55 patients) and 29% in paclitaxel-eluting stents (55 patients).[12] The ISAR-LEFT-MAIN study compared 305 patients receiving sirolimus-eluting stents and 302 patients receiving paclitaxel-eluting stents with a prospective randomized design.[47] At 1 year, major adverse events occurred in 13.6% of paclitaxel-eluting and 15.8% of sirolimus-eluting stent groups with 16.0% and 19.4% of restenosis, respectively (P = NS). The use of second-generation DES is now being evaluated.

COMPARISON WITH CORONARY ARTERY BYPASS SURGERY

Current guidelines for unprotected LMCA treatment, in which elective PCI for patients who are treatable with bypass surgery is a contraindication, are based mostly on 20-year-old clinical trials.[1–3] These studies demonstrated a definite benefit of survival for CABG in LMCA stenosis compared with medical treatment. However, application of these results to current practice seems inappropriate because the surgical technique and medical treatment in these studies is outdated by today's standards, and no adequately powered randomization studies between PCI and CABG have

been conducted. The lack of data on the current CABG procedure used in unprotected LMCA stenosis further precludes a theoretical comparison of the 2 revascularization strategies. **Table 2** lists the patient and lesion characteristics favoring PCI or CABG based on current expert opinion and evidence.

Several nonrandomized studies comparing the safety and efficacy of DES treatment of unprotected LMCA stenosis with CABG have been published (**Table 3**). Chieffo and colleagues[7] retrospectively compared the outcomes of 107 patients undergoing DES placement with 142 patients undergoing CABG. They showed that DES was associated with nonsignificant mortality benefits (odds ratio = 0.331, $P = .167$) and significantly lower incidence of composites of death or MI (0.260, $P = .0005$) and death, MI, or

---

Table 2
Features favoring PCI or CABG

Indications in Favor of PCI	
Absolute	• Suitable coronary anatomy for stenting with preserved left ventricular function ($\geq$40%) • Patient who refuses surgery
Relative	• Lesion restricted to the LMCA ostium or shaft • Isolated LMCA lesion • Bailout procedure (eg, dissection at the LMCA complicated during angiography or PCI) • Acute MI at the LMCA, in which emergent revascularization is necessary • Cardiogenic shock due to LMCA stenosis, in which emergent revascularization is necessary • Old age ($\geq$80 y) • Serious comorbid disease (eg, chronic lung disease, poor general performance) • Limited life expectancy of less than 1 y • Prior CABG • Coronary anatomy, unsuitable for CABG (eg, poor distal runoff)
Indications in favor of CABG	
Absolute	• Patient who refuses PCI • Contraindication to antiplatelet therapy including aspirin, heparin, and thieno-pyridine (ticlopidine or clopidogrel) • History of serious allergic reaction to stainless steel, drugs coved on DESs, and contrast agent • History of known coagulopathy or bleeding diathesis • Pregnant women
Relative	• Complex coronary anatomies at LMCA, unsuitable for stenting (eg, severe calcification, severe tortuosity) • Total occlusions at other major epicardial coronary arteries ($\geq$2) • Multivessel stenosis except LMCA • Decreased left ventricular dysfunction (<40%) • Extensive peripheral vascular disease, in which placement of guiding catheter or intra-aortic balloon pump is not likely to be performed • In-stent restenosis at the LMCA, in which repeat PCI is not likely to be performed

Abbreviations: CABG, coronary artery bypass graft surgery; LMCA, left main coronary artery; PCI, percutaneous coronary intervention.

Table 3
Comparison of DES to coronary artery bypass surgery for unprotected LMCA stenosis

	Chieffo et al[7]		Lee et al[9]		Palmerini et al[15]		Buszman et al[17]		Seung et al[21]	
Study design	Registry		Registry		Registry		Randomized study		Registry	
Treatment type	PCI with SES, PES	CABG	PCI with SES	CABG	PCI with SES	CABG	PCI with BMS, DES	CABG	PCI with BMS, DES	CABG
No. of patients	107	142	50	123	157	154	52	53	1102	1138
Age (y)	64	68	72	70	73[a]	69	61	61	62	64
Ejection fraction (%)	52	52	51	52	52	55	54	54	62	60
EuroSCORE or Parsonnet score (Lee)	4.4	4.3	18[a]	13	6[a]	5	3.3	3.5	NA	NA
Initial clinical outcomes	In-hospital		30 d		30 d		30 d		NA	
Death (%)	0	2	2	5	3.2	4.5	0	0	NA	NA
MI (%)	9	26	0	2	4.5	1.9	1.9	3.8	NA	NA
TVR (%)	0	2	0	1	0.6	0.6	1.9	0	NA	NA
Any MACE (%)	NA	NA	0	8	NA	NA	NA	NA	NA	NA
Cerebrovascular accident	0	1.4	2[a]	17	NA	NA	0	2	NA	NA
Long-term clinical outcomes	Cumulative after discharge		Kaplan-Meier		Cumulative		At 1 y		Kaplan-Meier at 3 y for propensity-matched cohort	
Mean follow-up (mo)	12	12	6	6	14	14	NA	NA	33.9	38.4
Death (%)	2.8	6.4	4	13	13.4	12.3	1.9	7.5	7.9	7.8
MI (%)	0.9	1.4	NA	NA	8.3	4.5	1.9	5.7	NA	NA
TVR (%)	19.6[a]	3.6	7	1	25.5[a]	2.6	28.8[a]	9.4	12.6	2.6
Cerebrovascular accident (%)	0.9	0.7	NA	NA	NA	NA	0	3.8	NA	NA
Any events (%)	NA	NA	11	17	NA	NA	NA	NA	NA	NA

Abbreviations: BMS, bare-metal stent; DES, drug-eluting stent; MACE, major adverse cardiac events including death, MI, and TVR; NA, not available; PCI, percutaneous coronary intervention; PES, paclitaxel-eluting stent; SES, sirolimus-eluting stent; TVR, target vessel revascularization.
[a] $P<.05$ for PCI versus CABG.

cerebrovascular accident (odds ratio = 0.385, P = .01) at 1-year follow-up. Conversely, CABG was correlated with a lower occurrence of target-vessel revascularization (3.6% vs 19.6%, P = .0001). These finding were supported by Lee and colleagues,[9] who studied 50 patients with DES placement and 123 patients with CABG. Although the DES group had a slightly higher surgical risk, the rate of mortality or MI at 30 days was comparable between the 2 treatments. At 1-year follow-up, the DES had nonsignificantly better clinical outcomes compared with CABG, reflected by overall survival (96% vs 85%) and survival freedom from death, MI, target vessel revascularization, or adverse cerebrovascular events (83% vs 75%). However, the survival freedom from repeat revascularization at 1 year remained nonsignificantly higher for CABG compared with DES (95% vs 87%). The results of a recent multicenter registry were in agreement with the previous 2 reports regarding the safety outcomes.[10] The PCI group treated with BMS or DES (60%) had a similar incidence of death or MI, but a higher incidence of TLR compared with the CABG group. A similarity in safety with the use of PCI compared with CABG was ascertained for older patients (age ≥75 years) by Palmerini and colleagues.[15] Recently, a randomized study comparing PCI (N = 52) versus CABG (N = 53) was undertaken for 105 patients with unprotected LMCA stenosis.[17] PCI was performed using BMS (65%) or DES (35%). The primary end point was the change in left ventricular ejection fraction 12 months after the intervention, and a significant increase in ejection fraction was noted only in the PCI group (3.3% ± 6.7% after PCI vs 0.5% ± 0.8% after CABG; P = .047). In contrast, 1 year after procedure, repeat revascularization was significantly lower in the CABG group (N = 5) than in the PCI group (N = 15), although the incidence of death or MI was comparable between the 2 groups. However, this study was still underpowered to assess the long-term clinical effectiveness of PCI compared with CABG.

Stronger evidence for the feasibility of PCI as an alternative to CABG comes from the recent large registry, the MAIN-COMPARE study.[21] This analyzed data from 2240 patients with unprotected LMCA disease treated at 12 medical centers in Korea. Of these, 318 were treated with BMS, 784 were treated with DES, and 1138 underwent CABG. To avoid bias due to the nonrandomized study design, a novel adjustment was performed using propensity-score matching in the overall population, and separate periods. In the first and second waves, BMS and DES, respectively, were exclusively used. The outcomes of stenting in the overall patients and each wave were compared with those of concurrent CABG. During 3 years of follow-up, patients treated with stenting were nearly 4 times as likely to need repeat revascularization compared with those who underwent CABG (hazard ratio, 4.76; 95% CI, 2.80–8.11). However, the rates of death (hazard ratio, 1.18; 95% CI, 0.77–1.80) and the combined rates of death, MI, and stroke (hazard ratio, 1.10; 95% CI, 0.75–1.62) were not significantly higher with stenting compared with CABG, as shown in **Fig. 2**. A similar pattern was observed in patients treated with DES or BMS. Most repeat revascularization in PCI patients was treated with repeat PCI instead of CABG. The recommendation for CABG for unprotected LMCA disease has been based mostly on the survival benefit, compared

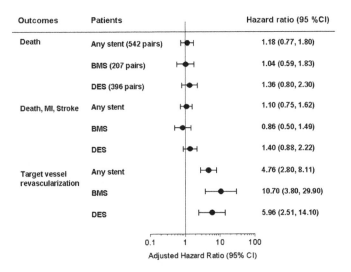

Outcomes	Patients	Hazard ratio (95 %CI)
Death	Any stent (542 pairs)	1.18 (0.77, 1.80)
	BMS (207 pairs)	1.04 (0.59, 1.83)
	DES (396 pairs)	1.36 (0.80, 2.30)
Death, MI, Stroke	Any stent	1.10 (0.75, 1.62)
	BMS	0.86 (0.50, 1.49)
	DES	1.40 (0.88, 2.22)
Target vessel revascularization	Any stent	4.76 (2.80, 8.11)
	BMS	10.70 (3.80, 29.90)
	DES	5.96 (2.51, 14.10)

0.1   1   10   100
Adjusted Hazard Ratio (95% CI)

Fig. 2. Hazard ratios for clinical outcomes after stenting as compared with CABG among propensity-matched patients from the MAIN-COMPARE registry.[21] Hazard ratios were measured between any stent versus any CABG (any stent), BMS versus contemporary CABG (BMS), and DES versus contemporary CABG (DES) after propensity-matching adjustment in each cohort.

with medical treatment, so the lack of a statistically significant difference in mortality may support PCI as an alternative option to bypass surgery. In addition, a current recommendation of routine angiographic surveillance at 6 to 9 months after PCI for unprotected LMCA stenosis might increase the use of unnecessary repeat revascularization due to the "oculostenotic" reflex.

The ultimate proof of the relative values of PCI versus CABG for unprotected LMCA stenosis clearly depends on the results of randomized clinical trials comparing the 2 treatment strategies. The trials will involve several technical considerations that could significantly alter angioplasty outcomes. The SYNTAX trial compared the outcomes of PCI with paclitaxel-eluting stents versus CABG for unprotected LMCA stenosis in a subgroup analysis from the randomized study cohort.[30] As shown in the subset of LMCA disease comprising 348 patients receiving CABG and 357 receiving PCI, PCI (15.8%) demonstrated equivalent 1-year clinical outcomes to CABG (13.7%, $P = .44$). The higher rate of repeat revascularization with PCI (11.8% vs 6.5%, $P = .02$) was offset by a higher incidence of stroke with CABG (2.7% vs 0.3%, $P = .01$). However, it should be noted that the analysis for LMCA disease was not the primary objective of the analysis but the post-hoc analysis, which is a hypothesis generating. Therefore, a further randomized study is warranted to provide confirmation of the question for a specific cohort of patients having unprotected LMCA stenosis. Another randomized study, the PRECOMBAT (PREmier of Randomized COMparison of Bypass Surgery versus AngioplasTy using Sirolimus-Eluting Stent in Patients with Left Main Coronary Artery Disease) trial, is being performed in Korea, randomizing 600 patients with unprotected LMCA patients with CABG or PCI with sirolimus-eluting stent. This study has a noninferiority design, with the primary end point of major adverse cardiac and cerebrovascular events at a mean of 2 years.

TECHNICAL ISSUES
Stenting Techniques

Stenting for ostial or body LMCA lesions seems simple, as do the other stenting techniques for non-LMCA coronary lesions. For instance, a brief and adequate stent expansion is required to get optimal stent expansion and to avoid ischemic complication. In ostial LMCA lesions, a coronary stent is generally positioned outside the LMCA for complete lesion coverage of the ostium. Stenting for bifurcation LMCA lesions, however, is more complex and technically demanding. In general, selection of appropriate stenting strategy is dependent on the plaque configuration surrounding the LMCA. However, despite recent randomized studies comparing single-stent versus 2-stent treatment of bifurcation coronary lesions,[54,55] the optimal stenting strategy for LMCA bifurcation lesions has not yet been determined. Current consensus is that a 2-stent strategy has no long-term advantages in terms of the incidence of any major cardiac events compared with a single-stent strategy. Therefore, a systemic 2-stent strategy for all LMCA bifurcation lesions, such as T-stenting, Kissing stenting, Crush technique, or Culotte technique is not generally recommended. Instead, a provisional stenting strategy should be considered as the first line treatment of LMCA bifurcations without significant side-branch stenosis.

IVUS

IVUS is considered to be a useful invasive diagnostic modality in determining anatomic configuration, selecting treatment strategy, and defining optimal stenting outcomes in the BMS or DES era.[56] Although a retrospective study reported that the clinical impact of IVUS-guided stenting for LMCA with DES did not show a significant clinical long-term benefit compared with the angiography-guided procedure,[57] the usefulness of IVUS-guided stenting may not be hampered by this underpowered retrospective study. The information gathered by IVUS may be crucial for the optimal stenting procedure in unprotected LMCA stenosis. Angiography has a limitation in assessing the true luminal size of LMCA, because the left main is often short and lacks a normal segment for comparison. Therefore, the severity of LMCA stenosis is often underestimated by the misinterpretation of the normal segment adjacent to focal stenosis. In addition to the assessment of an LMCA lesion before procedure, use of IVUS is helpful in getting an adequate expansion of DES, in preventing stent inapposition, and in achieving full lesion coverage with DES.

A recent subgroup analysis from the MAIN-COMPARE registry reported that IVUS guidance was associated with improved long-term mortality compared with conventional the angiography-guided procedure.[23] With an adjustment using propensity-score matching, for 201 matched pairs, there was a strong tendency of lower risk of 3-year mortality with IVUS guidance compared with angiography guidance (6.3% vs 13.6%, log rank $P = .063$, hazard ratio, 0.54; 95% CI, 0.28–1.03). In particular, for 145 pairs of patients receiving DES, the 3-year incidence of mortality was lower with IVUS guidance than with angiography guidance (4.7% vs 16.0%, log rank $P = .048$; HR, 0.39; 95% CI, 0.15–1.02). Mortality started to diverge beyond 1 year after the procedure. Therefore, despite the inherent limitations of nonrandomized registry design, this study indicates that IVUS guidance may play a role in reducing late stent thrombosis and subsequent long-term mortality. IVUS evaluations of stent underexpansion, incomplete lesion coverage, small stent area, large residual plaque, and inapposition have been found to predict stent thrombosis after DES placement.[58–62] Therefore, the authors strongly recommend the mandatory use of IVUS in PCI for unprotected LMCA.

Debulking Atherectomy

In the BMS era, debulking coronary atherectomy before stenting was widely used in an attempt to reduce restenosis by removal of the plaque burden. However, after the introduction of DES, the role of debulking was greatly diminished due to the dramatic benefit of restenosis reduction. A study suggested a viable role of debulking atherectomy, even in the DES era, for 99 coronary bifurcations.[63] Debulking in the main and side branches for the LMCA stenoses allowed single stenting in 60 of the 63 LMCA bifurcation stenoses. In the 1-year follow-up, no serious adverse event occurred. This study indicates that debulking may be preferable in LMCA bifurcations to aid the provisional single-stenting strategy. In addition, debulking still has a limited role to play in facilitating stent delivery. In a patient illustrated in **Fig. 3**, debulking was used to remove the plaque in the LMCA that was inhibiting advancement of the wire into the left anterior descending artery. Similarly, rotablator has been used before stenting when calcification in the proximal segment prevents stent delivery or a calcified target lesion is not sufficiently dilated. Therefore, although the data are limited, debulking atherectomy or rotablator still have a limited role, even in DES treatment, in improving lesion compliance.

Hemodynamic Support

Patients in an unstable hemodynamic condition need pharmacologic- or device-based hemodynamic support during the procedure for LMCA stenosis. Old age, MI, cardiogenic shock, and decreased left ventricular ejection fraction are common clinical conditions requiring elective or provisional hemodynamic support. Of the hemodynamic support devices (eg, include intra-aortic balloon pumps, percutaneous hemodynamic

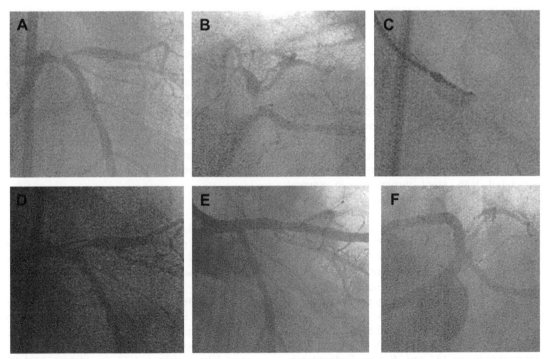

Fig. 3. Debulking coronary atherectomy followed by provisional stenting for a 71-year-old man. (*A, B*) Baseline angiograms. (*C*) Debulking due to a difficulty in advancement of wire into the left anterior descending artery. (*D*) Successful wiring. (*E, F*) Final angiograms after provisional stenting with three 2.5 × 33 mm, 3.0 × 23 mm, and 3.5 × 18 mm Cypher sirolimus-eluting stents (Cordis Corp, Johnson & Johnson, Warren, NJ).

support devices, or left ventricular assist devices), the intra-aortic balloon pump has been used most frequently. Although there is no doubt that provisional use of an intra-aortic balloon pump in patients with hemodynamic compromise is necessary for a successful procedure, the literature suggests that the prevalence of planned use of balloon pump varies widely. A study recently surveyed the role of intra-aortic balloon pump support in 219 elective LMCA interventions.[64] They used a prophylactic balloon pump for a broad range of patients with distal LMCA bifurcation lesion, a low ejection fraction of less than 40%, the use of debulking devices, unstable angina, and critical right coronary artery disease. Although the patients receiving elective intra-aortic balloon pump support had more complex clinical risk profiles, the rate of procedural complications was lower than for those not receiving its support (1.4% vs 9.3%, $P = .032$). Therefore, its elective use, at least, needs to be considered for patients with high-risk conditions, having multivessel disease, complex LMCA anatomy, low ejection fraction, or unstable presentations. New support devices, such as Tandem-Heart (CardiacAssist, Pittsburgh, PA) or the Impella Recover LP 2.5 System (Impella CardioSystems, Aachen, Germany), may benefit from improved implementing feasibility and complication rates.

Antithrombotics

Although the reported incidence of stent thrombosis in DES treatment of LMCA lesions was low,[19] a fear of stent thrombosis remains a major concern that prevents the more generalized use of DES. Therefore, careful administration of antiplatelet agents is important to prevent the occurrence of stent thrombosis. Premature discontinuation of clopidogrel has been strongly associated with stent thrombosis in several studies.[32,65] Therefore, as generally recommended, dual antiplatelet therapy, including aspirin and clopidogrel (or ticlopidine), should be maintained for 1 year. If the patients seem to be at high risk, a high loading dose (600 mg) or lifelong administration of clopidogrel needs to be considered. A recent study added the benefit of aggressive use of clopidogrel in the early period after DES implantation.[66] After stopping clopidogrel between 31 and 180 days, the hazard of cardiac death or MI was 4.20 ($P = .009$), compared with stopping between 181 and 36 days. Furthermore, in some Asian countries, adjunctive administration of cilostazol has been used for the purpose of reducing thrombotic complications.[67]

Aggressive use of antithrombotics should also be considered for complex lesion anatomy or unstable coronary condition. For example, as shown in the previous studies, the use of glycoprotein IIb/III inhibitor may play a role in reducing procedure-related thrombotic complications including death or MI.[68] However, the additive role of the glycoprotein IIb/IIa inhibitor, cilostzol, low–molecular weight heparin, direct thrombin inhibitor, or other new drugs in DES treatment of LMCA lesions needs to be investigated in future research. Until the evidence has accumulated, an aggressive combination of antithrombotic drugs before, during, or after the procedure, to avoid thrombotic complications for high risk patients, must be considered. Although high-risk features are not well defined, off-label use of DES (such as in diabetes mellitus, multiple stenting, long DES, chronic renal failure, or presentation with MI) is a good index of high-risk procedures.[69]

SUMMARY

Current studies, although limited by nonrandomized study design, small sample size, and short-term follow-up, have demonstrated the potential of DES for procedural and mid-term safety and effectiveness, compared with BMS or CABG. The authors believe that PCI with DES will progressively increase and can be recommended as a reliable alternative to bypass surgery for patients with unprotected LMCA stenosis, especially as the first-line therapy for ostial or shaft stenosis. Although bifurcation stenosis remains challenging for the percutaneous approach, further research on novel procedural techniques, new dedicated stent platforms, and optimal pharmacotherapies may improve outcomes. Upcoming randomized clinical trials comparing PCI with CABG for unprotected LMCA stenosis may soon demonstrate the long-term safety, durability, and efficacy of PCI.

REFERENCES

1. Takaro T, Hultgren HN, Lipton MJ, et al. The VA cooperative randomized study of surgery for coronary arterial occlusive disease II. Subgroup with significant left main lesions. Circulation 1976;54: III107–17.

2. Chaitman BR, Fisher LD, Bourassa MG, et al. Effect of coronary bypass surgery on survival patterns in subsets of patients with left main coronary artery disease. Report of the Collaborative Study in Coronary Artery Surgery (CASS). Am J Cardiol 1981;48: 765–77.

3. Park SJ, Mintz GS. Left main stem disease. Seoul: Informa Healthcare; 2006.

4. Chieffo A, Stankovic G, Bonizzoni E, et al. Early and mid-term results of drug-eluting stent implantation in unprotected left main. Circulation 2005; 111:791–5.

5. Park SJ, Kim YH, Lee BK, et al. Sirolimus-eluting stent implantation for unprotected left main coronary artery stenosis: comparison with bare metal stent implantation. J Am Coll Cardiol 2005;45:351–6.

6. Valgimigli M, van Mieghem CA, Ong AT, et al. Short- and long-term clinical outcome after drug-eluting stent implantation for the percutaneous treatment of left main coronary artery disease: insights from the Rapamycin-Eluting and Taxus Stent Evaluated At Rotterdam Cardiology Hospital registries (RESEARCH and T-SEARCH). Circulation 2005; 111:1383–9.

7. Chieffo A, Morici N, Maisano F, et al. Percutaneous treatment with drug-eluting stent implantation versus bypass surgery for unprotected left main stenosis: a single-center experience. Circulation 2006;113:2542–7.

8. Kim YH, Park SW, Hong MK, et al. Comparison of simple and complex stenting techniques in the treatment of unprotected left main coronary artery bifurcation stenosis. Am J Cardiol 2006;97:1597–601.

9. Lee MS, Kapoor N, Jamal F, et al. Comparison of coronary artery bypass surgery with percutaneous coronary intervention with drug-eluting stents for unprotected left main coronary artery disease. J Am Coll Cardiol 2006;47:864–70.

10. Palmerini T, Marzocchi A, Marrozzini C, et al. Comparison between coronary angioplasty and coronary artery bypass surgery for the treatment of unprotected left main coronary artery stenosis (the Bologna Registry). Am J Cardiol 2006;98:54–9.

11. Price MJ, Cristea E, Sawhney N, et al. Serial angiographic follow-up of sirolimus-eluting stents for unprotected left main coronary artery revascularization. J Am Coll Cardiol 2006;47:871–7.

12. Valgimigli M, Malagutti P, Aoki J, et al. Sirolimus-eluting versus paclitaxel-eluting stent implantation for the percutaneous treatment of left main coronary artery disease: a combined RESEARCH and T-SEARCH long-term analysis. J Am Coll Cardiol 2006;47:507–14.

13. Valgimigli M, Malagutti P, Rodriguez-Granillo GA, et al. Distal left main coronary disease is a major predictor of outcome in patients undergoing percutaneous intervention in the drug-eluting stent era: an integrated clinical and angiographic analysis based on the rapamycin-eluting stent evaluated at Rotterdam cardiology hospital (RESEARCH) and taxus-stent evaluated at Rotterdam cardiology hospital (T-SEARCH) registries. J Am Coll Cardiol 2006;47:1530–7.

14. Chieffo A, Park SJ, Valgimigli M, et al. Favorable long-term outcome after drug-eluting stent implantation in nonbifurcation lesions that involve unprotected left main coronary artery. A multicenter registry. Circulation 2007;116:158–62.

15. Palmerini T, Barlocco F, Santarelli A, et al. A comparison between coronary artery bypass grafting surgery and drug eluting stent for the treatment of unprotected left main coronary artery disease in elderly patients (aged ≥75 years). Eur Heart J 2007;28:2714–9.

16. Sheiban I, Meliga E, Moretti C, et al. Long-term clinical and angiographic outcomes of treatment of unprotected left main coronary artery stenosis with sirolimus-eluting stents. Am J Cardiol 2007;100:431–5.

17. Buszman PE, Kiesz SR, Bochenek A, et al. Acute and late outcomes of unprotected left main stenting in comparison with surgical revascularization. J Am Coll Cardiol 2008;51:538–45.

18. Biondi-Zoccai GGL, Lotrionte M, Moretti C, et al. A collaborative systematic review and meta-analysis on 1278 patients undergoing percutaneous drug-eluting stenting for unprotected left main coronary artery disease. Am Heart J 2008;155:274–83.

19. Chieffo A, Park S-J, Meliga E, et al. Late and very late stent thrombosis following drug-eluting stent implantation in unprotected left main coronary artery: a multicentre registry. Eur Heart J 2008;29:2108–15.

20. Kim YH, Dangas GD, Solinas E, et al. Effectiveness of drug-eluting stent implantation for patients with unprotected left main coronary artery stenosis. Am J Cardiol 2008;101:801–6.

21. Seung KB, Park DW, Kim YH, et al. Stents versus coronary-artery bypass grafting for left main coronary artery disease. N Engl J Med 2008;358:1781–92.

22. Tamburino C, Di Salvo ME, Capodanno D, et al. Are drug-eluting stents superior to bare-metal stents in patients with unprotected non-bifurcational left main disease? Insights from a multicentre registry. Eur Heart J 2009;30:1171–9.

23. Park SJ, Kim YH, Park DW, et al. Impact of intravascular ultrasound guidance on long-term mortality in stenting for unprotected left main coronary artery stenosis. Circ Cardiovasc Interv 2009; 2:167–77.

24. Palmerini T, Sangiorgi D, Marzocchi A, et al. Ostial and midshaft lesions vs. bifurcation lesions in 1111 patients with unprotected left main coronary artery stenosis treated with drug-eluting stents: results of the survey from the Italian Society of Invasive Cardiology. Eur Heart J 2009;30:2087–94.

25. Tamburino C, Di Salvo ME, Capodanno D, et al. Comparison of drug-eluting stents and bare-metal stents for the treatment of unprotected left main coronary artery disease in acute coronary syndromes. Am J Cardiol 2009;103:187–93.

26. Palmerini T, Marzocchi A, Tamburino C, et al. Two-year clinical outcome with drug-eluting stents versus bare-metal stents in a real-world registry of unprotected left main coronary artery stenosis from the

Italian Society of Invasive Cardiology. Am J Cardiol 2008;102:1463–8.

27. Kim YH, Park DW, Lee SW, et al. Long-term safety and effectiveness of unprotected left main coronary stenting with drug-eluting stent compared with bare-metal stent. Circulation 2009;120:400–7.

28. de Lezo JS, Medina A, Pan M, et al. Rapamycin-eluting stents for the treatment of unprotected left main coronary disease. Am Heart J 2004;148:481–5.

29. Meliga E, Garcia-Garcia HM, Valgimigli M, et al. Longest available clinical outcomes after drug-eluting stent implantation for unprotected left main coronary artery disease: the DELFT (Drug Eluting stent for LeFT main) registry. J Am Coll Cardiol 2008;51:2212–9.

30. Serruys PW, Morice MC, Kappetein AP, et al. Percutaneous coronary intervention versus coronary-artery bypass grafting for severe coronary artery disease. N Engl J Med 2009;360:961–72.

31. Patel MR, Dehmer GJ, Hirshfeld JW, et al. ACCF/SCAI/STS/AATS/AHA/ASNC 2009 Appropriateness criteria for coronary revascularization: a report by the American College of Cardiology Foundation Appropriateness Criteria Task Force, Society For Cardiovascular Angiography and Interventions, Society of Thoracic Surgeons, American Association for Thoracic Surgery, American Heart Association, and the American Society of Nuclear Cardiology. Endorsed by the American Society of Echocardiography, the Heart Failure Society of America, and the Society of Cardiovascular Computed Tomography. J Am Coll Cardiol 2009;53:530–53.

32. Iakovou I, Schmidt T, Bonizzoni E, et al. Incidence, predictors, and outcome of thrombosis after successful implantation of drug-eluting stents. JAMA 2005;293:2126–30.

33. Lagerqvist B, James SK, Stenestrand U, et al. Long-term outcomes with drug-eluting stents versus bare-metal stents in Sweden. N Engl J Med 2007;356:1009–19.

34. Spaulding C, Daemen J, Boersma E, et al. A pooled analysis of data comparing sirolimus-eluting stents with bare-metal stents. N Engl J Med 2007;356:989–97.

35. Stone GW, Moses JW, Ellis SG, et al. Safety and efficacy of sirolimus- and paclitaxel-eluting coronary stents. N Engl J Med 2007;356:998–1008.

36. Park D-W, Park S-W, Lee S-W, et al. Frequency of coronary arterial late angiographic stent thrombosis (LAST) in the first six months: outcomes with drug-eluting stents versus bare metal stents. Am J Cardiol 2007;99:774–8.

37. Farb A, Boam AB. Stent thrombosis redux–the FDA perspective. N Engl J Med 2007;356:984–7.

38. Arnett EN, Isner JM, Redwood DR, et al. Coronary artery narrowing in coronary heart disease: comparison of cineangiographic and necropsy findings. Ann Intern Med 1979;91:350–6.

39. Fisher LD, Judkins MP, Lesperance J, et al. Reproducibility of coronary arteriographic reading in the Coronary Artery Surgery Study (CASS). Cathet Cardiovasc Diagn 1982;8:565–75.

40. Isner JM, Kishel J, Kent KM, et al. Accuracy of angiographic determination of left main coronary arterial narrowing. Angiographic–histologic correlative analysis in 28 patients. Circulation 1981;63:1056–64.

41. Gerber TC, Erbel R, Gorge G, et al. Extent of atherosclerosis and remodeling of the left main coronary artery determined by intravascular ultrasound. Am J Cardiol 1994;73:666–71.

42. Abizaid AS, Mintz GS, Abizaid A, et al. One-year follow-up after intravascular ultrasound assessment of moderate left main coronary artery disease in patients with ambiguous angiograms. J Am Coll Cardiol 1999;34:707–15.

43. Fassa AA, Wagatsuma K, Higano ST, et al. Intravascular ultrasound-guided treatment for angiographically indeterminate left main coronary artery disease: a long-term follow-up study. J Am Coll Cardiol 2005;45:204–11.

44. Jasti V, Ivan E, Yalamanchili V, et al. Correlations between fractional flow reserve and intravascular ultrasound in patients with an ambiguous left main coronary artery stenosis. Circulation 2004;110:2831–6.

45. Pijls NH, Van Gelder B, Van der Voort P, et al. Fractional flow reserve. A useful index to evaluate the influence of an epicardial coronary stenosis on myocardial blood flow. Circulation 1995;92:3183–93.

46. Pijls NH, De Bruyne B, Peels K, et al. Measurement of fractional flow reserve to assess the functional severity of coronary-artery stenoses. N Engl J Med 1996;334:1703–8.

47. Mehilli J, Kastrati A, Byrne RA, et al. Paclitaxel-versus sirolimus-eluting stents for unprotected left main coronary artery disease. J Am Coll Cardiol 2009;53:1760–8.

48. Takagi T, Stankovic G, Finci L, et al. Results and long-term predictors of adverse clinical events after elective percutaneous interventions on unprotected left main coronary artery. Circulation 2002;106:698–702.

49. Marroquin OC, Selzer F, Mulukutla SR, et al. A comparison of bare-metal and drug-eluting stents for off-label indications. N Engl J Med 2008;358:342–52.

50. Tu JV, Bowen J, Chiu M, et al. Effectiveness and safety of drug-eluting stents in Ontario. N Engl J Med 2007;357:1393–402.

51. Tan WA, Tamai H, Park SJ, et al. Long-term clinical outcomes after unprotected left main trunk percutaneous revascularization in 279 patients. Circulation 2001;104:1609–14.

52. Kim YH, Ahn JM, Park DW, et al. EuroSCORE as a predictor of death and myocardial infarction after unprotected left main coronary stenting. Am J Cardiol 2006;98:1567–70.

53. Valgimigli M, Malagutti P, Rodriguez Granillo GA, et al. Single-vessel versus bifurcation stenting for the treatment of distal left main coronary artery disease in the drug-eluting stenting era. Clinical and angiographic insights into the Rapamycin-Eluting Stent Evaluated at Rotterdam Cardiology Hospital (RESEARCH) and Taxus-Stent Evaluated at Rotterdam Cardiology Hospital (T-SEARCH) registries. Am Heart J 2006;152:896–902.

54. Colombo A, Moses JW, Morice MC, et al. Randomized study to evaluate sirolimus-eluting stents implanted at coronary bifurcation lesions. Circulation 2004;109:1244–9.

55. Steigen TK, Maeng M, Wiseth R, et al. Randomized study on simple versus complex stenting of coronary artery bifurcation lesions: the Nordic bifurcation study. Circulation 2006;114:1955–61.

56. Mintz GS, Nissen SE, Anderson WD, et al. American College of Cardiology clinical expert consensus document on standards for acquisition, measurement and reporting of intravascular ultrasound studies (IVUS). A report of the American College of Cardiology Task Force on Clinical Expert Consensus Documents. J Am Coll Cardiol 2001;37:1478–92.

57. Agostoni P, Valgimigli M, Van Mieghem CAG, et al. Comparison of early outcome of percutaneous coronary intervention for unprotected left main coronary artery disease in the drug-eluting stent era with versus without intravascular ultrasonic guidance. Am J Cardiol 2005;95:644–7.

58. Sonoda S, Morino Y, Ako J, et al. Impact of final stent dimensions on long-term results following sirolimus-eluting stent implantation: serial intravascular ultrasound analysis from the Sirius Trial. J Am Coll Cardiol 2004;43:1959–63.

59. Marco A. Costa OSGMMZPSGTAB. Synergistic use of sirolimus-eluting stents and intravascular ultrasound for the treatment of unprotected left main and vein graft disease. Catheter Cardiovasc Interv 2004;61:368–75.

60. Fujii K, Carlier SG, Mintz GS, et al. Stent underexpansion and residual reference segment stenosis are related to stent thrombosis after sirolimus-eluting stent implantation: an intravascular ultrasound study. J Am Coll Cardiol 2005;45:995–8.

61. Cook S, Wenaweser P, Togni M, et al. Incomplete stent apposition and very late stent thrombosis after drug-eluting stent implantation. Circulation 2007;115:2426–34.

62. Okabe T, Mintz GS, Buch AN, et al. Intravascular ultrasound parameters associated with stent thrombosis after drug-eluting stent deployment. Am J Cardiol 2007;100:615–20.

63. Tsuchikane EAT, Tamai H, Igarashi Y, et al. The efficacy of pre drug eluting stent debulking by directional atherectomy for bifurcated lesions: a multicenter prospective registry (PERFECT Registry). J Am Coll Cardiol 2007;49(Suppl 2):15B.

64. Briguori C, Airoldi F, Chieffo A, et al. Elective versus provisional intraaortic balloon pumping in unprotected left main stenting. Am Heart J 2006;152:565–72.

65. Park DW, Park SW, Park KH, et al. Frequency of and risk factors for stent thrombosis after drug-eluting stent implantation during long-term follow-up. Am J Cardiol 2006;98:352–6.

66. Palmerini T, Marzocchi A, Tamburino C, et al. Temporal pattern of ischemic events in relation to dual antiplatelet therapy in patients with unprotected left main coronary artery stenosis undergoing percutaneous coronary intervention. J Am Coll Cardiol 2009;53:1176–81.

67. Lee SW, Park SW, Hong MK, et al. Triple versus dual antiplatelet therapy after coronary stenting: impact on stent thrombosis. J Am Coll Cardiol 2005;46:1833–7.

68. Cura FA, Bhatt DL, Lincoff AM, et al. Pronounced benefit of coronary stenting and adjunctive platelet glycoprotein IIb/IIIa inhibition in complex atherosclerotic lesions. Circulation 2000;102:28–34.

69. Tina L, Pinto Slottow RW. Overview of the 2006 food and drug administration circulatory system devices panel meeting on drug-eluting stent thrombosis. Catheter Cardiovasc Interv 2007;69:1064–74.

Drug-Eluting Stents: Issues of Late Stent Thrombosis

Gilles Lemesle, MD, Gabriel Maluenda, MD,
Sara D. Collins, MD, Ron Waksman, MD*

KEYWORDS

- Drug-eluting stent • Stent thrombosis
- Percutaneous coronary intervention

Compared with bare metal stents (BMSs), drug-eluting stents (DESs) have shown a clear and constant reduction in the rate of in-stent restenosis after percutaneous coronary intervention (PCI).[1–4] Nevertheless, the emergence of DESs has raised concerns regarding the occurrence of late and very late stent thrombosis[5,6] related to delayed strut endothelialization and potential prothrombotic characteristics of the DES itself.[7,8]

Since September 2006 (European Society of Cardiology, World Congress of Cardiology in Barcelona, Spain) and the controversy about the use of DESs and the risk of late events,[5,6] despite much discussion no clear-cut conclusion can be drawn on the potential increased risk of late and very late stent thrombosis with DESs. Although results for early stent thrombosis seem clear and show no difference between DESs and BMSs, results for late and very late stent thrombosis are more debated. In addition, the time of dual antiplatelet therapy is usually longer for DESs than for BMSs in different randomized clinical trials. To enable consistent and reliable information on the use of both stent types, the Academic Research Consortium (ARC) has published the definition of stent thrombosis.[9] New generations of DESs with novel polymers, antiproliferative drugs, and improved platforms are now approved and available for use.

This article reviews safety issues of different DESs, with focus on late and very late stent thrombosis.

ARC DEFINITION OF STENT THROMBOSIS

The lack of consensus among clinical trials on the definition of stent thrombosis has led to disparities in reports of stent thrombosis and, in particular, has prevented comparison of stent thrombosis rates between studies. To address this issue, the ARC definition of stent thrombosis was established[9] and stent thrombosis was categorized according to (1) the timing after initial PCI and (2) the evidence of stent thrombosis (**Box 1**).

Timing of Stent Thrombosis

Stent thrombosis is considered acute when it occurs between 0 and 24 hours after stent implantation; subacute, between 24 hours and 30 days; late, between 30 days and 1 year; and very late, after 1 year. Acute or subacute stent thrombosis can also be termed early stent thrombosis.

Definite Stent Thrombosis

Definite stent thrombosis is defined by the presence of an angiographic confirmation of stent thrombosis (the presence of a thrombus that originates in the stent or in the segment 5 mm proximal or distal to the stent) associated with the presence of at least 1 of the following criteria within a 48-hour window: (1) acute onset of ischemic symptoms at rest, (2) new ischemic electrocardiographic changes that suggest acute ischemia or typical rise and fall in cardiac biomarkers, or by

Division of Cardiology, Department of Internal Medicine, Washington Hospital Center, 110 Irving Street, NW, Suite 4B-1, Washington, DC 20010, USA
* Corresponding author.
E-mail address: ron.waksman@medstar.net (R. Waksman).

cardiology.theclinics.com

Definite stent thrombosis

- Angiographic confirmation of stent thrombosis associated with the presence of at least 1 of the following criteria within a 48-hour window

  - Acute onset of ischemic symptoms at rest
  - New ischemic electrocardiographic changes that suggest acute ischemia or typical rise and fall in cardiac biomarkers

- Or pathologic confirmation (autopsy) of stent thrombosis

  - Probable stent thrombosis

- Any unexplained death within the first 30 days after stent implantation
- Or any myocardial infarction (MI) related to documented acute ischemia in the territory of the implanted stent without angiographic confirmation of stent thrombosis and in the absence of any other obvious cause, irrespective of the time after the index procedure.

Possible stent thrombosis

- Any unexplained death from 30 days after intracoronary stenting until the end of follow-up

the presence of a pathologic confirmation of stent thrombosis (evidence of recent thrombus within the stent determined at autopsy or via examination of tissue retrieved after thrombectomy). The incidental angiographic documentation of stent occlusion in the absence of clinical signs or symptoms is not considered a confirmed stent thrombosis (silent occlusion).

Probable Stent Thrombosis

Probable stent thrombosis is defined as unexplained death within the first 30 days after stent implantation or any myocardial infarction (MI) related to documented acute ischemia in the territory of the implanted stent without angiographic confirmation of stent thrombosis and in the absence of any other obvious cause, irrespective of the time after the index procedure.

Possible Stent Thrombosis

Possible stent thrombosis is defined as any unexplained death from 30 days after intracoronary stenting until the end of follow-up.

INCIDENCE OF LATE AND VERY LATE STENT THROMBOSIS
Late Stent Thrombosis

According to recent studies and meta-analyses, the incidence of late stent thrombosis seems to be similar for DESs and BMSs, at around 0.5%.[10–16] The cumulative event rates for both types of stents are consequently around 1.5% at 1 year after PCI. Nevertheless, the duration of the use of dual antiplatelet therapy was usually longer for DESs compared with BMSs in these studies (3 or 6 months vs 1 month), making it difficult to draw any conclusions on outcome.

Spaulding and colleagues[13] reported a cumulative rate of stent thrombosis of 0.8% for BMSs versus 1.8% for sirolimus-eluting stents (SESs) (P = .53) at 1 year using the ARC definition of stent thrombosis in a meta-analysis of the 4 Cypher stent (Cordis Corporation, Bridgewater, NJ, USA) trials (RAVEL [Randomized Study with the Sirolimus-eluting Velocity Balloon-Expandable Stent], SIRIUS [SIRolImUS-coated Bx Velocity balloon-expandable stent in the treatment of patients with de novo coronary artery lesions], E-SIRIUS [The European Sirolimus-Eluting Stent in De Novo Native Coronary Lesions], and C-SIRIUS [Canadian Sirolimus-Eluting Stent in Coronary Lesions), which included 1748 patients.

Using the per-protocol definition of stent thrombosis, Stone and colleagues[14] reported in their meta-analysis of 9 trials (RAVEL, SIRIUS, E-SIRIUS, C-SIRIUS and TAXUS stent [Boston Scientific Inc, Natick, MA, USA] I–V), which included 3513 patients, a cumulative rate of stent thrombosis of 0.6% for BMSs versus 1.2% for SESs (P = .2) and 0.9% for BMSs versus 1.3% for paclitaxel-eluting stents (PESs) (P = .3). By using the ARC definition of stent thrombosis, Mauri and colleagues,[11] in their meta-analysis of the same 9 trials, reported a cumulative rate of stent thrombosis of 1.7% for BMSs versus 1.5% for SESs (P = .7) and 1.4% for BMSs versus 1.8% for PESs (P = .52). Jensen and colleagues,[17] in their registry of 12,395 patients, reported a cumulative rate of stent thrombosis of 2% for BMSs versus 1.6% for SESs (P = .5) and 1.4% for BMSs versus 1.8% for PESs (P = .52). Stettler and colleagues[12] performed a meta-analysis of 38 trials and reported an incidence of stent thrombosis of 1% for BMSs, 1.1% for PESs, and 1.1% for SESs (P = .62). These analyses show that stent type was not a predictor of late stent thrombosis when the ARC definition was used.

Very Late Stent Thrombosis

Because of the overall rarity of this event, the incidence of very late stent thrombosis is poorly described and authors disagree about the potential increased risk of very late stent thrombosis after DES implantation. According to newer registries,[18–20] the incidence of very late stent thrombosis seems to range between 0.4% and 0.6% per year after DES implantation in real world practice, which is seemingly higher than the rate observed in the randomized clinical trials.[10–16] By contrast, no registry data reflect the real incidence of very late stent thrombosis after BMS implantation.

This question was addressed by many meta-analyses of different randomized trials that compared DESs with BMSs. The conclusion of these meta-analyses seems to be directly driven by the type of definition used for stent thrombosis (**Fig. 1**). The meta-analyses using the ARC definition did not show any significant difference between DESs and BMSs with regard to the rate of very late stent thrombosis.[11–13] By contrast, most of the meta-analyses using the per-protocol definitions[10–12,14–16] showed a higher risk of very late stent thrombosis in the DES groups. Consequently, no clear-cut conclusions can be drawn. In the analyses using the per-protocol definitions, when rates of very late stent thrombosis were similar to those reported in the meta-analyses using the ARC definition in the DES groups, the rates of very late stent thrombosis in the BMS groups were much lower for some unexplained reasons (**Table 1**).

Several limits of these meta-analyses should be addressed. Firstly, the follow-up at 4 or 5 years was largely incomplete. For example, the larger meta-analysis published by Stettler and colleagues[12] reported a 4-year follow-up of 45% for the BMS group, less than 20% for the paclitaxel group, and less than 25% for the sirolimus group. Secondly, except the meta-analysis published by Stettler and colleagues,[12] others could not determine a difference between the incidence of very late BMS and very late DES thrombosis. Consequently, the low frequency of this event makes it very difficult to be definitive. For instance, to design an adequately powered clinical trial (power of 80%) to show even a doubling of the very late stent thrombosis rate with DESs, the trial would have to enroll approximately 5500 patients (2750 in each group) with a long-term follow-up (at least 4 years), assuming a baseline rate of 0.6% per year in the DES group.

The use of DESs has not been associated with an increase in overall mortality.[12–14,21–23] This discordance may be explained by a reduction in

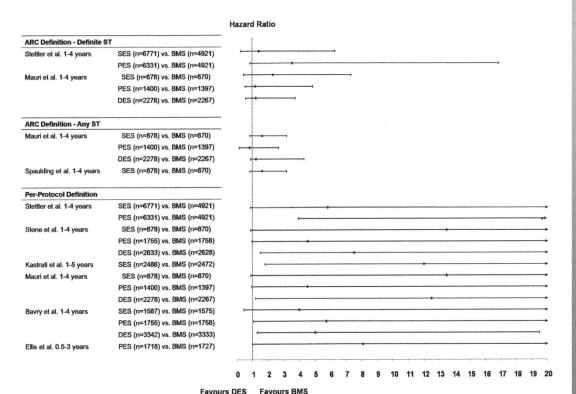

Fig. 1. Comparison between DESs and BMSs in very late stent thrombosis. *Data from* Refs.[10–16]

Table 1
Comparison of very late stent thrombosis incidences between DESs and BMSs and according to the definition used, either the ARC or the per-protocol definitions

Very late Stent Thrombosis	Hazard Ratio	95% Confidence Interval	Cumulative Incidence (%)		
			DES	BMS	P value
ARC definition—definite ST					
Stettler et al 1–4 y[12]					
SES (n = 6771) vs BMS (n = 4921)	1.43	0.27–6.24	nc	nc	ns
PES (n = 6331) vs BMS (n = 4921)	3.57	0.86–16.85	nc	nc	ns
Mauri et al 1–4 y[11]					
SES (n = 878) vs BMS (n = 870)	2.33	0.45–7.34	0.7	0.3	ns
PES (n = 1400) vs BMS (n = 1397)	1.2	0.55–4.89	0.6	0.5	ns
DES (n = 2278) vs BMS (n = 2267)	1.25	0.6–3.76	0.5	0.4	ns
ARC definition—any ST					
Mauri et al 1–4 y[11]					
SES (n = 878) vs BMS (n = 870)	1.65	0.85–3.2	2.9	1.7	ns
PES (n = 1400) vs BMS (n = 1397)	0.85	0.17–2.67	1.8	2.1	ns
DES (n = 2278) vs BMS (n = 2267)	1.26	0.88–4.31	1.9	1.5	ns
Spaulding et al 1–4 y[13]					
SES (n = 878) vs BMS (n = 870)	1.65	0.85–3.2	2.8	1.7	ns
Per-protocol definition					
Stettler et al 1–4 y[12]					
SES (n = 6771) vs BMS (n = 4921)	5.82	0.88–76.89	nc	nc	ns
PES (n = 6331) vs BMS (n = 4921)	20.02	3.92–221.7	nc	nc	0.001
Stone et al 1–4 y[14]					
SES (n = 878) vs BMS (n = 870)	13.5	0.9–122	0.6	0	0.025
PES (n = 1755) vs BMS (n = 1758)	4.54	0.98–21.03	0.7	0.2	ns
DES (n = 2633) vs BMS (n = 2628)	7.5	1.5–125	0.6	0.08	0.004
Kastrati et al 1–5 y[10]					
SES (n = 2486) vs BMS (n = 2472)	12	1.8–120	0.6	0.05	0.02
Mauri et al 1–4 y[11]					
SES (n = 878) vs BMS (n = 870)	13.5	0.9–122	0.6	0	0.025
PES (n = 1400) vs BMS (n = 1397)	4.52	0.97–21.03	0.6	0.2	ns
DES (n = 2278) vs BMS (n = 2267)	12.5	1.22–80.75	0.5	0.04	0.006
Bavry et al 1–4 y[15]					
SES (n = 1587) vs BMS (n = 1575)	3.99	0.45–35.62	0.4	0	ns
PES (n = 1755) vs BMS (n = 1758)	5.72	1.08–32.45	0.6	0	0.049
DES (n = 3342) vs BMS (n = 3333)	5.02	1.29–19.52	0.5	0	0.02
Ellis et al 0.5–3 y[16]					
PES (n = 1718) vs BMS (n = 1727)	8.09	1.01–64.67	0.5	0.06	0.021

Abbreviations: nc, not communicated; ns, not significant; ST, stent thrombosis.

the rate of complications related to repeat revascularization. It is clear that the use of DESs is associated with a decrease in the rate of repeat revascularization.[1–4]

NEW GENERATION OF DESS

New DESs have been approved for use by the Food and Drug Administration, the zotarolimus-eluting stent (ZES, Endeavor [Medtronic, Minneapolis, MN, USA]) and the everolimus-eluting stent (EES, Xience V, [Abbott Laboratories, Abbott Park, IL, USA] or Promus [Boston Scientific Inc, Natick, MA, USA]). To date, little data on late and, especially, very late stent thrombosis are available for these 2 new DESs, and most of these data have not yet been published.

The early 9-month results of the Endeavor II trial,[24] which included 1197 patients and compared ZESs with BMSs, showed similar incidences of stent thrombosis in both groups, 0.5% versus 1.2% in the ZES and BMS groups, respectively (P = not significant [ns]). No cases of late stent thrombosis were indexed in both groups. Similarly, the results of the Endeavor III trial,[25] which included 436 patients and compared ZESs to SESs, showed no occurrence of stent thrombosis in both groups at 2 years. In the Endeavor IV trial[26] (Leon MB, unpublished data, 2007), which included 1548 patients and compared ZESs with PESs, the results showed no difference at 1 year between both groups in any stent thrombosis (0.8% vs 0.1% in the ZES and PES groups, respectively [P = ns]) or in late stent thrombosis (0.4% vs 0% in the ZES and PES groups, respectively [P = ns]). But the early results of the SORT OUT III (a prospective randomized comparison of zotarolimus-eluting stents and sirolimus-eluting stents in patients with coronary artery disease) trial[27] (Lassen J, unpublished data, 2008), which included 2334 patients and compared ZESs with SESs, and the results of Western Denmark Heart Registry[28] (Thuesen L, unpublished data, 2008), which included 6122 patients and compared ZESs with SESs, were in contrast with the other studies. In the SORT OUT III trial,[27] the use of ZESs was significantly associated with a higher rate of stent thrombosis at 9 months (hazard ratio [HR], 4.62; 95% confidence interval [CI], 1.33–16.1). There was a trend for a higher rate of stent thrombosis at 28 months in the Western Denmark Heart Registry in the ZES group (HR, 2.06; 95% CI, 0.77–5.51).[28] Nevertheless, at the time, the difference between the 2 groups in these studies seems to be essentially driven by the rate of early stent thrombosis for some unexplained reasons.

Data on EESs are even less. In the SPIRIT II trial,[29] which included 300 patients and compared EESs with PESs, only 2 cases of stent thrombosis were indexed (1 in each group) with an available follow-up of only 6 months. The results of the SPIRIT III trial,[30,31] which included 1002 patients and compared EESs with PESs, showed a low rate of stent thrombosis between 1 and 2 years, defined as very late stent thrombosis, 0.3% versus 1.0% in the EES and PES groups, respectively (P = ns).

Pending more data and especially more detailed data on the SORT OUT III trial and the Western Denmark Heart Registry, no clear-cut conclusions can be drawn on the safety of these 2 new devices.

CORRELATES OF LATE AND VERY LATE STENT THROMBOSIS
Clinical Correlates of Stent Thrombosis

Many predictors have been identified for late and very late stent thrombosis after DES implantation. These include acute coronary syndrome at index presentation,[18,32,33] left ventricular ejection fraction,[34] diabetes mellitus,[18,34] renal failure,[33–35] total stent length,[32,33,36] number of stents used,[18] bifurcation lesions,[34,35] side branch occlusion,[36] stent under-expansion and/or malapposition,[37] and use of brachytherapy[34] (**Box 2**).

Discontinuation of Antiplatelet Therapy

The association between cessation of antiplatelet therapy and early stent thrombosis is clear.[33–35,38] It is the strongest predictor of early stent thrombosis. Iakovou and colleagues[34] reported a relative risk of 161.17 in this situation. The current European and North American guidelines,[39,40] which

---

Box 2
Predictors for late and very late stent thrombosis

Acute coronary syndrome at index presentation

Diabetes mellitus

Chronic renal failure

Left ventricular ejection fraction

Antiplatelet therapy discontinuation?

Bifurcation

Total stent length

Number of stents

Stent under-expansion or malapposition

DES use?

Brachytherapy

highlight the need for dual antiplatelet therapy during the first 4 weeks after PCI even with BMSs, are derived directly from those results.

By contrast, the real place of antiplatelet therapy cessation in late and very late stent thrombosis remains to be determined. Several studies seem to have identified cessation of antiplatelet therapy (especially clopidogrel) as a predictor of late stent thrombosis in cases of DES use, which reported a relative risk of stent thrombosis between 24.79 and 57.13.[33,34] Stone and colleagues[41] have reported a trend for fewer very late stent thrombosis episodes in patients still taking thienopyridines compared with those who discontinued its use at 1 year. Other studies have reported contradictory results and have not found any link between discontinuation of antiplatelet therapy and incidence of late or very late stent thrombosis.[42,43] In a large European multicenter study, thienopyridine discontinuation after 6 months in patients with DESs was not a risk factor for subsequent stent thrombosis.[42] Thus, no clear-cut conclusions can be drawn, especially on any potential link between antiplatelet therapy cessation and very late stent thrombosis. The European and North American guidelines recommend pursuing the dual antiplatelet therapy 1 year after a DES implantation,[39,40] but there is no recommendation after this time period.

Histopathologic Correlates of Late Stent Thrombosis

Several authors have reported pathologic findings for late stent thrombosis. In addition to the often evocated delayed strut endothelialization,[7,8] Farb and colleagues[44] suggested other pathologic mechanisms of late and very late stent thrombosis based on autopsy data. Among the causes suggested are in-stent restenosis, chronic inflammation, and atherosclerosis progression proximal or distal to the stent. In in-stent restenosis, the severe narrowing caused by neointima formation might be a leading cause for clot formation and late or very late stent thrombosis. Such findings were reported in several cases. In others, coronary angiograms showed intimal dissection in the non-stented arterial edges. Coronary atherosclerosis is a diffused disease, and the number of vulnerable thin-cap atheromas increases with the number of coronary risk factors. A plaque rupture that occurs in close proximity to the stent can extend to the adjacent stented segment and present as late stent thrombosis. Farb and colleagues[44] suggested that stenting of highly necrotic and inflammatory plaques might also lead to late or very late stent thrombosis.

OUTCOME

Stent thrombosis is well known as a severe complication after PCI. Nonfatal acute MI is the most frequent clinical presentation of stent thrombosis (70%–80% of cases).[45,46] Moreover, 10% to 30% of patients presenting with definite stent thrombosis will die in hospital.[45,46] Cutlip and colleagues[47] have reported a 1-month mortality rate of 20%, whereas Orford and colleagues[48] reported a 6-month mortality rate of 48% after definite stent thrombosis. Stent thrombosis can also lead to unexplained sudden deaths. In addition, 15% to 39% of patients who presented with a stent thrombosis and who were successfully treated experienced a recurrent MI within the first month.[35,49,50] These recurrent MIs are most often related to recurrent stent thrombosis.[49]

Some authors have reported that late and very late stent thrombosis seem to have a less severe prognosis than early stent thrombosis.[51] This fact may be explained at least in part by the occurrence of 2 successive MIs within 30 days in patients with early stent thrombosis, leading to a higher rate of cardiogenic shock. When a stent thrombosis occurs, the index PCI was the most often performed in the context of a MI (50%–70% of cases), and acute MI is a well-known predictor for stent thrombosis. Therefore, patients presenting with an early stent thrombosis suffer 2 successive MIs without any time to recover between both events. Moreover, it is possible that some patients who have late or very late stent thrombosis after DES implantation have also developed in-stent restenosis before the event and suffered from ongoing ischemia, which then led to the development of collaterals.[52–54] Nathoe and colleagues[55] have shown the prognostic value of the presence of collateral circulation in patients presenting with an MI. Collaterals may minimize the damage to the myocardium at the time of the event and result in better prognosis.

PREVENTIVE TREATMENT OF STENT THROMBOSIS

The basis of preventive treatment for stent thrombosis is, above all, to perform the best PCI possible, including good expansion and apposition of the stent. In this context, the role of intravascular ultrasound must be highlighted. To avoid all mechanical predictors for stent thrombosis, this technique that allows a better stent apposition is systematically recommended by some authors.[56,57]

Antiplatelet therapy for the preventive treatment for early stent thrombosis is relatively well codified.

However, as mentioned earlier, the situation is more confusing for late and very late stent thrombosis. Guidelines currently recommend a 12-month dual antiplatelet therapy after DES implantation.[39,40] Some authors[33,34] suggest that this association must be pursued for more than 12 months, but no strong data regarding the safety and benefit of such a prescription are currently available. Consequently, for each patient the risk/benefit balance must be analyzed with caution.

SUMMARY

If the rates of early and late stent thrombosis seem to be similar between BMSs and DESs, there are still serious doubts on a potential increase in the rate of very late stent thrombosis after DES implantation compared with BMS. Nevertheless, the use of DESs seems not to be associated with an increase in overall mortality. New generations of DESs are available; however, few data regarding the rate of very late stent thrombosis were reported. Thus, pending results of larger studies, no conclusion can be drawn regarding their long-term safety. Many predictors of late and very late stent thrombosis have been identified. Yet, the optimal duration of dual antiplatelet therapy remains unknown in this setting.

REFERENCES

1. Morice MC, Serruys PW, Barragan P, et al. Long-term clinical outcomes with sirolimus-eluting coronary stents: five-year results of the RAVEL trial. J Am Coll Cardiol 2007;50:1299–304.

2. Moses JW, Leon MB, Popma JJ, et al. Sirolimus-eluting stents versus standard stents in patients with stenosis in a native coronary artery. N Engl J Med 2003;349:1315–23.

3. Stone GW, Ellis SG, Cox DA, et al. One-year clinical results with the slow-release, polymer-based, paclitaxel-eluting TAXUS stent: the TAXUS-IV trial. Circulation 2004;109:1942–7.

4. Weisz G, Leon MB, Holmes DR Jr, et al. Two-year outcomes after sirolimus-eluting stent implantation: results from the Sirolimus-Eluting Stent in de Novo Native Coronary Lesions (SIRIUS) trial. J Am Coll Cardiol 2006;47:1350–5.

5. Camenzind E, Steg PG, Wijns W. Stent thrombosis late after implantation of first-generation drug-eluting stents: a cause for concern. Circulation 2007;115:1440–55 [discussion: 1455].

6. Nordmann AJ, Briel M, Bucher HC. Mortality in randomized controlled trials comparing drug-eluting vs. bare metal stents in coronary artery disease: a meta-analysis. Eur Heart J 2006;27:2784–814.

7. Finn AV, Joner M, Nakazawa G, et al. Pathological correlates of late drug-eluting stent thrombosis: strut coverage as a marker of endothelialization. Circulation 2007;115:2435–41.

8. Joner M, Finn AV, Farb A, et al. Pathology of drug-eluting stents in humans: delayed healing and late thrombotic risk. J Am Coll Cardiol 2006;48:193–202.

9. Cutlip DE, Windecker S, Mehran R, et al. Clinical end points in coronary stent trials: a case for standardized definitions. Circulation 2007;115:2344–51.

10. Kastrati A, Mehilli J, Pache J, et al. Analysis of 14 trials comparing sirolimus-eluting stents with bare-metal stents. N Engl J Med 2007;356:1030–9.

11. Mauri L, Hsieh WH, Massaro JM, et al. Stent thrombosis in randomized clinical trials of drug-eluting stents. N Engl J Med 2007;356:1020–9.

12. Stettler C, Wandel S, Allemann S, et al. Outcomes associated with drug-eluting and bare-metal stents: a collaborative network meta-analysis. Lancet 2007;370:937–48.

13. Spaulding C, Daemen J, Boersma E, et al. A pooled analysis of data comparing sirolimus-eluting stents with bare-metal stents. N Engl J Med 2007;356:989–97.

14. Stone GW, Moses JW, Ellis SG, et al. Safety and efficacy of sirolimus- and paclitaxel-eluting coronary stents. N Engl J Med 2007;356:998–1008.

15. Bavry AA, Kumbhani DJ, Helton TJ, et al. Late thrombosis of drug-eluting stents: a meta-analysis of randomized clinical trials. Am J Med 2006;119:1056–61.

16. Ellis SG, Colombo A, Grube E, et al. Incidence, timing, and correlates of stent thrombosis with the polymeric paclitaxel drug-eluting stent: a TAXUS II, IV, V, and VI meta-analysis of 3,445 patients followed for up to 3 years. J Am Coll Cardiol 2007;49:1043–51.

17. Jensen LO, Maeng M, Kaltoft A, et al. Stent thrombosis, myocardial infarction, and death after drug-eluting and bare-metal stent coronary interventions. J Am Coll Cardiol 2007;50:463–70.

18. Daemen J, Wenaweser P, Tsuchida K, et al. Early and late coronary stent thrombosis of sirolimus-eluting and paclitaxel-eluting stents in routine clinical practice: data from a large two-institutional cohort study. Lancet 2007;369:667–78.

19. Pinto Slottow TL, Steinberg DH, Roy PK, et al. Observations and outcomes of definite and probable drug-eluting stent thrombosis seen at a single hospital in a four-year period. Am J Cardiol 2008;102:298–303.

20. Vaknin-Assa H, Assali A, Ukabi S, et al. Stent thrombosis following drug-eluting stent implantation. A single-center experience. Cardiovasc Revasc Med 2007;8:243–7.

21. Holmes DR Jr, Moses JW, Schofer J, et al. Cause of death with bare metal and sirolimus-eluting stents. Eur Heart J 2006;27:2815–22.

22. Marzocchi A, Saia F, Piovaccari G, et al. Long-term safety and efficacy of drug-eluting stents: two-year results of the REAL (REgistro AngiopLastiche dell'Emilia Romagna) multicenter registry. Circulation 2007;115:3181–8.

23. Shishehbor MH, Goel SS, Kapadia SR, et al. Long-term impact of drug-eluting stents versus bare-metal stents on all-cause mortality. J Am Coll Cardiol 2008; 52:1041–8.

24. Fajadet J, Wijns W, Laarman GJ, et al. Randomized, double-blind, multicenter study of the Endeavor zotarolimus-eluting phosphorylcholine-encapsulated stent for treatment of native coronary artery lesions: clinical and angiographic results of the ENDEAVOR II trial. Circulation 2006;114:798–806.

25. Kandzari DE, Leon MB, Popma JJ, et al. Comparison of zotarolimus-eluting and sirolimus-eluting stents in patients with native coronary artery disease: a randomized controlled trial. J Am Coll Cardiol 2006;48:2440–7.

26. Leon MB. Endeavor IV: a randomized comparison of a Zotarolimus-eluting stent and a Paclitaxel-eluting stent in patients with coronary artery disease. Washington, DC: TCT Congress; 2007. Available at: http://www.tctmd.com/Show.aspx?id=7700. Accessed March 1, 2009.

27. Lassen J. SORT OUT III: a prospective randomized comparison of Zotarolimus-eluting and Sirolimus-eluting stents in patients with coronary artery disease. Washington, DC: TCT Congress; 2008. Available at: http://www.crtonline.org/flash.aspx?PAGE_ID=5820. Accessed March 1, 2009.

28. Thuesen L. Western Denmark Heart Registry: large-scale registry examining safety and effectiveness of Zotarolinus-eluting and Sirolimus-eluting stents in patients with coronary artery disease. Washington, DC: TCT Congress; 2008. Available at: http://www.crtonline.org/flash.aspx?PAGE_ID=5818. Accessed March 1, 2009.

29. Serruys PW, Ruygrok P, Neuzner J, et al. A randomized comparison of an everolimus-eluting stent with a paclitaxel-eluting stent: the SPIRIT II trial. EuroIntervention 2006;2:286–94.

30. Stone GW, Midei M, Newman W, et al. Randomized comparison of everolimus-eluting and paclitaxel-eluting stents. Two-year clinical follow-up from the Clinical Evaluation of the Xience V Everolimus Eluting Coronary Stent System in the Treatment of Patients with de novo Native Coronary Artery Lesions (SPIRIT) III trial. Circulation 2009;119(5):680–6.

31. Stone GW, Midei M, Newman W, et al. Comparison of an everolimus-eluting stent and a paclitaxel-eluting stent in patients with coronary artery disease: a randomized trial. JAMA 2008;299:1903–13.

32. de la Torre-Hernandez JM, Alfonso F, Hernandez F, et al. Drug-eluting stent thrombosis: results from the multicenter Spanish registry ESTROFA (Estudio ESpanol sobre TROmbosis de stents FArmacoactivos). J Am Coll Cardiol 2008;51:986–90.

33. Park DW, Park SW, Park KH, et al. Frequency of and risk factors for stent thrombosis after drug-eluting stent implantation during long-term follow-up. Am J Cardiol 2006;98:352–6.

34. Iakovou I, Schmidt T, Bonizzoni E, et al. Incidence, predictors, and outcome of thrombosis after successful implantation of drug-eluting stents. JAMA 2005;293:2126–30.

35. Kuchulakanti PK, Chu WW, Torguson R, et al. Correlates and long-term outcomes of angiographically proven stent thrombosis with sirolimus- and paclitaxel-eluting stents. Circulation 2006;113: 1108–13.

36. Pfisterer M, Brunner-La Rocca HP, Buser PT, et al. Late clinical events after clopidogrel discontinuation may limit the benefit of drug-eluting stents: an observational study of drug-eluting versus bare-metal stents. J Am Coll Cardiol 2006;48:2584–91.

37. Cook S, Wenaweser P, Togni M, et al. Incomplete stent apposition and very late stent thrombosis after drug-eluting stent implantation. Circulation 2007; 115:2426–34.

38. Jeremias A, Sylvia B, Bridges J, et al. Stent thrombosis after successful sirolimus-eluting stent implantation. Circulation 2004;109:1930–2.

39. Silber S, Albertsson P, Aviles FF, et al. Guidelines for percutaneous coronary interventions. The Task Force for Percutaneous Coronary Interventions of the European Society of Cardiology. Eur Heart J 2005;26:804–47.

40. Smith SC Jr, Feldman TE, Hirshfeld JW Jr, et al. ACC/AHA/SCAI 2005 Guideline Update for Percutaneous Coronary Intervention-Summary Article: a Report of the American College of Cardiology/American Heart Association Task Force on Practice Guidelines (ACC/AHA/SCAI Writing Committee to Update the 2001 Guidelines for Percutaneous Coronary Intervention). J Am Coll Cardiol 2006;47: 216–35.

41. Stone GW, Ellis SG, Colombo A, et al. Effect of prolonged thienopyridine use after drug-eluting stent implantation (from the TAXUS landmark trials data). Am J Cardiol 2008;102:1017–22.

42. Airoldi F, Colombo A, Morici N, et al. Incidence and predictors of drug-eluting stent thrombosis during and after discontinuation of thienopyridine treatment. Circulation 2007;116:745–54.

43. De Luca G, Cassetti E, Marino P. Impact of duration of clopidogrel prescription on outcome of DES as compared to BMS in primary angioplasty: a meta-regression analysis of randomized trials. J Thromb Thrombolysis 2008;27(4):365–78.

44. Farb A, Burke AP, Kolodgie FD, et al. Pathological mechanisms of fatal late coronary stent thrombosis in humans. Circulation 2003;108:1701–6.

45. Lemesle G, Delhaye C, Bonello L, et al. Stent thrombosis in 2008: Definition, predictors, prognosis and treatment. Arch Cardiovasc Dis 2008;101:769–77.

46. Kereiakes DJ, Choo JK, Young JJ, et al. Thrombosis and drug-eluting stents: a critical appraisal. Rev Cardiovasc Med 2004;5:9–15.

47. Cutlip DE, Baim DS, Ho KK, et al. Stent thrombosis in the modern era: a pooled analysis of multicenter coronary stent clinical trials. Circulation 2001;103:1967–71.

48. Orford JL, Lennon R, Melby S, et al. Frequency and correlates of coronary stent thrombosis in the modern era: analysis of a single center registry. J Am Coll Cardiol 2002;40:1567–72.

49. Lemesle G, Sudre A, Modine T, et al. High incidence of recurrent in stent thrombosis after successful treatment of a first in stent thrombosis. Catheter Cardiovasc Interv 2008;72:470–8.

50. Wenaweser P, Rey C, Eberli FR, et al. Stent thrombosis following bare-metal stent implantation: success of emergency percutaneous coronary intervention and predictors of adverse outcome. Eur Heart J 2005;26:1180–7.

51. Lemesle G, de Labriolle A, Bonello L, et al. Clinical manifestation and prognosis of early- versus late stent thrombosis of drug-eluting stents. J Interv Cardiol 2009;22:228–33.

52. Nakae I, Fujita M, Fudo T, et al. Relation between preexistent coronary collateral circulation and the incidence of restenosis after successful primary coronary angioplasty for acute myocardial infarction. J Am Coll Cardiol 1996;27:1688–92.

53. Newman PE. The coronary collateral circulation: determinants and functional significance in ischemic heart disease. Am Heart J 1981;102:431–45.

54. Sabri MN, DiSciascio G, Cowley MJ, et al. Coronary collateral recruitment: functional significance and relation to rate of vessel closure. Am Heart J 1991;121:876–80.

55. Nathoe HM, Koerselman J, Buskens E, et al. Determinants and prognostic significance of collaterals in patients undergoing coronary revascularization. Am J Cardiol 2006;98:31–5.

56. Gerber R, Colombo A. Does IVUS guidance of coronary interventions affect outcome? A prime example of the failure of randomized clinical trials. Catheter Cardiovasc Interv 2008;71:646–54.

57. Roy P, Steinberg DH, Sushinsky SJ, et al. The potential clinical utility of intravascular ultrasound guidance in patients undergoing percutaneous coronary intervention with drug-eluting stents. Eur Heart J 2008;29:1851–7.

Adjunct Therapy in STEMI Intervention

Sameer Mehta, MD, MBA[a],*, Carlos E. Alfonso, MD[b],
Estefania Oliveros, MD[c], Faisal Shamshad, MD[d],
Ana I. Flores, MD[e], Salomon Cohen, MD[f],
Esther Falcão, MD[g]

KEYWORDS

• STEMI • Thrombectomy • Left ventricular assist device

The pathophysiology of acute myocardial infarction (AMI) has been well studied, and it has been related to underlying atherosclerosis with superimposed acute thrombotic occlusion of an epicardial coronary artery.[1] The benefit of early revascularization in ST-elevation myocardial infarction (STEMI) is well established, resulting in smaller infarcts and less acute and long-term clinical events, including recurrent myocardial infarction (MI) and death.[2,3] The ultimate goal of revascularization should be to establish reperfusion as quickly as possible.[4,5] Primary angioplasty is superior to thrombolysis and has become the preferred revascularization strategy and standard of care in centers and communities in which it is available.[3] Percutaneous coronary angioplasty with stenting has similar mortality and repeat infarction rates at 30 days and 1 year to percutaneous balloon angioplasty alone, but it has superior long-term results with less restenosis and need for target lesion revascularization.[2–4]

Percutaneous coronary intervention (PCI) for AMI involves a unique subset of patients and presents particular challenges in dealing with STEMI interventions.[4,5] Some of the special challenges in STEMI interventions include the management of thrombus burden, hemodynamic instability, and cardiogenic shock, and the long-term preservation and salvage of the myocardium and myocardial function.

Thrombus is the sine qua non of AMI, and, as such, one of the challenges of STEMI interventions is dealing with this thrombus burden. Evidence of distal embolization is seen as often as 15% of the time during primary PCI (PPCI). No-reflow, similar to distal embolization, is an adverse prognostic marker after percutaneous coronary intervention. Distal embolization and no-reflow are associated with less angiographic success (70% vs 90%); reduced myocardial blush and ST-segment resolution (STR) after PCI; larger enzymatic infarct size; lower left ventricular ejection fraction (LVEF) at discharge (42% vs 51%); and higher long-term mortality (44% vs 9%).[6] Distal embolization is related to reduced myocardial reperfusion, more extensive myocardial damage, and a poor prognosis. Although angioplasty and stenting are effective in reestablishing flow, the need for adjunctive

[a] University of Miami – Miller School of Medicine, Mercy Medical Center, 55 Pinta Road, Miami, FL 33133, USA
[b] Cardiovascular Division, Miller School of Medicine, University of Miami, Room 1129, Clinical Research Building, 1120 NW 14th Street, Miami, FL 33136, USA
[c] School of Medicine, Central University of Venezuela, Los Naranjos, Avenue Sur 7 Qta Gabriela, Caracas, Venezuela
[d] Columbia University Division of Cardiology at Mount Sinai Medical Center, 20 Berkshire Way, East Brunswick, NJ 08816, USA
[e] School of Medicine, Universidad Autonoma de Guadalajara, Serdan # 640 Col Esterito 23020, La Paz, B.C.S, Mexico
[f] School of Medicine, Universidad Anáhuac, Lomas Country Ave Club de Golf # 3 Torre A - 1501, Huixquilucan, Edo Mexico 52787, Mexico
[g] Federal University of Ceara, Rua torquato Aguiar # 55-1600 – Meireles, Fortaleza, Ceara 60115010, Brazil
* Corresponding author.
E-mail address: mehtas@bellsouth.net (S. Mehta).

Cardiol Clin 28 (2010) 107–125
doi:10.1016/j.ccl.2009.09.005
0733-8651/09/$ – see front matter © 2010 Elsevier Inc. All rights reserved.

interventions to prevent or treat distal embolization and no-reflow is recognized.[6] Pharmacologic strategies, including anticoagulation and antiplatelet therapy, such as aspirin, clopidogrel, and glycoprotein IIb/IIIa inhibitors, are critical. Adjunctive mechanical devices and pharmacotherapy at the time of PCI can potentially decrease the rates of adverse events after PPCI.[7]

MECHANICAL ADJUNCTS FOR PPCI

Adjunctive mechanical devices fall into 2 categories: thrombectomy and/or aspiration catheters and distal protection wires, filters, or balloons (**Box 1** and **Fig. 1**). Overall, results of their use has demonstrated only marginal superiority over conventional PPCI in randomized clinical trials.[7,9,14,15] Although most individual trials were small, a meta-analysis of 21 randomized trials concluded that adjunctive devices showed a significantly higher thrombolysis in myocardial infarction (TIMI) 3 flow (89.4% vs 87.1%,); higher myocardial blush grade (MBG) 3 (48.8% vs 36.5%); less distal embolization (6.0% vs 9.3%); but with no observed benefit in 30-day mortality (2.5% vs 2.6%).[9]

Thrombectomy and Aspiration Catheters

There have been various published clinical trials using thrombectomy and/or aspiration catheters in patients with acute STEMI (**Table 1**). AngioJet (Possis Medical, Inc, Minneapolis, MN, USA) was one of the first thrombectomy devices available and was evaluated clinically in the AngioJet Rheolytic Thrombectomy in Patients Undergoing Primary Angioplasty for Acute Myocardial Infarction (AIMI) trial.[12,16] Although it was an effective thrombectomy tool, it demonstrated no clinical benefit and a trend toward increased infarct size. The results may be due to the complexities of the device, which may be too time-consuming to use in the urgent setting of a STEMI. The Randomized Evaluation of the Effect of Mechanical Reduction of Distal Embolization by Thrombus-Aspiration in Primary and Rescue Angioplasty (REMEDIA) trial compared thrombus aspiration with the Diver CE (Invatec, Brescia, Italy) before PCI versus conventional PPCI in STEMI.[15] There was no difference in clinical outcomes or peak creatine kinase, muscle and brain (CK-MB) elevation but a significant improvement in perfusion grades and in STR (68.0% vs 44.9% and 58.0% vs 36.7%, respectively); significant difference in the secondary endpoint of direct stenting (66% vs 24.4%); and a trend toward less distal embolization, slow flow, or no-reflow (22% vs 34.7%).

More recently, several simple, yet efficient, aspiration catheters have emerged. They have

---

Box 1
Mechanical adjunctive devices for thrombectomy or distal embolic protection

1. - Aspiration thrombectomy catheters
   a) AngioJet (Possis Medical, Inc, Minneapolis, MN, USA))
   b) Export catheter (Medtronic, Inc, Minneapolis, MN, USA)
   c) Pronto catheter (Vascular Solutions, Inc, Minneapolis, MN, USA)
   d) Rescue (Boston Scientific SCIMED, Inc, Maple Grove, MN, USA)
   e) X-sizer (eV3 Endovascular, Inc Peripheral Vascular, Plymouth; MN, USA)
2. - Distal embolic protection filters and balloons
   a) FilterWire-EZ (Boston Scientific, Santa Clara, CA, USA)
   b) GuardWire (Medtronic, Inc; Minneapolis, MN, USA)
   c) SpiderFX (eV3 Endovascular, Inc Peripheral Vascular, Plymouth, MN, USA)
   d) AngioGuard XP Filter (Cordis Corporation, Miami Lakes, FL, USA)
3. - Proximal protection devices
   a) Proxis (St Jude Medical, St Paul, MN, USA)
   b) Rinspirator System (eV3 Endovascular, Inc Peripheral Vascular, Plymouth; MN, USA)

---

a low-profile with good tractability and rely on negative pressure for aspiration, without adding significant procedural time to the intervention. The Dethrombosis to Enhance Acute Reperfusion in Myocardial Infarction (DEAR-MI) Trial enrolled 160 STEMI patients treated with aspiration catheters; it failed to demonstrate morbidity and mortality benefits, but it showed significant improvement in myocardial perfusion and STR in the aspiration cohort.[17] The Thrombectomy With Export Catheter in Infarct-Related Artery During Primary Percutaneous Coronary Intervention (EXPIRA) and EXPORT trials evaluated the Export catheter (Medtronic, Inc, Minneapolis, MN) in PPCI. Similar to DEAR-MI, these trials demonstrated improvement in surrogate markers, including myocardial perfusion grades (MBG 3) and resolution of STR. The recently published Thrombus Aspiration During Percutaneous Coronary Intervention in Acute Myocardial Infarction (TAPAS) trial is the largest randomized trial to date evaluating thrombus aspiration in PPCI for STEMI.[18] It randomized 1071 patients and demonstrated effective manual thrombus aspiration in 73% in the treatment group. There was a trend toward less major adverse cardiac events (MACE) at 30 days (risk ratio, 0.72; 95% confidence interval [CI], 0.48 to 1.08; P = .12)

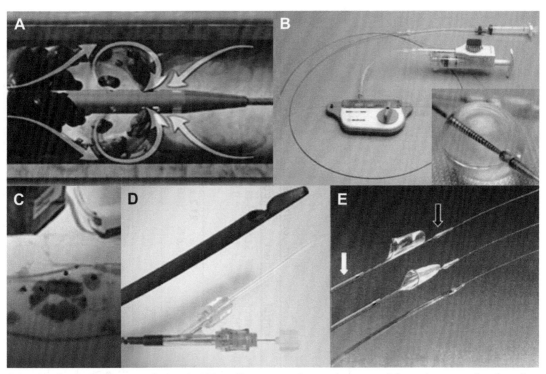

Fig. 1. Mechanical adjunctive devices in STEMI. There are various catheters used for active or passive thrombectomy including (A) the AngioJet rheolytic thrombectomy catheter, which uses an active jet of saline and aspiration to retrieve thrombus. Alternatively, distal protection devices can consist of distal balloons, such as the GuardWire (B), or distal filter devices. Aspiration of thrombus is common (C), and for cases with small thrombus load, a simple negative pressure aspiration catheter, such as the Pronto catheter (D), is one of various aspiration catheters available. As opposed to the GuardWire, distal protective filters, such as the FilterWire (E), are distal mesh nets of various materials and pore sizes that allow blood flow to continue but catch any distally embolized material.

and a benefit in surrogate markers of MPG and STR.[18]

Overall, although most trials of aspiration or thrombectomy failed to show any significant morbidity or mortality benefit, they demonstrate significant improvement in STR, improved MBG, and TIMI flow.[12,17] There was a decreased incidence of no-reflow and/or distal embolization consistently across all the trials where it was evaluated. In addition, an increased proportion of patients underwent direct stenting after thrombectomy. In the TAPAS trial, the surrogate end points of MBG and the electrocardiographic variables of reperfusion were associated with the rates of death and major adverse cardiac events. At 30 days, the rate of death in patients with an MBG of 0 or 1, 2, and 3 was 5.2%, 2.9%, and 1.0%, respectively (P = .003), and the rate of adverse events was 14.1%, 8.8%, and 4.2%, respectively (P<.001). Similarly, for patients with STR of less than 30%, 30% to 70%, and more than70%, the rates of death were 8.6%, 3.6%, and 0.7%, and

MACE events were 15.2%, 10.3%, and 4.8%, respectively.[18]

Distal and Proximal Protection Devices

For thrombotic, saphenous vein graft (SVG) interventions, distal protection demonstrates improved clinical outcomes with a reduction in the rate of no-reflow. However, results of distal embolic protection for AMI (**Table 2**) have been variable. The large multicenter, randomized Enhanced Myocardial Efficacy and Recovery by Aspiration of Liberated Debris (EMERALD) Trial demonstrated no significant improvements in the primary end points of myocardial reperfusion or infarct size with the use of the distal balloon occlusion and aspiration system, GuardWire, despite the removal of visible debris in a high proportion of patients (73%).[19] The Drug Elution and Distal Protection in ST-Elevation Myocardial Infarction (DEDICATION) trial randomized 626 patients to distal protection using a filter wire (FilterWire-EZ), or a SpiderFX protection

Table 1
Randomized controlled trials of aspiration and thrombectomy catheters in STEMI

Device	N	TIMI Flow Post-PCI Treat	Control	MBG Treat	Control	STR Treat	Control	MACE Treat	Control	Infarct Size/EF Treat	Control	No-Reflow Treat	Control	Distal Emboli Treat	Control
Napodano et al[8] X-sizer	92	93.5%	97.7%	71.70%	36.90%	82.60%	52.20%	Death:6.5% CHF:10.9% MI: 2.2% stroke 0	Death:6.5% CHF:21.7% MI: 2.2% Stroke 0	EF: 51.0 ± 7.7	EF: 48.7 ± 0.9	2.2%	10.8%	4.3%	15.2%
Antoniucci et al[9] AngioJet	100	18.2 ± 7.7	22.5 ± 11	—	—	90%	72%	Death:0 MI:0 CVA:2%	Death:0 MI: 0 CVA: 0	13.0 ± 11.6%	21.2 ± 18.0%	—	—	—	—
X AMINE ST trial X-sizer	201	2.96 ± 0.20	2.89 ± 0.31	31.2	30.4	67.80%	52.60%	30 d: 9	30 d:7	—	—	3.0%	9.9%	2.1%	10.0%
REMEDIA Diver CE (Invatec, Brescia, Italy)	99	69%	51%	46%	24.50%	46%	24.5	Death 6% MI:4% CVA: 2%	Death: 6.2% MI: 4.1% CVA: 2.1%	—	—	8.3%	12.2%	8.0%	17.8%
Dudek et al[10] Rescue catheter	72	89%	80%	54%	38%	68%	25%	—	—	—	—	—	—	—	—
De Luca et al[11] Diver CE	78	36.8%	—	81.60%	13.1%	8.60%	55.30%	—	10.50%	—	—	—	—	—	—
AIMI AngioJet	480	91.8%	97.0%	—	—	6.70%	—	6.70%	1.70%	—	—	—	—	—	—

Trial	Catheter	N														
NON STOP	Rescue catheter	258	—	—	—	—	—	90%	72%	—	—	13.0 ± 11.6	21.2 ± 18.0	—	—	—
Beran et al[12]	X-sizer	61	90%	84%	—	—	—	2.78 ± 3.05	6.15 ± 6.32	6.10%	—	—	—	—	6.10%
DEAR-MI	Pronto catheter	148	89%	78%	88%	44%	—	68%	50%	0	—	15	3%	15%	5%	19%	0
Kaltoft et al[13]	Rescue catheter	215	—	—	—	—	44%	37%	2%	2%	15	7.5	—	—	—
VAMPIRE	TVAC	355	87.5%	80.6%	46%	20.5%	40%	39%	14.0%	21.0%	EF: 57.4%	EF: 56.8%	—	3.1%
EXPORT	Export catheter	250	82%	76.90%	73.5	64.8	35.8	25.4	5.8	4.7	—	3.3	10.1	9.3	16.8
EXPIRA	Export catheter	175	100	97.4	70.3	28.7	80	37.5	10.3	4.5	—	NR	NR	NR
TAPAS	Export catheter	1071	86	82.5	82.9	73.7	56.6	44.2	6.8	9.4	—	—	—	—

Various thrombectomy and aspiration catheters have been studied in the setting of STEMI. Most trials were too small to detect a benefit in morbidity, mortality, or MACE. Instead the primary endpoints were various parameters and surrogate markers of reperfusion, including TIMI myocardial flow postangioplasty, MBG, resolution of ST-segment elevation, or infarct size, as determined by EF, myocardial SPECT perfusion imaging, or enzymatic infarct size. The primary endpoints are *italicized* and values in **bold** reached statistical significance with $p < 0.05$. (*Adapted from* Mehta S. Textbook of STEMI interventions. Miami (FL): HMP Communications; 2008 p. 126–7; with permission).

Abbreviations: AIMI, AngioJet Rheolytic Thrombectomy in Patients Undergoing Primary Angioplasty for Acute Myocardial Infarction; CVA, cerebrovascular accident; CHF, chronic heart failure; DEAR-MI, Dethrombosis to Enhance Acute Reperfusion in Myocardial Infarction; EF, ejection fraction; EXPIRA, Thrombectomy With Export Catheter in Infarct-Related Artery During Primary Percutaneous Coronary Intervention; MACE, major adverse cardiac events; MI, myocardial infarction; REMEDIA, Randomized Evaluation of the Effect of Mechanical Reduction of Distal Embolization by Thrombus-Aspiration in Primary and Rescue Angioplasty; SPECT, single photon emission computed tomography; TAPAS, Thrombus Aspiration During Percutaneous Coronary Intervention in Acute Myocardial Infarction Study; TVAC, TransVascular Aspiration Catheter (TVAC; Nipro, Osaka, Japan); VAMPIRE, vacuum aspiration thrombus removal; X-AMINE, X-sizer in AMI for negligible embolization and optimal ST resolution.

Table 2
Randomized controlled trials of distal protection devices in STEMI

Trial	Device	n	TIMI-3 Flow Post-PCI		MBG 3		STR		MACE		Infarct Size/EF		No-Reflow		Distal Emboli	
			Treat	Control	Treat	Control	Treat	Control	Treat	Control	Treat	Control	Treat	Control	Treat	Control
EMERALD	GuardWire	501	—	—	60.1%	52.7%	62.2%	60.6%	—	—	SPECT: 17.1%	SPECT: 14.3%	—	—	—	—
PROMISE	FilterWire	200	—	—	31.2	30.4	67.80%	52.60%	—	—	—	—	3.0%	9.9%	**2.1%**	**10.0%**
DIPLOMAT	AngioGuard	60	—	—	—	—	80%	73%	3.3%	8%	—	—	—	—	—	—
PREPARE	Proxis	284	93%	87%	81%	83%	81%	74%	4%	7%	—	—	—	—	10%	14%
DEDICATION	FilterWire or SpiderFX	626	**95%**	**85%**	—	—	76%	72%	5.4%	3.2%	WMI: 1.7 Trop: 4.8	WMI: 1.7 Trop: 5	—	—	—	—

Most trials of distal protection devices in the setting of STEMI failed to demonstrate a benefit for distal protection versus conventional PPCI in STEMI. These trials evaluated various surrogate markers as primary endpoints, including MBG and resolution of ST-segment elevation. The primary endpoints are *italicized* and values in **bold** reached statistical significance with p<.05.

Abbreviations: DEDICATION, Drug Elution and Distal Protection in ST-Elevation Myocardial Infarction; DIPLOMAT, Distal Protection Combined With PTCA in AMI Patients; EMERALD, Enhanced Myocardial Efficacy and Recovery by Aspiration of Liberated Debris; PREPARE, Proximal Embolic Protection in AMI and Resolution of ST-elevation; PROMISE, PCI Treatment of Myocardial Infarction for Salvage of Endangered Myocardium; PTCA, percutaneous transluminal coronary angioplasty; Trop, troponin; WMI, wall motion index.

device, versus standard PPCI without distal protection.[20] It found no significant difference in the primary endpoint of STR (76% vs 72%, P = .29) or in cardiac biomarker elevation or left ventricular (LV) wall motion index, and found a higher major adverse cardiac and cerebrovascular event rate (5.4% vs 3.2%, P = .17) with distal protection.[20]

As compared with the distal protection devices, the Proxis device is a catheter that occludes proximal blood flow. The PCI is performed with occlusive flow, after which aspiration theoretically removes any embolic debris and improves flow. In the setting of STEMI, use of the Proxis device demonstrated an initial benefit in STR; however, this benefit was not maintained over time with a late catch-up in the control group.

In their entirety, the results of the current trials evaluating the effect of distal and or proximal protection in PPCI for STEMI suggest that routine use of embolic protection devices cannot be advocated during PCI treatment of patients with STEMI.[19,20]

Laser Therapy

Excimer laser coronary angioplasty (ELCA) has been evaluated for the treatment of coronary atherosclerosis in multiple scenarios, including in-stent restenosis, chronic occlusions, and AMI. In AMI, ELCA has proven safe and effective in debulking and dissolving thrombotic lesions in STEMI, particularly lesions with extensive thrombus burden.[21]

Recommended Use of Aspiration, Thrombectomy, and Other Specialty Catheters in STEMI

Floating thrombus is observed in about a quarter of patients with AMI at angiography, with angiographic signs of high thrombus burden present from 32% to 63% of patients. Patients with occluded arteries and higher thrombus grades seem to benefit most from aspiration and atherectomy techniques to debulk lesions before angioplasty and stenting.[22] An objective quantification of thrombus load has been previously proposed. Angiographic markers of high thrombus/embolic burden include a complete vessel occlusion with a cut-off pattern, an angiographic thrombus with the greatest linear dimension more than 3 times the reference luminal diameter, a persistent stasis of contrast medium distal to the obstruction, and a reference luminal diameter of 4.0 mm or more. The rate of no-reflow is significantly increased in the presence of a cut-off sign or large angiographic thrombus (52%) versus the absence of

either sign (10% and 4%, respectively). IVUS evidence of a floating thrombus is also a significant predictor of distal embolization.[22] The thrombus burden as assessed on the initial angiogram or by intravascular ultrasonography (IVUS) should guide the subsequent interventional strategy, reviewed in **Fig. 2**. Thrombus burden is dynamic and should be reassessed continuously.

As illustrated in the Single Individual Community Experience Registry for Primary PCI (SINCERE) database in **Fig. 2**, good procedural and clinical success was obtained using a thrombus-guided interventional strategy.[22] Based on this strategy, if the extent of thrombus is small (thrombus grade 0–1), direct angioplasty and stenting may be sufficient. This is demonstrated in the example shown in **Fig. 3**. Conversely, as shown in **Fig. 4**, if more significant thrombus burden is present (thrombus grade 2–3), initial aspiration with an aspiration catheter is usually prudent; apart from decreasing distal embolization and no-reflow, it may also facilitate subsequent stenting. Although most aspiration catheters are similar in form and function, there are a few practical tips regarding their use, enumerated in **Box 2**. If a very large thrombus burden is present (thrombus grade 4–5), as demonstrated in **Fig. 5**, aspiration may be insufficient and rheolytic thrombectomy with an AngioJet catheter may be warranted.[22] In such procedures with voluminous thrombus, the authors believe that the AngioJet is a superb device for debulking these lesions.[22] The newer AngioJet catheters have smaller profiles and are more user-friendly.[22] Rheolytic thrombectomy is most effective with a fresh clot whereas organized thrombus is more resistant to debulking. Although not yet validated, the authors believe that a strategy to guide adjunctive therapy for STEMI based on thrombus burden, as depicted in **Fig. 2** and **Table 3**, makes good clinical and practical sense.

INTRACORONARY PHARMACOTHERAPY

Adjunctive pharmacologic therapy is crucial for the success of PPCI. Pharmacotherapy starts at the initial patient encounter, when the patient should initially receive aspirin, and it continues in the ER, catheterization laboratory, and in the postprocedure period.[23] Adjunct systemic treatment, including anticoagulant and antiplatelet treatment is also vital. However, for conciseness, this article is confined to direct local intracoronary (IC) therapies delivered in the catheterization laboratory.

Slow or no-reflow phenomenon continues to be a serious complication after PPCI and results in poor short- and long-term outcomes.[24] Although

Grade	Thrombus Definition	Angiographic Examples	Mehta Classification	Technical Tips of Use	
				Aspiration Catheter	Angio Jet
0	No cine angiographic characteristics of thrombus present		Direct Stent +/- Pre dilatation	- Most effective with fresh clot; organized thrombus is more resistant to debulking.	- Can be used from the radial route. Although LAD and some LCX may not need a TPM, I place TPM's in all Angiojet procedures.
1	Possible thrombus present. Angiography demonstrates reduced contrast density, haziness, irregular lesion contour or a smooth convex 'meniscus' at the site of total occlusion suggestive but not diagnostic of thrombus	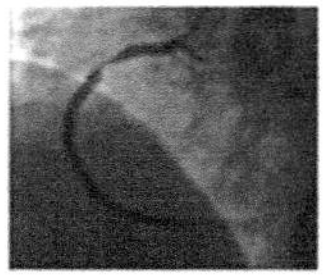 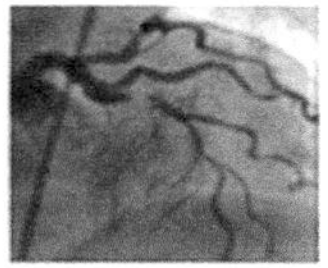	Direct Stent +/- Pre dilatation	- Different profiles, push-ability, tractability and aspiration rates. - All are 6F-compatable - It is useful to stock and be familiar with the use of at least one.	- Often, multiple passes will be required. Try to pause after every 2-3 passes to enable hemodynamics to be restored, to optimize guide wire and guiding catheter support and to evaluate the results.
2	Thrombus present-small size: Definite thrombus with greatest dimensions less than or equal to ½ vessel diameter	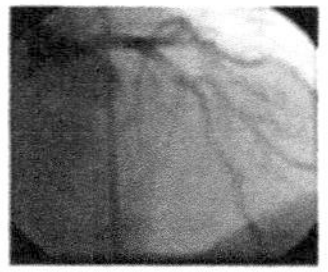 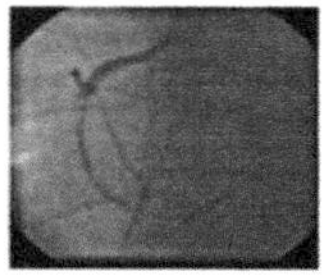	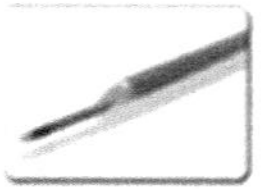 Aspiration thrombectomy	- Flush catheter lumen well before use as it facilitates better tracking over the wire.	- Often, just the first passage will restore adequate flow

Fig. 2. Strategy based on thrombus grade for management of the STEMI lesion: Mehta classification.

3	Thrombus present- moderate size: Definite thrombus but with greatest linear dimension greater than ½ but less than 2 vessel diameters	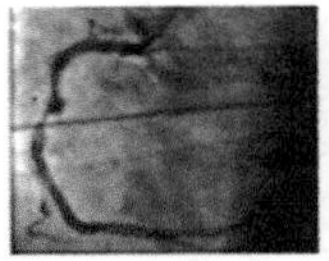 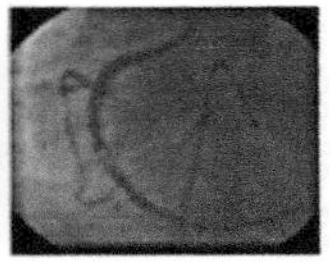	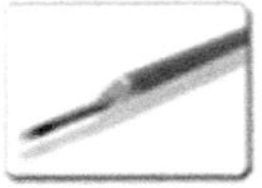 Aspiration thrombectomy	- Avoid kinking the catheter – advance slowly over the initial, softer portion of the catheter. - Monitor distal tip of the guide wire as the aspiration catheter is advanced – it is not uncommon for the guide wire to advance during this maneuver - Advance the aspiration catheter through the entire length of occlusive disease.	-Resistant and stubborn thrombus will require more distal advancement that must be done more carefully. - Avoid advancing in severe tortuousity and in vessels <2mm -Since the Angiojet is used for large thrombus burden and high thrombus grade, consider Abciximab as adjunctive therapy
4	Thrombus present- large size: As in Grade 3 but with the largest dimension greater than or equal to 2 vessel diameters	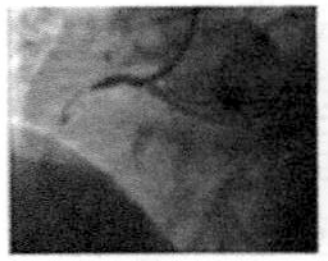 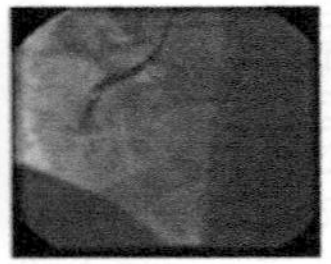	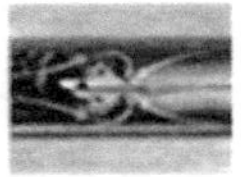 Angio Jet		
5	Total occlusion	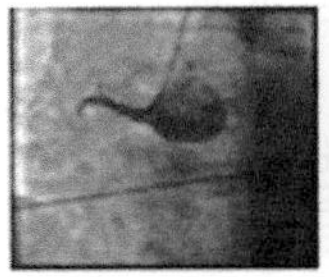 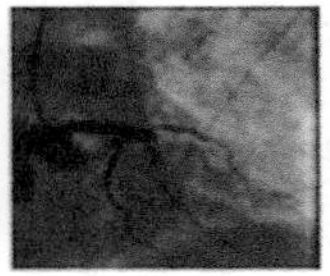	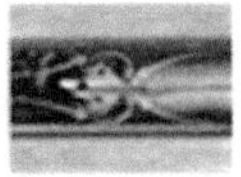 Angio Jet		

Fig. 2. (continued)

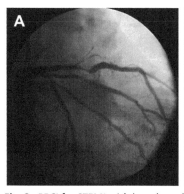 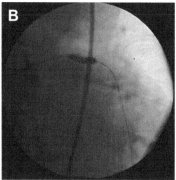 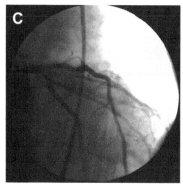

Fig. 3. PPCI for STEMI with low thrombus burden. Lesions with low-grade thrombus can be treated safely without more complex catheters or procedures. The angiograms shown here are from a patient who presented with an acute anterior wall ST-elevation MI. The initial angiogram demonstrated a critical mid-LAD culprit lesion with a low grade 0–1 thrombus burden (A). The lesion was stented directly with a 3.5 mm drug-eluting stent (B), with a door-to-balloon time of 56 minutes and final angiography demonstrating TIMI 3 flow (C). LAD, left anterior descending coronary artery.

its precise mechanisms remains unclear, there is burgeoning evidence suggesting that no-reflow is related to microcirculatory dysfunction that occurs at the level of the resistance arterioles. This occurs despite the use of aspiration catheters, with less than 50% of patients achieving MBG greater than 2 and STR greater than 70%. The incidence of distal embolization, slow-flow, or no-reflow remains as high as 20% in some cases.[22,24] Cannulating the infarct-related artery with the guide catheter permits IC delivery of drugs to alter vascular tone, reestablishes microvascular perfusion, limits reperfusion injury, diminishes final infarct size, and ultimately improves clinical outcomes.[23–25] Despite higher local concentrations with direct IC versus intravenous (IV) delivery, drug delivery via the guide catheter may not be adequate if epicardial coronary flow is inadequate. Mechanisms of direct IC drug delivery include

infusion via a distal over-the-wire balloon, infusion catheters, or infusion balloons.[23–25] The medications administered can be broadly divided into metabolic, vasodilators, and anticoagulants/antiplatelet therapies.[22] Vasodilators that have been tried include nitroprusside, adenosine, diltiazem, verapamil, nicardipine, and clevidipine.[22–25] IC delivery may also be used for abciximab, to obtain higher local concentrations and glycoprotein IIb/IIIa inhibition (**Table 4**).[26]

Adenosine

Reperfusion injury may play a significant role in myocardial injury after PPCI.[23] Adenosine has been studied as a cardio-protective agent, because it may have a role in ischemic preconditioning and has been shown to replenish high-energy phosphate, inhibit oxygen free radical

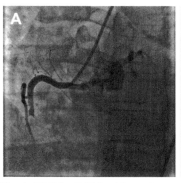 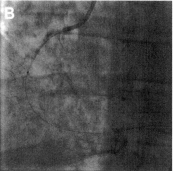 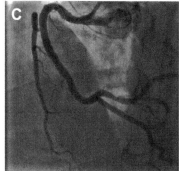

Fig. 4. PPCI for STEMI with moderate thrombus burden. Lesions with moderate-grade thrombus are best treated with aspiration thrombectomy devices before definitive treatment and stenting. This angiogram shows a moderate thrombus (grade 3) in a patient with ST-elevation in leads DII-III. The first angiogram demonstrates a mid-RCA culprit lesion with a moderate-grade thrombus (A). The lesion was treated with an aspiration catheter (B) followed by angioplasty and stenting with a 4.0 mm bare-metal stent with a door-to-balloon time of 61 minutes with great results (C). RCA, right coronary artery.

Box 2
Practical tips for the use of aspiration catheters

1. Flush catheter lumen well before use to facilitate better tracking over the wire
2. Slowly advance the initial portion to avoid kinking the catheter
3. Monitor the distal tip with advancement of the aspiration catheter
4. Advance the aspiration catheter through the entire length of occlusive disease
5. Maintain aspiration for a longer duration in the dense portion of the thrombus
6. Maintain aspiration rate (ie, negative pressure) during advancement and withdrawal of the catheter
7. Watch the guide catheter as the aspiration catheter is withdrawn from the artery
   a. If the guide catheter gets sucked in, it may cause trauma to a proximal vessel (eg, left main)
   b. Consider releasing the negative pressure while withdrawing the catheter
8. If no suction of blood, despite appropriate preparation and lesion selection
   a. the aspiration lumen may be plugged with thrombus
   b. withdraw the catheter under negative pressure, flush the catheter, and repeat
9. Additional passes may be needed for bulky thrombus
10. If thrombus burden is unchanged after 2 passes with the appropriate device, consider switch to a more aggressive thrombectomy device (ie, AngioJet or laser)

---

formation, inhibit neutrophil activity, and improve microvascular function. Animal models of ischemia and acute injury previously suggested a beneficial role for adenosine in reducing ischemic injury and infarct size. However, the results of human studies have been equivocal. In the initial Acute Myocardial Infarction Study of Adenosine (AMISTAD) trial of adenosine (administered as a 3-hour IV infusion at 70 mcg/kg/min) as an adjunct to thrombolysis for AMI, the subset of patients with large anterior MI demonstrated a benefit with smaller infarct size at 5–12 days by single photon emission computed tomography (SPECT) imaging. In the larger 2118-patient follow-up AMISTAD II study, although the median infarct size was diminished 57% with 70 mcg/kg/min adenosine infusion, there was no improvement in clinical outcomes in patients with STEMI undergoing reperfusion therapy.[23]

Nitroglycerin

Nitric oxide is a potent vasodilator in the resistance arteriolar circulation and plays a significant role in coronary blood flow through the microcirculation. Nitroglycerin (NTG) is a nitric oxide donor, and functions as a potent venodilator and arterial vasodilator. As such, NTG is often administered IC for vasodilatory effects. In patients with slow or no-reflow, after elective PCI and PPCI, IC NTG has been used to improve epicardial and microvascular perfusion with mixed results. To derive nitric oxide, NTG has to be metabolized by the vascular wall. Unlike large nonresistance vessels, the smaller resistance arterioles are unable to metabolize NTG into nitric oxide. Therefore, the effect of NTG on the microvascular circulation and its role in the treatment of no-reflow, may be limited.[22,23]

Nitroprusside

Unlike NTG, nitroprusside serves as a direct donor of nitric oxide without requiring intracellular metabolism. Selective IC nitroprusside administration is safe, generally well-tolerated, and superior to NTG for improving final epicardial blood flow

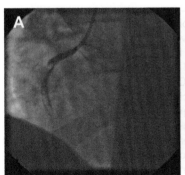
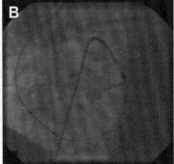
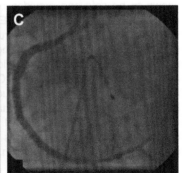

Fig. 5. PPCI for STEMI with large thrombus burden. Lesions with high-grade thrombus may require some thrombectomy before definitive treatment and stenting. The initial angiogram of this patient, who presented with an acute inferior wall ST-elevation MI, demonstrated a large amount of thrombus (grade 3–4) (*A*). An AngioJet catheter (*B*) was initially used for rheolytic thrombectomy and after angioplasty and stenting, the final angiographic result was excellent (*C*).

Table 3
Procedural characteristics from SINCERE database (n = 420)

Procedural Characteristics	N (%)
Stenting	394 (94.4%)
PTCA/thrombectomy only	26 (5.6%)
Direct stenting	122 (29%)
Initial thrombectomy/aspiration	298 (71%)
Devices used	
Aspiration catheters	184 (44.6%)
Export	151/232 (64.6%)
QuickCat (Kensey Nash Corporation, Exton, PA)	42/232 (18.2%)
Pronto	37 (16.2%)
AngioJet	66 (15.7%)
Closure device	344 (82.5%)
IC nitroprusside	298 (71.3%)
Procedural results	
Procedure success rate	96.6%
TIMI 3 Flow	399 (95%)
MBG 3	352 (84%)
Sub-acute stent thrombosis	2 (0.47%)
In-hospital mortality	14 (3.4%)

The SINCERE database is an ongoing, prospectively collected database of all PPCI for STEMI performed by a single, experienced, interventional cardiologist, starting from January of 2005 to September 2009, it includes 441 STEMI interventions. Review of the procedural characteristics demonstrates a significant use of adjunctive treatments, including thrombectomy and aspiration catheters, and IC nitroprusside. Overall there is a high procedure success rate with blush grade 3 achieved in 84% of patients.

Abbreviations: IC, intracoronary; PTCA, percutaneous transluminal coronary angioplasty; SINCERE, single individual community experience registry.

and microvascular circulation in patients with AMI undergoing PPCI.[25] If administered before balloon angioplasty, IC nitroprusside may decrease rates of no-reflow, increase myocardial blush scores, and shorten procedure times. In cases of impaired flow during coronary interventions , combination therapy of adenosine and nitroprusside has been shown to be safe and provides better improvement in coronary flow and MACE as compared with IC adenosine alone. IC nitroprusside at doses of 50 to 200 μg has shown promising results for the reduction and treatment of no-reflow when given alone or with IC adenosine.[22,25] Compared with adenosine, IC nitroprusside produces an equivalent but more prolonged coronary hyperemic response, and it improves clinical outcomes at 6 months as reflected by reductions in recurrent MI and target vessel revascularization.[25]

Calcium Channel Blockers

IC verapamil has been shown to prevent no-reflow in some patients. IC nicardipine was effective in the treatment of prophylactic no-reflow and

non–Q-wave myocardial infarction during elective SVG graft intervention. Although small trials suggest that there may be a role for prophylactic IC calcium channel blockers, there is no randomized trial to support this strategy.

Abciximab

Systemic inhibition of glycoprotein IIb/IIIa receptors with intravenous abciximab administration is an established therapy to improve coronary microcirculation and reduce MACE in AMI, as an adjunct to a planned PCI.[26,33] IC abciximab bolus administration is associated with high local concentrations and a high degree of platelet inhibition, which may improve dissolution of thrombi and myocardial microcirculation and reduce no-reflow and infarct size. In a randomized trial of IC bolus administration of abciximab in PPCI, 154 patients were randomized to IC abciximab versus standard intravenous abciximab.[31] IC abciximab was superior to standard intravenous treatment with smaller infarct size, extent of microvascular obstruction, and perfusion. There was also a trend toward

Table 4
Clinical trials demonstrating use of intracoronary drugs for STEMI

Trial	Medication	N	Treatment Protocol vs Control	TIMI-3 Flow Post-PCI		MBG 3		STR		MACE		Infarct Size		No-Reflow	
				Treat	Control	Treat	Control	Treat	Control	Treat	Control	Treat	Control	Treat	Control
Marzilli et al[27]	Adenosine	54	IC adenosine vs. saline	100%	70%	—	—	—	—	18%	48%	—	—	4%	26%
Claeys et al[28]	Adenosine	279	IC adenosine	89%	87%	—	—	81%	65%	4%	6.5%	—	—	—	—
AMISTAD	Adenosine	236	IV adenosine vs placebo	—	—	—	—	—	—	—	—	**15%**	**45.5%**	—	—
AMISTAD II	Adenosine	2118	IV adenosine vs placebo	—	—	—	—	—	—	**11.8**	**10.2%**	**11%**	**26%**	—	—
Hang et al[29]	Verapamil	50	IC verapamil	90%	86%	—	—	—	—	0%	6%	—	—	—	—
Amit et al[25]	Nitroprusside	98	IC nitroprusside vs placebo	86.4%	81.4%	28%	29.5%	68.9%	67.3%	6.3%	20%	—	—	—	—
Shinozaki et al[30]	Nitroprusside	120	IC nitroprusside	59%	53%	49%	33%	—	—	0%	0%	—	—	—	—
Thiele et al[31]	Abciximab	154	IC abciximab vs IV abciximab	84.4%	85.7%	72.7%	66.2%	77.8%	70%	**5.2%**	**15.6%**	**15.1%**	**23.4%**	12%	35%
Bellandi et al[32]	Abciximab	45	IC abciximab vs IV abciximab	100%	87%	95.5%	65.2%	86.4%	52.2%	—	—	**13.5%**	**21.4%**	—	—

Trials of adjunctive pharmacotherapy for STEMI. In the AMISTAD and AMISTAD II trials, adenosine was given as a 3-hour infusion after thrombolysis. In small studies, IC abciximab demonstrated an additional benefit over IV abciximab in infarct size reduction. Infarct size was measured by myocardial SPECT perfusion imaging, enzymatic infarct size, or by % of myocardium assessed by MRI as in the Leipzig Trial. The primary endpoints are *italicized* and values in **bold** reached statistical significance with p <0.05.
Abbreviations: AMISTAD, Acute Myocardial Infarction Study of Adenosine; IV, intravenous.

a lower rate of MACE after IC abciximab (5.2% vs 15.6%; $P = .06$; relative risk, 0.33; 95% CI, 0.09 to 1.05).[31]

Recommended Use of IC Medications in STEMI

Particular subgroups of STEMI patients may benefit more from IC vasodilators and antiplatelet agents. These include patients with large anterior MI, large thrombus burden, residual thrombus, side-branch involvement, and those that demonstrate slow or no-reflow. The authors prefer to use IC nitroprusside in a method described in **Box 3**. With the use of IC vasodilators, caution should be exercised, because systemic effects, such as hypotension or heart block may be observed.[22] Although drops in blood pressure are generally transient and self-limited, in the case of severe hypotension, phenylephrine (Neo-synephrine) can be administered intravenously. Adenosine may be particularly useful for patients with limited hemodynamic reserve. IC adenosine can cause transient heart block. Having the patient cough or perform Valsalva maneuvers may be beneficial, and a prophylactic temporary pacemaker is rarely needed.

HEMODYNAMIC SUPPORT FOR SHOCK IN STEMI

Cardiogenic shock (CS), although infrequent, is present in approximately 15% of patients presenting with AMI and carries a poor prognosis.[25] The clinical deterioration of patients with AMI and CS has been described as a downward spiral in which progressively decreased coronary blood flow causes a decrease in cardiac output and resultant

---

Box 3
Use of IC nitroprusside for STEMI interventions

1. Ensure that the stent has been well deployed
2. Remove the guide wire that, itself, is a nidus from thrombus
3. Systolic BP should be greater than 100 at least, but the higher the better
4. Nitroprusside prepared in a dose of 100 ug/ml
5. Use in an incremental bolus of 50 ug, as high as the patient tolerates—mean dose used in SINCERE database was 200 ug
6. For hypotension, the authors use 100 to 200 ug bolus of phenylephrine (Neo-synephrine)
7. You can expect blush grade improvement by one grade on the average
8. To demonstrate blush, use the left anterior oblique view for the left coronary artery and use right anterior oblique, for the right coronary artery.

---

hypotension with progressively more cardiac ischemia and dysfunction, eventually resulting in left ventricular failure and death. A mortality rate up to 60% has been reported in medically stabilized patients in the SHOCK trial registry.[34] Early reperfusion therapy is the standard of care for patients presenting with acute STEMI associated with CS, and it is preferably achieved by PPCI. Early revascularization provides a survival benefit at 6 months; however, CS complicating AMI remains the leading cause of death, with mortality rates remaining as high as 50%.[35]

Intra-aortic Balloon Pump

Intra-aortic counter pulsation therapy with an intra-aortic balloon pump (IABP) reduces afterload and may be effective in improving reperfusion in high-risk infarct patients treated with primary angioplasty.[34–36] Despite theoretical benefits, routine use of IABP after primary angioplasty has not been demonstrated to improve myocardial salvage or clinical outcomes in high-risk infarct patients without CS. A meta-analysis by Sjauw and colleagues[35] of 7 randomized trials of IABP, which included thrombolysis, PPCI, or no reperfusion therapy and involved 1009 patients, corroborated the findings of these individual studies with no significant benefit on 30-day survival or on left ventricular ejection fraction. Moreover, for high-risk patients with STEMI, IABP was associated with an increase in stroke incidence and bleeding. Therefore, given the lack of a demonstrable benefits, IABP should be reserved for patients with severe hemodynamic compromise and in CS (in the SHOCK trial, 86% of patients were treated with an IABP). Currently, IABP therapy in STEMI is mainly indicated as an adjunctive therapy to revascularization in CS that is not quickly reversed by pharmacological therapy, and it is a class IB recommendation in the current American College of Cardiology (ACC)/American Heart Association (AHA) guidelines.[35]

Given the lack of randomized trials, Sjauw and colleagues performed a second meta-analysis of all studies comparing IABP therapy with no IABP therapy in STEMI complicated by CS. This analysis examined 9 cohort studies of patients with STEMI and CS (n = 10,529). In patients treated with thrombolysis, IABP was associated with an 18% decrease in 30-day mortality; however, in patients treated with PPCI, IABP was associated with a 6% increase in 30-day mortality.[35] Another retrospective study of 23,180 patients from the National Registry of Myocardial Infarction (NRMI) 2 evaluated patients with AMI complicated by CS. The overall mortality among patients with CS was

70%, with an extraordinarily high 78% mortality rate among patients who received no reperfusion therapy. IABP was used in 31% of the cohort, and, when augmenting thrombolytic therapy, resulted in a significant reduction in mortality to 49% with an odds ratio (OR) of 0.82, (95% CI 0.72–0.93). Mortality among patients who had AMI with CS and underwent primary percutaneous transluminal coronary angioplasty was 42%. IABP in this cohort was not associated with a reduction in mortality, and, in fact, was associated with higher in-hospital mortality, 47% (OR 1.26, 95% CI 1.07–1.50).[35]

Percutaneous LV Assist Devices

Surgically implantable LV assist devices (LVADs) have been shown to provide more effective circulatory support.[37–39] However, in the setting of STEMI complicated by CS, the applicability of this therapy is limited. Therefore, the development of percutaneous LVADs has been of great interest. More recently, the TandemHeart (CardiacAssist, Inc, Pittsburgh, PA, USA)and the Impella 2.5LP and the Impella 5.0LP (Abiomed, Inc, Danvers, MA, USA) have been introduced (**Fig. 6**).

TandemHeart

The TandemHeart percutaneous ventricular assist device (pVAD) is an extracorporeal, dual-chambered, and centrifugal, continuous-flow pump, and it has 2 large cannulas designed as a left atrial to femoral artery bypass system for short-term mechanical LV support. In small trials comparing IABP with TandemHeart in STEMI patients with CS, hemodynamic parameters improved significantly in patients who were supported by the Tandem Heart pVAD, albeit with a high complication rate. Complications observed included tamponade, major bleeding, critical limb ischemia, sepsis, and arrhythmias. The most important factors contributing to these complications are likely to be the highly invasive and complex insertion procedure and the extracorporeal support method, combined with full high anticoagulation. Finally, although the TandemHeart device is capable of delivering effective mechanical LV and circulatory support, the complexity of the device and its high complication rate may impede its widespread use. Nevertheless, it may be useful in specific circumstances.[22,36–38]

Impella

The Impella LP2.5 and the Impella LP5.0 are catheter-mounted, micro axial blood pumps that are positioned across the aortic valve and designed for short-term LV support.[37] The Impella LP2.5 can provide up to 2.5 L/min of cardiac output and can be positioned percutaneously via a 13 French arterial sheath. The Impella LP5.0 is more effective in LV unloading and hemodynamic support, but it requires surgical implantation. The PROTECT I trial demonstrated the feasibility of minimally invasive circulatory support using the Impella 2.5 system in 20 patients with significant

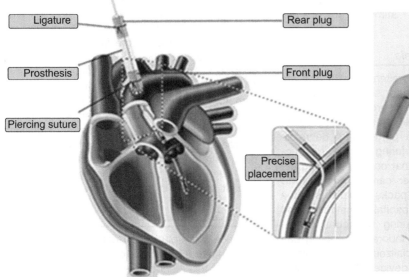
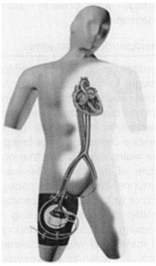

Fig. 6. LV assist device. The Impella ventricular device is shown on the left and the Tandem Heart ventricular device is shown on the right.

comorbidities and reduced LV systolic function, undergoing high-risk PCI.[39] The MACH 2 trial demonstrated that prolonged Impella 2.5LP support as an adjunctive therapy to PPCI (n = 10) in patients with large anterior STEMI resulted in an improvement in mean LVEF. The ISAR-SHOCK trial randomized 26 patients presenting with STEMI and CS to PPCI with Impella LP2.5 support or IABP therapy. Impella LP2.5 was safe and feasible, increased cardiac output, and reduced blood lactate levels, although overall 30-day mortality remained high (46%) in both groups.[36] The left ventricular unloading decreases LV pressures and myocardial wall stress, improves endocardial perfusion, and may ultimately improve long-term LV remodeling, recovery of LV function, and clinical outcomes, particularly in large anterior wall MI, associated with cardiogenic shock.[36,37] Currently, the Impella versus IABP reduces infarct size (IMPRESS) in STEMI trial is underway and will compare mechanical support using IABP versus Impella LP2.5 in STEMI patients with early signs of CS.

OTHER MODALITIES AND FUTURE THERAPIES FOR INFARCT SIZE MODIFICATION AND MYOCARDIAL REGENERATION

Long-term outcomes after PPCI are strongly influenced by the preservation of LV myocardium and function. LVEF is the strongest clinical predictor of subsequent clinical events. Although the benefit of early reperfusion is clear, realistically, there is a limit to how quickly this can be accomplished. Therefore, there are various strategies that have been developed and tested to reduce myocardial damage and possibly stimulate myocardial regeneration.

Therapeutic Hypothermia

A subgroup of patients presenting with AMI are brought to the hospital after suffering a cardiac arrest. In these patients, neurologic recovery is as important as cardiac reperfusion and recovery. Therapeutic hypothermia portends to decrease cerebral damage by interfering with the destructive molecular cascade that occurs following the return of circulation after cardiac arrest. EMS personnel can apply ice packs to patients in the field or at the referring hospital or institution and cooling is continued during transport. At the receiving catheterization laboratory, cooling can be maintained with specialized cooling devices, such as the Arctic Sun device (Medivance, Inc, Louisville, CO, USA), to a target core temperature of 91.4°F, which is then maintained for 24 hours. The Hypothermia after Cardiac Arrest (HACA)

study demonstrated that therapeutic hypothermia significantly improved survival and neurologic outcomes in patients with an out-of-hospital cardiac arrest due to ventricular fibrillation (VF) or ventricular tachycardia (VT). The "Cool It" MI Trial included 51 patients with pulseless electrical activity (PEA) or asystole (non-HACA criteria) and 52 patients with VF/VT (HACA criteria). Fifty percent of these patients presented with STEMI, and 40% had evidence of cardiogenic shock.[40] In the "Cool It" MI trial, the survival rate was 73% for patients meeting HACA criteria and 39% for higher-risk non-HACA criteria patients. There was an improvement in neurological outcomes in "Cool It" MI, which may be due to earlier initiation of cooling protocols and prehospital cooling. For each hour that therapeutic hypothermia was delayed, the relative risk of death increased by 25%.[40]

Supersaturated Oxygen Therapy

The TherOx SSO2 (TherOx Inc, Irvine, CA) is a catheter-based device designed to deliver supersaturated oxygen (SSO_2) therapy IC. The Acute Myocardial Infarction with Hyperoxemic Oxygen Therapy (AMIHOT) and AMIHOT-II studies evaluated the effect of SSO_2 therapy on infarct size beyond that achieved by PPCI. A total of 222 patients in the SSO_2 cohort received SSO_2 for 90 minutes, whereas the remaining 79 were in the standard therapy cohort; it demonstrated a reduction in the primary endpoint of absolute infarct size, measured by Tc-99m-sestamibi SPECT. Despite the reduction in infarct size, the rate of 30-day MACE was no different, 3.8% in both groups. There was also nonsignificant increase in mortality in the SSO_2 group, and adverse events were more frequent in the treatment group (5.4%, SSO_2 group vs 3.8%, control).[41] Among high-risk patients with anterior AMI undergoing successful PCI within 6 hours of symptom onset, infusion of SSO_2 into the myocardial infarct territory results in a significant reduction in infarct size. A clinically significant decrease in clinical endpoints has yet to be demonstrated, and FDA approval of the device has been placed on hold until such a clinical benefit is proven by further studies.

Stem Cell Therapy for AMI

Stem cells are pluripotent cells with the ability to differentiate into various cell lines that may hold promise for regeneration of viable myocardial tissue in postinfarct patients. In 13 trials, there was a variable improvement in LVEF ranging from 3.1% to 18%, with modest decrease in rates of death, reinfarction, and revascularization.[22] Adult mesenchymal stem cells (MSCs) have been demonstrated to improve ejection fraction and cardiac remodeling in patients with a prior MI. Indeed, various stem cell types including autologous, unmanipulated bone marrow mononuclear cells, purified hematopoietic stem cells (HSCs) expressing CD133 or CD34 markers, unselected peripheral blood stem cells, mesenchymal stem cells, or circulating progenitor cells have been used with moderate success. In the setting of AMI, it may be hypothesized that the ideal stem cell population should be readily available, capable of being delivered IC, have good uptake into the myocardium, and demonstrate clinical efficacy and safety.[42] The ongoing OSIRIS Phase I trial seeks to determine the safety and efficacy of 3 different dose levels of allogeneic bone-marrow–derived MSCs compared with placebo, in patients who have had an AMI. At 6 months, key safety data showed a significantly lower rate of arrhythmias in the cell-treated group. MRI data at 1 year demonstrated a progressive reduction in end systolic volume and increase in ejection fraction in the cell-treated group. Although prior trials have suggested a modest benefit with little toxicity, clinical trials are still necessary and ongoing to determine the most appropriate cell type, dose, method, and timing of delivery for the use of HSCs for recovery of myocardial function.[42,43]

SUMMARY

Excluding patients with cardiogenic shock at presentation, PPCI for AMI has decreased mortality rates to as low as 3% and 5.3% at 30 days and 1 year, respectively.[2–5] Given the improved clinical results that have been achieved with early revascularization and PPCI, it may be difficult for any one intervention to demonstrate a large absolute risk reduction of hard clinical endpoints in all-comers. However, benefits in various surrogate markers, such as LVEF, infarct size, TIMI flow, and myocardial perfusion grade, may be associated with improved overall clinical outcomes. The treatment of AMI has evolved into a multifactorial pursuit involving early revascularization, myocardial endocardial perfusion, and long-term clinical treatment.[22] In the catheterization laboratory, it is essential to develop a thrombus-driven strategy for the management of STEMI, with the provisional use of various adjunctive devices and medications to establish adequate epicardial and myocardial perfusion and to limit reperfusion injury. Hypothermic therapy may be an option for the subgroup of patients suffering from an out-of-hospital arrest, particularly if instituted early in the event.[40] LV support devices should be available and tailored to provide the necessary LV unloading and hemodynamic support in the high-risk patients.[27,28] Given the high mortality rate, the greatest strides may be possible in the future within the high-risk group of patients. Long-term regeneration of myocardium with stem cell therapy holds some promise and clinical trials are ongoing.[42,43]

REFERENCES

1. Burke AP, Virmani R. Pathophysiology of acute myocardial infarction. Med Clin North Am 2007; 91(4):553–72.
2. Grines C, Browne K, Marco J, et al. A comparison of immediate angioplasty with thrombolytic therapy for acute myocardial infarction. The Primary Angioplasty in Myocardial Infarction Study Group. N Engl J Med 1993;328(10):673–9.
3. Keeley Ellen C, Boura Judith A, Grines Cindy L. Primary angioplasty versus intravenous thrombolytic therapy for acute myocardial infarction: a quantitative review of 23 randomized trials. Lancet 2003;361: 13–20.
4. Antman EM, Anbe DT, Armstrong PW, et al. ACC/AHA guidelines for the management of patients with ST-elevation myocardial infarction: a report of the American College of Cardiology/American Heart Association Task Force on Practice Guidelines (Committee to Revise the 1999 Guidelines for the Management of patients with acute myocardial infarction). Circulation 2004;110:192–292.
5. Van de Werf F, Ardissino D, Betriu A, et al. Management of acute myocardial infarction in patients presenting with ST-segment elevation: the Task Force on the Management of Acute Myocardial Infarction of the European Society of Cardiology. Eur Heart J 2003;24:28–66.
6. Henriques JPS, Zijistra F, Ottervanger JP, et al. Incidence and clinical significance of distal embolization during primary angioplasty for AMI. Eur Heart J 2002;23:1112–7.
7. De Luca G, Suryapranata H, Stone GW, et al. Adjunctive mechanical devices to prevent distal embolization in patients undergoing mechanical revascularization for acute myocardial infarction: a meta-analysis of randomized trials. Am Heart J 2007;153(3):343–53.
8. Napodano M, Pasquetto G, Sacca S, et al. Intracoronary thrombectomy improves myocardial reperfusion in patients undergoing direct angioplasty for acute myocardial infarction. J Am Coll Cardiol 2003;42:1395–402.
9. Antoniucci D, Valenti R, Migliorini A, et al. Comparison of rheolytic thrombectomy before direct infarct

artery stenting versus direct stenting alone in patients undergoing percutaneous coronary intervention for acute myocardial infarction. Am J Cardiol 2004;93:1033–5.

10. Dudek D, Mielecki W, Legutko J, et al. Percutaneous thrombectomy with the RESCUE system in acute myocardial infarction. Kardiol Pol 2004;61: 523–33.

11. De Luca L, Sardella G, Davidson CJ, et al. Impact of intracoronary aspiration thrombectomy during primary angioplasty on left ventricular remodelling in patients with anterior ST elevation myocardial infarction. Heart 2006;92:951–7.

12. Beran G, Lang I, Schreiber W, et al. Intracoronary thrombectomy with the X-sizer catheter system improves epicardial flow and accelerates ST-segment resolution in patients with acute coronary syndrome: a prospective, randomized, controlled study. Circulation 2002;105:2355–60.

13. Kaltoft T, Bøttcher M, Nielsen SS, et al. Routine thrombectomy in percutaneous coronary intervention for acute ST-segment-elevation myocardial infarction: a randomized, controlled trial. Circulation 2006;114:40–7.

14. Lefevre T, Garcia E, Reimers B, et al. X AMINE ST Investigators. X-sizer for thrombectomy in acute myocardial infarction improves ST-segment resolution: results of the X-sizer in AMI for negligible embolization and optimal ST resolution (X AMINE ST) trial. J Am Coll Cardiol 2005;46:246–52.

15. Burzotta F, Trani C, Romagnoli E, et al. Manual thrombus-aspiration improves myocardial reperfusion: the randomized evaluation of the effect of mechanical reduction of distal embolization by thrombus-aspiration in primary and rescue angioplasty (REMEDIA) trial. J Am Coll Cardiol 2005;46:371–6.

16. Ali A, Cox D, Dib N, et al. Rheolytic thrombectomy with percutaneous coronary intervention for infarct size reduction in acute myocardial infarction: 30-day results from a multicenter randomized study. J Am Coll Cardiol 2006;48:244–52.

17. Colombo P, Silva P, Bigi R, et al. Thrombus aspiration improves coronary flow and myocardial reperfusion in acute myocardial infarction: final results of the DEAR-MI (Dethrombosis to Enhance Acute Reperfusion in Myocardial Infarction) study. Am J Cardiol 2005;96(Suppl):74H.

18. Svilaas T, Vlaar P, van der Horst I, et al. Thrombus aspiration during primary percutaneous intervention. N Engl J Med 2008;358:557–67.

19. Stone GW, Webb J, Cox DA, et al. Enhanced Myocardial Efficacy and Recovery by Aspiration of Liberated Debris (EMERALD) Investigators. Distal microcirculatory protection during percutaneous coronary intervention in acute ST-segment elevation myocardial infarction: a randomized controlled trial. JAMA 2005;293:1063–72.

20. Kelbaek H, Terkelsen C, Helqvist S, et al. Randomized comparison of distal protection versus conventional treatment in primary percutaneous coronary intervention: the drug elution and distal protection in ST-elevation myocardial infarction (DEDICATION) trial. J Am Coll Cardiol 2008;51(9):899–905.

21. Topaz O, Ebersole D, Das T, et al. Excimer laser angioplasty in acute myocardial infarction (the CARMEL multicenter trial). Am J Cardiol 2004;93:694–701.

22. Mehta S, Briceno R, Alfonso C, et al. Lessons from the Single INdividual Community Experience REgistry for Primary PCI (SINCERE) Database. In: Kappur R, editor. Textbook of STEMI interventions. Miami (FL): HMP Communications; 2008. p. 130–67.

23. Mahaffey KW, Puma JA, Barbagelata NA, et al. Adenosine as an adjunct to thrombolytic therapy for acute myocardial infarction: results of a multicenter, randomized, placebo-controlled trial: the Acute Myocardial Infarction STudy of ADenosine (AMISTAD) trial. J Am Coll Cardiol 1999;34: 1711–20.

24. Wang HJ, Lo PH, Lin JJ, et al. Treatment of slow/no-reflow phenomenon with intracoronary nitroprusside injection in primary coronary intervention for acute myocardial infarction. Catheter Cardiovasc Interv 2004;63:171.

25. Amit G, Cafri C, Yaroslavtsev S, et al. Intracoronary nitroprusside for the prevention of the no-reflow phenomenon after primary percutaneous coronary intervention in acute myocardial infarction. A randomized, double-blind, placebo-controlled clinical trial. Am Heart J 2006;152(5):887 e9–14.

26. Stone GW, Grines CL, Cox DA, et al. Comparison of angioplasty with stenting, with or without abciximab, in acute myocardial infarction. N Engl J Med 2002; 346:957–66.

27. Marzilli M, Orsini E, Marraccini P, et al. Beneficial effects of intracoronary adenosine as an adjunct to primary angioplasty in acute myocardial infarction. Circulation 2000;101:2154.

28. Claeys MJ, Bosmans J, De Ceuninck M, et al. Effect of intracoronary adenosine infusion during coronary intervention on myocardial reperfusion injury in patients with acute myocardial infarction. Am J Cardiol 2004;94:9–13.

29. Hang CL, Wang CP, Yip HK, et al. Early administration of intracoronary verapmil improves myocardial perfusion during percutaneous coronary interventions for acute myocardial infarction. Chest 2005;128:93–8.

30. Shinozaki N, Ichinose H, Yahikozawa K, et al. Selective intracoronary administration of nitroprusside before balloon dilatation prevents slow reflow during percutaneous coronary intervention in patients with acute myocardial infarction. Int Heart J 2007;48: 423–33.

31. Thiele H, Schindler K, Friedenberger J, et al. Intracoronary compared with intravenous bolus abciximab application in patients with ST-elevation myocardial infarction undergoing primary percutaneous coronary intervention: the randomized Leipzig immediate percutaneous coronary intervention abciximab IV versus IC in ST-elevation myocardial infarction trial. Circulation 2008;118:49–57.

32. Bellandi F, Maioli M, Gallopin M, et al. Increase of myocardial salvage and left ventricular function recovery with intracoronary abciximab downstream of the coronary occlusion in patients with acute myocardial infarction treated with primary coronary intervention. Catheter Cardiovasc Interv 2004;62: 186–92.

33. Antoniucci D, Rodriguez A, Hempel A, et al. A randomized trial comparing primary infarct artery stenting with or without abciximab in acute myocardial infarction. J Am Coll Cardiol 2003;42: 1879–85.

34. Hochman JS, Buller CE, Sleeper LA, et al. Cardiogenic shock complicating acute myocardial infarction—etiologies, management and outcome: a report from the SHOCK trial registry. J Am Coll Cardiol 2000;36:1063–70.

35. Sjauw KD, Engström AE, Vis MM, et al. A systematic review and meta-analysis of intra aortic balloon pump therapy in ST-elevation myocardial infarction: should we change the guidelines? Eur Heart J 2009;30:459–68.

36. Thiele H, Sick P, Boudriot E, et al. Randomized comparison of intra-aortic balloon support with a percutaneous left ventricular assist device in patients with revascularized acute myocardial infarction complicated by cardiogenic shock. Eur Heart J 2005;26:1276–83.

37. Dixon SR, Henriques JPS, Mauri L, et al. A prospective feasibility trial investigating the use of the Impella 2.5 system in patients undergoing high-risk percutaneous coronary intervention (The PROTECT I trial). JACC Cardiovasc Interv 2009;2:91–6.

38. Sjauw KD, Remmelink M, Baan J Jr, et al. Left ventricular unloading in acute STEMI patients is safe and feasible and provides acute and sustained left ventricular recovery. The AMC MACH 2 study. J Am Coll Cardiol 2008;51:1044–6.

39. Seyfarth M, Sibbing D, Bauer I, et al. A randomized clinical trial to evaluate the safety and efficacy of a percutaneous left ventricular assist device versus intra-aortic balloon pumping for the treatment of cardiogenic shock caused by myocardial infarction. J Am Coll Cardiol 2008;52:1584–8.

40. Swanson L. Cool It: therapeutic hypothermia for cardiac arrest in patients with ST-elevation myocardial infarction and unique benefits with combined treatment. Presented at: American College of Cardiology Scientific Session. Orlando, FL, March 31, 2009.

41. O'Neill WW. Acute Myocardial Infarction with Hyperoxemic Therapy (AMIHOT): a prospective, randomized trial of intracoronary hyperoxemic reperfusion after percutaneous coronary intervention. J Am Coll Cardiol 2007;50:397–405.

42. Burt R, Loh Y, Pearce W, et al. Clinical applications of blood-derived and marrow-derived stem cells for nonmalignant diseases. JAMA 2008;299(8): 925–36.

43. Zohlnhöfer D, Dibra A, Koppara T, et al. Stem cell mobilization by granulocyte colony-stimulating factor for myocardial recovery after acute myocardial infarction. J Am Coll Cardiol 2008;51: 1429–37.

Stem Cell Therapy for the Treatment of Acute Myocardial Infarction

Jonathan H. Dinsmore, PhD[a], Nabil Dib, MD, MSc[b,c],*

KEYWORDS
- Stem cell • Myocardial infarction • Therapy
- Myocardial regeneration

The last decade has been accompanied by great optimism and interest in the concept of cell or tissue regeneration in the postinfarction myocardium. However, despite the promise, progress has been slow. Data derived from multiple controlled studies in hundreds of patients' postmyocardial infarction have shown hints of potential benefit[1–22] but not of the magnitude anticipated. The complexity and hurdles to repair the damaged myocardium have been more daunting than originally estimated.

Part of the challenge has been due to the lack of systematic data from preclinical animal models on which to base clinical trials. Basics such as cell dose, preferred cell source, and route of delivery had not been adequately compared and optimized before the initiation of multiple human studies.[2,16,18] The first studies, all small and open labeled, showed some promise. Revolutionary observations emerging from basic research efforts on the ability of cells to undergo fate changes and morph into "repair all" cells were also promising. What were once thought to be lineage-restricted hematopoietic and mesenchymal stem cells were shown to behave like pluripotent stem cells forming vascular endothelium, cardiomyocytes, vascular smooth muscle, skeletal muscle, hepatocytes, pancreatic islets, and even neuronal cells in the brain.[23–25] The concept emerged that these adult stem cells need to be placed only in the appropriate environment where local cues would guide their commitment to regenerate damaged tissues. Embryologists had showed long ago that such phenomena existed in species such as the newt that could regenerate whole limbs and damaged myocardium. However, it was not until recently that further studies would again reestablish the lineage restrictions of these adult stem cells in mammalians.[25–28] The revisionist theories that had spurned the initiation of so many human clinical trials were being reversed, leaving the field needing to reexamine and reinterpret the present and future work on myocardial regeneration. There is a rich body of work conducted at clinical centers in Europe, Asia, and the United States that have involved more than 700 patients, with follow-up in some studies now reaching the 5-year point. The results from these studies have been viewed largely as positive rather than as disappointing. The challenge ahead will be to use what has been learned to guide future directions for study.

This article takes a fresh look at the progress in myocardial regeneration. The authors look at the postmyocardial environment for cues that may guide repair, and they look closely at the clinical data for evidence of cardiac regeneration. This evidence is used for suggestions on how to best proceed with future work.

[a] Children's Hospital Boston, 300 Longwood Avenue, Boston, MA 02115, USA
[b] Cardiovascular Research, Catholic Health Care West (CHW), Mercy Gilbert and Chandler Medical Centers, Phoenix, AZ 85297, USA
[c] Clinical Cardiovascular Cell Therapy, San Diego Medical Center, University of California, San Diego, USA
* Corresponding author. Clinical Cardiovascular Cell Therapy, 9350 Campus Point Drive, Suite 1D, La Jolla, CA 92037-1300.
E-mail address: ndib@cardiostem.com (N. Dib).

Cardiol Clin 28 (2010) 127–138
doi:10.1016/j.ccl.2009.09.004

MYOCARDIAL EVENTS POST INFARCTION

In the moments leading up to and during acute myocardial infarction (MI), heart muscle suffers ischemic damage that increases with postocclusion time. Early reperfusion mediated through drug or catheter intervention relieves the ischemic stress, but not without cost. On reperfusion, massive oxidative stress is placed on the tissue, with a dramatic increase in formation of reactive oxygen species (ROS) and a concomitant destruction of myocardial tissue.[29–32] ROS directly damage the cell membrane, causing cell death[32] and a massive release of intracellular Ca^{2+} stores, which in turn cause shutdown of gap junctions[33] and intracellular communication. There is also a stimulated release of inflammatory cytokines such as tumor necrosis factor-α, interleukin-1β (IL-1β), and interleukin-6 (IL-6).[29,34–36] These inflammatory cytokines then activate matrix metalloproteinases that degrade the extracellular matrix signaling proliferation of fibroblasts, resulting in collagen deposition and eventual scar formation.[37,38] Also activated is the expression of extracellular adhesion proteins, intracellular adhesion molecule-1, selectins, and integrins, which attract circulating neutrophils, macrophages, and mast cells.[29,39,40] Finally, expression of matricellular proteins such as osteopontin, osteonectin, tenascin, and thrombospondin are induced, affecting alterations in vasculogenesis.[38,41–43] This change in the extracellular environment is critical for the infiltration of inflammatory cells to remove cellular debris and to further release modulatory cytokines. The combination of ROS and inflammatory cytokines adversely affects Ca^{2+} homeostatsis,[29] with ROS causing lipid peroxidation and the opening of voltage-sensitive Ca^{2+} channels, release of Ca^{2+} from intracellular stores, and inhibition of Ca^{2+} uptake by sarcoplasmic reticulum Ca^{2+} ATPase.

The postinfarct period can be described in 3 phases that lead to the eventual resolution of the ischemic event and the formation of scar tissue: the inflammatory phase just described, the proliferative phase, and the consolidation phase. During the proliferative phase, resident cardiac fibroblasts are stimulated to proliferate and undergo differentiation to an array of phenotypes that include formation of myofibroblasts that can assume many of the appearances of cardiomyocytes, but function differently. The myofibroblasts are a main contributor to the compensatory cardiac hypertrophy that occur post-MI.[44] Fibroblast proliferation drives the reparation mechanisms at the infarct site, with increased matrix synthesis providing for continued phagocytosis by invading macrophages and for the stimulation of angiogenesis to reestablish blood supply for oxygenation and provision of cellular nutrients.[29,31,45–47] The proliferative phase then gives way to consolidation whereby synthesized collagen begins to undergo cross-linking, reduction in proliferation, regression of inflammatory cells, and arterioles leaving behind the predominantly acellular scar—appropriate collagen maturation being necessary for buttressing the ventricular wall against intraventricular pressure.[45] Interference with effective deposition of a dense collagen matrix has been shown to be detrimental to heart function, resulting in a weakened myocardial scar susceptible to rupture and contributing to arrhythmia formation.[37,45,48,49]

The sequence of events is common to all species, but there is a marked difference in the time required for these events. In the mouse, the consolidation phase is well underway by 1 week to 10 days post-MI. However, in the dog heart, consolidation does not begin for at least 4 to 6 weeks.[39,45] The time course in humans is delayed even further. Considering strategies for cardiac regeneration, the timing of administration of cells is an important variable. All human studies have administered cells within approximately 1 week of the MI (**Table 1**), when there is still an active inflammatory environment. At this time, the environment would most likely not promote cardiomyocyte growth and integration, but would more likely favor fibroblast or inflammatory cell fates. More likely than not, the environment would be toxic to any cells other than those specifically adapted to function there.[32,47,50] A later time point may not be any more favorable, with the consolidation mechanisms also selecting against appropriate cardiomyocyte differentiation or survival. The most appropriate animal model is the dog or other larger animal because the time course of infarct is more similar. A careful and detailed time course for cell survival and repair has never been performed in a large animal model. The work has relied on mouse models. Direct testing of this variable in humans is not advised, because repair mechanisms need to combine the functional and comparative anatomic analyses that can only be performed by detailed postmortem tissue histology. This is a very time-intensive and cost-intensive testing process, but an approach invaluable if the field is to advance based on scientific principles. Unfortunately, the mechanisms that ensure effective myocardial scar formation are contrary to the environment needed for muscle regrowth and repair.

Thus arises one of the conundrums of the regenerative process: balancing the need for short-term stabilization and reinforcement of the heart wall

Table 1
Cell purification and injection procedure

Study	Selection/Purification	Injection Procedure	Time Post-MI	Injection Media	Viability	Postinfusion Viability
Bartunek, 2005[3]	CD133+ antibody selected	3 × 3 min × 3.3 mL	12 d	Saline + 1% HSA	NR	NR
Meyer, 2006[12]	Gelatin-polysuccinate sedimentation	NR	5 d	Saline + 5% autol serum	NR	NR
Janssens, 2006[8]	Ficoll	3 × 3 min × 3.3 mL	4 d	Saline + 5% autol serum	NR	NR
Lunde, 2006[10]	Ficoll	NR	6 d	Saline + autol plasma	95%	NR
Shachinger, 2006[15]; Dill, 2009 substudy[6]	Ficoll	3 × 3 min × 3.3 mL	3–6 d	X-VIVO 10 media + 20% autol serum	98%	NR
Kang, 2006[9]	G-CSF mobilized PBMC/apharesis	Single infusion/no occlusion	7 d	NR	NR	NR
Meluzin, 2008[11]	Ficoll + O/N culture	7 × 3 min × 3 mL	5–9 d	CellGro medium	NR	NR
Penicka, 2007[14]	Gelatin-polysuccinate sedimentation	4–5 × 2.5–4 min × 5 mL	4–11 d	Saline	94%–99%	NR
Tatsumi, 2007[19]	Apharesis	3 × 3 min × 3.3 mL	2–3 d	NR	NR	NR
Huikuri, 2008[7]	Ficoll	NR—intermittent balloon inflation	2–6 d	Saline + 50% autol serum	NR	NR
Tendera, 2009[20]	Ficoll & antibody selection	3 × 3 min × 3.3 mL	7 d	Saline	98%	NR
Yousef, 2009[22]	Ficoll	4 × 4 min × NR: added dobutamine and microsphere injections before cell injection	7 d	Saline	93%	NR
Cao, 2009[4]	Ficoll	4 × 1 min × 2.5 mL	7 d	Saline	98%	NR

versus providing an inviting environment for re-growth of cardiac muscle cells. Regrowth of cardi-omyocytes is a complicated process that involves first, proliferation and second, gap-junction forma-tion,[33] myofibrillar development, and integration with the surviving myocardium[49]—mechanisms that are adversely affected by the stresses produced in the infarct compromised heart. Like-wise, any cells administered to repair the heart within the first month after infarct will encounter an environment that is profibrotic and unlikely to contain instructive signals for myocardial growth and repair.[32,40,41,44,46] In many respects, the cell best suited to repair the myocardium after an infarct is a committed cell such as the skeletal muscle myoblast—naturally induced to proliferate and repair damaged muscle in an inflammatory environment.[51] Perhaps clinicians need to rethink the requirements for a successful cardiac repair post-MI and consider that the ideal cell may not be the cardiomyocyte progenitor, but a cell that is better adapted to thrive within the post-MI milieu. The significance of the cell type chosen for post-MI repair will become more significant as the results of the human clinical studies per-formed to date and the cells used in those studies are examined.

CLINICAL TRIALS

A Lin⁻c-kit⁺ subset of bone marrow cells from male donor mice injected into the peri-infarct zone of the female recipient mice within a few hours after infarct were the first adult stem cells re-ported to survive, repair, and differentiate into car-diomyocytes in an acute MI.[52] Cell survival was shown by the presence of Y-chromosome–posi-tive cardiomyocytes in female donor hearts and by fluorescence imaging of enhanced green fluo-rescent protein from the transgenic male donor mice.[52] This study caused an almost immediate rush to test this procedure in patients even though no systematic investigation as to optimal dose, best delivery route, best cell source, or most appropriate time after infarct for maximum benefit had been undertaken.[2,16,18] Similarly, there was no elaboration of the mechanical pathway by which the introduced stem cells mediated repair, this being assumed to be through direct cellular replacement. However, this mechanism would eventually be shown to be incorrect,[27,53] and in fact the mechanism by which cardiac repair is mediated is still undefined.

To date, more than 15 published clinical trials, both open label and placebo controlled, using bone marrow stem cells (BMSC), have been con-ducted since 2001 (**Tables 2** and **3**).[54] From those

studies, a mean improvement of 3% to 4% in left ventricular ejection fraction (LVEF) in treated versus control patients was observed.[54–56] Although the observed increase in LVEF was statistically significant in their respective meta-analyses,[54–56] the clinical benefit of small changes to LVEF that already are in the normal range (40%–60%) are difficult to estimate. The measure of change in LVEF to assess heart function is not a standard or accepted end point for cardiac effi-cacy studies, although its use in these early studies is understandable as an objective measure of change. Unfortunately, in all studies the standard cardiovascular assessment measures that were examined in addition to LVEF failed to show statistical significance. One of the challenges that lies ahead is to determine if there are any efficacy measures from these initial studies that can be used in future prospec-tive, double-blind studies as an end point for regulatory approval. Most likely, the answer is no, which means that further studies are needed to identify appropriate efficacy measures. A few preclinical studies in MI models have used exer-cise capacity as a measure of efficacy.[57] More preclinical work with end points relevant to future human studies would be welcome, and will prob-ably become a requirement to justify entry into the clinic.

Cell-based therapies present challenges to the interpretation of clinical data unique to this area of study. For all other types of therapies including most gene therapies, the therapy of choice can be monitored systemically for blood levels, clear-ance rate, and half-life, allowing dose-response relationships to be determined and verified. Such measures are lacking for cell-based thera-pies. Noninvasive imaging using MRI to track survival and migration of prelabeled cells was a promising approach, but with further study has been shown to be unreliable.[58] Other approaches that have relied on genetic approaches to label cells have also been shown to be susceptible to artifact.[59,60] In addition, the purity of a small molecule drug product can be measured and quantified to high precision, and the manufacturing procedures standardized for consistent production, but this cannot be done readily for cells.

The delivery route and mechanism provide unique challenges for cells, and not nearly so for other therapeutics. The device and rate of delivery are critical for cells, and can have profound impact on the viability and therefore efficacy. Likewise, short-term storage of cells before administration to the patient can also adversely affect viability. Such variables as these confound

Table 2
Planned human clinical trials involving stem cells for acute myocardial infarction

Study Name	N	Delivery Route	Cell Type/Dose	End Point	Control
TIME	120	NS	Bone marrow mononuclear cells 3 or 7 d post-MI	LVEF at 6 mo	Randomized, double-blind media vs cells
Late TIME	87	NS	Bone marrow mononuclear cells 2 or 3 wk post-MI	LVEF at 6 mo	Randomized, double-blind media vs cells
BMSC Infusion following MI	60	Intracoronary	Bone marrow mononuclear cells	Primary: safety; secondary LVEF at 6 mo	No
REGEN-AMI	102	Intracoronary	Bone marrow mononuclear cells	Change in LVEF over 1 y	Saline vs cells
REVITALIZE	30	Intracoronary	Bone marrow mononuclear cells 3–14 d post-MI	LVEF at 4 mo	No
Prochymal following acute MI	220	Intravenous	Allogeneic human mesenchymal stem cells (Prochymal) within 7 d post-MI	LVESV	Randomized, double-blind media vs cells
Cultured MSC in AMI	20	Intravenous	Allogeneic bone marrow derived human mesenchymal stem cells within 2 d post-MI	Primary safety; secondary perfusion defect and infarct size	Plasmalyte A
Allogeneic mesenchymal precursor cells (MPCs) in acute MI	25	Transendocardial	25, 75, and 150 × 106 MPCs	Safety	Randomized: MPC in 20 patients; injection alone in 5
SELECT-AMI	60	Intracoronary	5 × 106 CD133+ bone marrow cells 5–10 d post-MI	Safety and myocardial thickening	Intracoronary saline

Data from Clintrials.gov. Available at: http://clinicaltrials.gov/. Accessed July 20, 2009.

Table 3
Clinical studies for acute MI

Study	N	Single or Multicenter	Sham Injection	Stem Cell Isolation from Control Patients	Difference Between Treatment vs Control in LVEF (%), Time Measured
Bartunek, 2005[3]	34	Single	No	No	3%, 4 mo
Meyer, 2006[12]	60	Single	No	No	6%, 6 mo; 3%, 18 mo
Janssens, 2006[8]	67	Single	Yes	Yes	0%, 4 mo
Lunde, 2006[10]	97	Single	No	No	1%, 6 mo
Schachinger, 2006[15], Dill, 2009 substudy[6]	204	Multi	Yes	Yes	2%, 4 mo
Dill, 2009 substudy[6]					2%, 12 mo: substudy
Kang, 2006[9]	50	Single	No	No	5%, 6 mo
Meluzin, 2008[11]	60	Single	No	No	6%, 3 mo; 7%, 6 mo; 7%, 12 mo
Tatsumi, 2007[19]	54	Single	No	No	6%, 6 mo
Huikuri, 2008[7]	80	Single	No	No	5%, 6 mo
Tendera, 2009[20]	200	Multi	No	No	3%, 6 mo
Yousef, 2009[22]	124	Single	No	No	6%, 3 mo; 6%, 12 mo; 6%, 5y
Cao, 2009[4]	86	Single	No	No	2%, 6 mo; 3%, 12 mo; 3%, 4y

interpretation of study outcomes when there is not a strict set of standards imposed to ensure that the final product delivered to the patient is comparable across patients. Very little similarity is seen when the published reports of BMSC are compared with studies for bone marrow harvest procedures or volumes collected, time from collection to administration, media used for delivery and storage, delivery rates and devices, or for total cell dose, and for no study is there an examination of the effects of storage in delivery media on cell viability (see **Table 1**). Furthermore, careful comparisons of cells isolated by different methods show differences in performance.[61,62] There is a degree of comparability across studies for the procedure used for cell delivery, but even this varies in its particulars across studies (see **Table 1**). Therefore, a meta-analysis for therapeutic effect is nearly impossible, as there are no reliable measures that can assure the same drug or cell product is being used or that there are no elements of the delivery technique that influence outcome.[54–56]

The most common technique for stem cell delivery is through an intracoronary injection with the deployment of a balloon catheter to occlude blood flow temporarily to allow time for cells to transmigrate into the myocardium (see **Table 1**). Studies that examined the effects of temporary occlusion and concomitant ischemia on myocardial cells revealed a preconditioning phenomenon.[32,63,64] Therefore, transient ischemia has beneficial effects on the myocardial function and survival. The procedure used to deliver stem cells causes transient ischemia and therefore might nonspecifically affect improved cardiac function when compared with controls in whom no procedure was performed (**Table 4**). A close inspection of studies in **Table 4** reveals an interesting association between positive outcome and the procedure used for the introduction of cells. For the studies of Meluzin and colleagues[11] and Yousef and colleagues,[22] there were clear distinctions in the procedures used, with one study using an increased number of occlusions during cell delivery[11] and the other including an additional dobutamine stimulation plus a microsphere injection to promote cell incorporation.[22] Both studies had amongst the highest benefit observed in LVEF improvement, being more or less 6% of those reported. However, neither study incorporated a matched control group such that the benefit could be ascribed to enhanced cell uptake versus an alternative mechanism such as preconditioning. Such studies highlight the difficulties in interpreting early clinical studies.

FUTURE CLINICAL STUDIES

Given some of the deficiencies in early clinical studies, which were in part due to restrictions imposed on any early clinical study, subsequent studies were designed to overcome these weaknesses. Judging from a listing of the studies that have been filed for further testing (see **Table 2**) there is still a need for more rigorous design. Reliance on LVEF as a measure for efficacy needs to be changed. There is little justification or precedence for LVEF as an appropriate end point. Furthermore, there is the continued use of a post-MI time closely matched to prior studies. Trials with stem cell therapies are complex and costly. Consequently, the trials are usually slow to recruit patients, and to complete enrollment and follow-up. Therefore, by the time results from today's planned studies became available many years would have passed. Therefore, now is the appropriate time to make some radical change in the path that is being followed.

PLACEBO CONTROLS

Growing evidence is emerging to support the increased impact of placebo effects in surgical devices or therapies that require an invasive procedure for their use.[65–67] In addition, cardiovascular studies[68,69] have been associated with some unusually large placebo effects (20%–30% change). These 2 placebo-related influences on outcome must be considered in planning and conducting any trial relating to cardiac regeneration. Early studies should not be faulted for the choice of conducting open label studies or using the best medical therapy controls, but any study that is to rigorously test the effects of cells versus placebo must have control for all aspects of the cell isolation procedure, cell injection, and postinjection follow-up. This necessity means that studies have to be prospectively randomized to start with, and that the treatment and evaluation teams cannot be blinded to the randomization. After randomization, subjects should undergo cell isolation regardless of the treatment assignment; the clinical pharmacist too should be blinded to the treatment assignment. The cell delivery procedure must be performed in the same manner regardless of the treatment group. In some cases, sham procedures may need to be employed whereby procedural risks do not justify actual injections. In such cases, the surgical team must create an experience for the patient that is indistinguishable from that for treatment counterparts. Only in trials with such rigorous controls can the effects of placebo be minimized.

Table 4
Cell types used for cardiac regeneration

Cell Type	Source	Cell Survival: Preclinical/ Human Sudies
BMSC	Bone marrow	No/No
EPC	Blood and bone marrow	No/No
Myoblasts	Skeletal muscle	Yes/Yes
Mesenchymal stem cells	Bone marrow	No/No
Embryonic stem cells	Embryo/inner cell mass	Yes/ND
iPS cells	Fibroblasts	Yes/ND
Isl1+ Cardiac stem cells	Fetal and adult heart	ND

From an examination of the studies conducted to date and described here, only 2 of 12 employed such rigorous methods. Not surprisingly, studies that have controlled for factors such as whether bone marrow isolation and injections of saline were performed in control patients show a more or less 2% nonsignificant difference in LVEF between treatment and control.[8,15]

The issue of placebo effects in myocardial repair studies is not new to trials with stem cells. Similar difficulties were encountered in angiogenesis studies conducted with gene or protein therapeutic strategies.[68,70] Preclinical animal studies had shown promise for this approach, which led to human clinical studies that showed benefits in patients during the initial studies. However, subsequent double-blind placebo controlled studies failed to confirm the initial positive results, the extent of improvement in the placebo group being the confounding result.[68,70] Not only did placebo controls show improvements in objective measures such as cardiac output and perfusion imaging, but also in exercise capacity and quality of life measures. The ability to detect improvements in cardiac viability measures and contractility that extends to a 3-year follow-up is surprising, and underscores the need for prospective trial designs that control for potential placebo effects.

CELL TYPES PRESENT AND FUTURE: WHAT IS BEST FOR MYOCARDIAL REPAIR

Many different types of cells have been examined for the ability to repair the infarcted myocardium (see **Table 3**), but the choice of cell type has been dramatically influenced by reports of bone marrow, fat, mesenchymal, and endothelial precursor cells capable of transdifferentiation into cardiomyocytes.[71] However, transdifferention is dependent on tissue instructive signals, and the post-MI environment is unlikely to contain those signals. There has been success using fetal cardiomyocytes, but these cells are not readily obtained in the quantities needed for widespread use. Cardiomyocytes differentiated from embryonic stem cells in vitro are a potential source, but are complicated by immunologic barriers to transplanting cells from an unrelated donor. Induced pluripotent stem (iPS) cells may be a viable alternative, but this technology is still in its early stages of investigation. Autologous skeletal muscle myoblasts have been used successfully in animal models and are an interesting approach that needs to be reconsidered, but the number of cells required and the mode of delivery need to be tested more completely before applying them in an acute MI setting. Finally, there are approaches that use administering agents, which can stimulate endogenous cells within the heart to proliferate and repair, but when to stimulate such cells is not clear. Before drawing conclusions about the utility of cell therapy for cardiac repair, it is useful to examine the different cells and results from the use of these cells in various clinical trials. The focus here is on clinical trial results versus preclinical studies, as the clinical data are more instructive at this time.

For various immunologic reasons, autologous stem cell transplantation is the favored approach. By far, use of BMSC has been the choice of favor (see **Tables 3** and **4**). Yet, there are significant questions as to whether these cells have the greatest potential for repair. Similar results were obtained with endothelial progenitor cells (EPC) that were isolated from circulating blood cells (see **Tables 3** and **4**). Within 1 to 3 months of administering either BMSC or EPC, significant improvement was noted in cardiac pumping efficiency (ejection fraction) of the patients with cell transplants, when compared with the patients who did not receive such cell transfusions. These small prospective pilot studies suggests that autotransplantation with stem cells contained in the bone marrow can significantly reduce the risk and extent of MI, but carry numerous caveats.

Recent reports have identified a new autologous stem cell derived directly from the heart. Lineage-tracing experiments have shown that Isl1-expressing cells can differentiate into endothelial, endocardial, smooth muscle, conduction system, right ventricular, and atrial myogenic lineages during the development of the embryonic heart.[72–74] Isl1-expressing cells are also present in the adult mammalian heart, but they are limited to the right atrium, are found in smaller numbers than in embryonic heart, and have an unknown physiologic role. The identification of various cell types with cardiogenic potential has stimulated interest in improving cardiac function by mobilizing endogenous stem cells and progenitor cells without removing and expanding the cells ex vivo. Like stem cells or progenitor cells in other tissues, cardiac stem cells reside in clusters consistent with the existence of cardiac niches. The factors that attract these cells out of their putative niches to an injury site remain to be defined.

NEXT STEPS

Through nearly a decade of human clinical studies, a significant body of research results has accumulated regarding the utility of adult stem cells for post-MI cardiac regeneration. The data do not support a magnitude of repair and recovery approaching that observed in preclinical animal models. Therefore, continued studies in humans should be carefully designed and controlled to better eliminate approaches that do not deserve further study. This does not mean that further human studies should not be pursued. Rather, lessons from prior tissue regeneration studies should be modeled.[75,76] A better coordinated and systematic preclinical experimental base needs to be established to identify critical variables that may affect outcomes. No data exist showing that one cell source compared with another provides any significant advantage. With many more stem cells continuing to be identified, the need for critical comparisons continues to be a high priority. The tools for studying cell survival, migration, and differentiation continue to expand in such a way that future preclinical studies will be more informative for future clinical studies. Standardization of techniques for cell delivery and cell preparation are important for future success. In the end analysis, progress will be made incrementally. The promise for cell therapy continues to be significant, but the challenges ahead are also significant. With a critical analysis of work completed, future advances can be made without unduly repeating past principles. The immense complexity of biologic systems makes the challenge for tissue repair a difficult one, and one for fertile future research.

REFERENCES

1. Assmus B, Honold J, Schachinger V, et al. Transcoronary transplantation of progenitor cells after myocardial infarction. N Engl J Med 2006;355(12):1222–32.
2. Assmus B, Schachinger V, Teupe C, et al. Transplantation of Progenitor Cells and Regeneration Enhancement in Acute Myocardial Infarction (TOPCARE-AMI). Circulation 2002;106(24):3009–17.
3. Bartunek J, Vanderheyden M, Vandekerckhove B, et al. Intracoronary injection of CD133-positive enriched bone marrow progenitor cells promotes cardiac recovery after recent myocardial infarction: feasibility and safety. Circulation 2005;112(Suppl 9):I178–83.
4. Cao F, Sun D, Li C, et al. Long-term myocardial functional improvement after autologous bone marrow mononuclear cells transplantation in patients with ST-segment elevation myocardial infarction: 4 years follow-up. Eur Heart J 2009;30(16):1986–94.
5. Dib N, Michler RE, Pagani FD, et al. Safety and feasibility of autologous myoblast transplantation in patients with ischemic cardiomyopathy: four-year follow-up. Circulation 2005;112(12):1748–55.
6. Dill T, Schachinger V, Rolf A, et al. Intracoronary administration of bone marrow-derived progenitor cells improves left ventricular function in patients at risk for adverse remodeling after acute ST-segment elevation myocardial infarction: results of the Reinfusion of Enriched Progenitor cells And Infarct Remodeling in Acute Myocardial Infarction study (REPAIR-AMI) cardiac magnetic resonance imaging substudy. Am Heart J 2009;157(3):541–7.
7. Huikuri HV, Kervinen K, Niemela M, et al. Effects of intracoronary injection of mononuclear bone marrow cells on left ventricular function, arrhythmia risk profile, and restenosis after thrombolytic therapy of acute myocardial infarction. Eur Heart J 2008;29(22):2723–32.
8. Janssens S, Dubois C, Bogaert J, et al. Autologous bone marrow-derived stem-cell transfer in patients with ST-segment elevation myocardial infarction: double-blind, randomised controlled trial. Lancet 2006;367(9505):113–21.
9. Kang HJ, Lee HY, Na SH, et al. Differential effect of intracoronary infusion of mobilized peripheral blood stem cells by granulocyte colony-stimulating factor on left ventricular function and remodeling in

patients with acute myocardial infarction versus old myocardial infarction: the MAGIC Cell-3-DES randomized, controlled trial. Circulation 2006; 114(Suppl 1):I145–51.

10. Lunde K, Solheim S, Aakhus S, et al. Intracoronary injection of mononuclear bone marrow cells in acute myocardial infarction. N Engl J Med 2006;355(12): 1199–209.

11. Meluzin J, Janousek S, Mayer J, et al. Three-, 6-, and 12-month results of autologous transplantation of mononuclear bone marrow cells in patients with acute myocardial infarction. Int J Cardiol 2008; 128(2):185–92.

12. Meyer GP, Wollert KC, Lotz J, et al. Intracoronary bone marrow cell transfer after myocardial infarction: eighteen months' follow-up data from the randomized, controlled BOOST (BOne marrOw transfer to enhance ST-elevation infarct regeneration) trial. Circulation 2006;113(10):1287–94.

13. Pagani FD, DerSimonian H, Zawadzka A, et al. Autologous skeletal myoblasts transplanted to ischemia-damaged myocardium in humans. Histological analysis of cell survival and differentiation. J Am Coll Cardiol 2003;41(5):879–88.

14. Penicka M, Horak J, Kobylka P, et al. Intracoronary injection of autologous bone marrow-derived mononuclear cells in patients with large anterior acute myocardial infarction: a prematurely terminated randomized study. J Am Coll Cardiol 2007;49(24): 2373–4.

15. Schachinger V, Erbs S, Elsasser A, et al. Intracoronary bone marrow-derived progenitor cells in acute myocardial infarction. N Engl J Med 2006;355(12): 1210–21.

16. Stamm C, Westphal B, Kleine HD, et al. Autologous bone-marrow stem-cell transplantation for myocardial regeneration. Lancet 2003;361(9351):45–6.

17. Strauer BE, Brehm M, Zeus T, et al. Regeneration of human infarcted heart muscle by intracoronary autologous bone marrow cell transplantation in chronic coronary artery disease: the IACT Study. J Am Coll Cardiol 2005;46(9):1651–8.

18. Strauer BE, Brehm M, Zeus T, et al. Repair of infarcted myocardium by autologous intracoronary mononuclear bone marrow cell transplantation in humans. Circulation 2002;106(15):1913–8.

19. Tatsumi T, Ashihara E, Yasui T, et al. Intracoronary transplantation of non-expanded peripheral blood-derived mononuclear cells promotes improvement of cardiac function in patients with acute myocardial infarction. Circ J 2007;71(8):1199–207.

20. Tendera M, Wojakowski W, Ruzyllo W, et al. Intracoronary infusion of bone marrow-derived selected CD34+CXCR4+ cells and non-selected mononuclear cells in patients with acute STEMI and reduced left ventricular ejection fraction: results of randomized, multicentre Myocardial Regeneration by Intracoronary Infusion of Selected Population of Stem Cells in Acute Myocardial Infarction (REGENT) Trial. Eur Heart J 2009;30(11):1313–21.

21. Wollert KC, Meyer GP, Lotz J, et al. Intracoronary autologous bone-marrow cell transfer after myocardial infarction: the BOOST randomised controlled clinical trial. Lancet 2004;364(9429):141–8.

22. Yousef M, Schannwell CM, Kostering M, et al. The BALANCE Study: clinical benefit and long-term outcome after intracoronary autologous bone marrow cell transplantation in patients with acute myocardial infarction. J Am Coll Cardiol 2009; 53(24):2262–9.

23. Beltrami AP, Barlucchi L, Torella D, et al. Adult cardiac stem cells are multipotent and support myocardial regeneration. Cell 2003;114(6):763–76.

24. Bjorklund A, Svendsen C. Stem cells. Breaking the brain-blood barrier. Nature 1999;397(6720): 569–70.

25. Vassilopoulos G, Wang PR, Russell DW. Transplanted bone marrow regenerates liver by cell fusion. Nature 2003;422(6934):901–4.

26. Alvarez-Dolado M, Pardal R, Garcia-Verdugo JM, et al. Fusion of bone-marrow-derived cells with Purkinje neurons, cardiomyocytes and hepatocytes. Nature 2003;425(6961):968–73.

27. Murry CE, Soonpaa MH, Reinecke H, et al. Haematopoietic stem cells do not trans-differentiate into cardiac myocytes in myocardial infarcts. Nature 2004;428(6983):664–8.

28. Wagers AJ, Sherwood RI, Christensen JL, et al. Little evidence for developmental plasticity of adult hematopoietic stem cells. Science 2002;297(5590): 2256–9.

29. Frangogiannis NG, Smith CW, Entman ML. The inflammatory response in myocardial infarction. Cardiovasc Res 2002;53(1):31–47.

30. Hori M, Nishida K. Oxidative stress and left ventricular remodelling after myocardial infarction. Cardiovasc Res 2009;81(3):457–64.

31. Pasotti M, Prati F, Arbustini E. The pathology of myocardial infarction in the pre- and post-interventional era. Heart 2006;92(11):1552–6.

32. Vanden Hoek TL, Becker LB, Shao Z, et al. Reactive oxygen species released from mitochondria during brief hypoxia induce preconditioning in cardiomyocytes. J Biol Chem 1998;273(29):18092–8.

33. Severs NJ, Bruce AF, Dupont E, et al. Remodelling of gap junctions and connexion expression in diseased myocardium. Cardiovasc Res 2008;80(1): 9–19.

34. Frangogiannis NG, Mendoza LH, Lindsey ML, et al. IL-10 is induced in the reperfused myocardium and may modulate the reaction to injury. J Immunol 2000; 165(5):2798–808.

35. Gwechenberger M, Mendoza LH, Youker KA, et al. Cardiac myocytes produce interleukin-6 in culture

and in viable border zone of reperfused infarctions. Circulation 1999;99(4):546–51.

36. Wanner GA, Muller PE, Ertel W, et al. Differential effect of anti-TNF-alpha antibody on proinflammatory cytokine release by Kupffer cells following liver ischemia and reperfusion. Shock 1999;11(6):391–5.

37. Lindsey ML, Mann DL, Entman ML, et al. Extracellular matrix remodeling following myocardial injury. Ann Med 2003;35(5):316–26.

38. Schellings MW, Pinto YM, Heymans S. Matricellular proteins in the heart: possible role during stress and remodeling. Cardiovasc Res 2004;64(1): 24–31.

39. Dewald O, Ren G, Duerr GD, et al. Of mice and dogs: species-specific differences in the inflammatory response following myocardial infarction. Am J Pathol 2004;164(2):665–77.

40. Frangogiannis NG, Lindsey ML, Michael LH, et al. Resident cardiac mast cells degranulate and release preformed TNF-alpha, initiating the cytokine cascade in experimental canine myocardial ischemia/reperfusion. Circulation 1998;98(7): 699–710.

41. Frangogiannis NG, Ren G, Dewald O, et al. Critical role of endogenous thrombospondin-1 in preventing expansion of healing myocardial infarcts. Circulation 2005;111(22):2935–42.

42. Schellings MW, Vanhoutte D, Swinnen M, et al. Absence of SPARC results in increased cardiac rupture and dysfunction after acute myocardial infarction. J Exp Med 2009;206(1):113–23.

43. Shimazaki M, Nakamura K, Kii I, et al. Periostin is essential for cardiac healing after acute myocardial infarction. J Exp Med 2008;205(2):295–303.

44. Frangogiannis NG, Michael LH, Entman ML. Myofibroblasts in reperfused myocardial infarcts express the embryonic form of smooth muscle myosin heavy chain (SMemb). Cardiovasc Res 2000;48(1): 89–100.

45. Dobaczewski M, Bujak M, Zymek P, et al. Extracellular matrix remodeling in canine and mouse myocardial infarcts. Cell Tissue Res 2006;324(3): 475–88.

46. Frangogiannis NG. The immune system and cardiac repair. Pharm Res 2008;58(2):88–111.

47. Richard V, Murry CE, Reimer KA. Healing of myocardial infarcts in dogs. Effects of late reperfusion. Circulation 1995;92(7):1891–901.

48. Weinheimer CJ, Toeniskoetter PD, Conversano A, et al. Pretreatment with buflomedil enhances ventricular function by reducing the dysfunctional area after transient coronary artery occlusion. Cardiovasc Res 1992;26(5):470–5.

49. Trueblood NA, Xie Z, Communal C, et al. Exaggerated left ventricular dilation and reduced collagen deposition after myocardial infarction in mice lacking osteopontin. Circ Res 2001;88(10):1080–7.

50. Pasceri V, Patti G, Di Sciascio G. Prevention of myocardial damage during coronary intervention. Cardiovasc Hematol Disord Drug Targets 2006; 6(2):77–83.

51. Prisk V, Huard J. Muscle injuries and repair: the role of prostaglandins and inflammation. Histol Histopathol 2003;18(4):1243–56.

52. Orlic D, Kajstura J, Chimenti S, et al. Bone marrow cells regenerate infarcted myocardium. Nature 2001;410(6829):701–5.

53. Balsam LB, Wagers AJ, Christensen JL, et al. Haematopoietic stem cells adopt mature hematopoietic fates in ischaemic myocardium. Nature 2004; 428(6983):668–73.

54. Reffelmann T, Konemann S, Kloner RA. Promise of blood- and bone marrow-derived stem cell transplantation for functional cardiac repair: putting it in perspective with existing therapy. J Am Coll Cardiol 2009;53(4):305–8.

55. Lipinski MJ, Biondi-Zoccai GG, Abbate A, et al. Impact of intracoronary cell therapy on left ventricular function in the setting of acute myocardial infarction: a collaborative systematic review and meta-analysis of controlled clinical trials. J Am Coll Cardiol 2007;50(18):1761–7.

56. Singh S, Arora R, Handa K, et al. Stem cells improve left ventricular function in acute myocardial infarction. Clin Cardiol 2009;32(4):176–80.

57. Jain M, DerSimonian H, Brenner DA, et al. Cell therapy attenuates deleterious ventricular remodeling and improves cardiac performance after myocardial infarction. Circulation 2001;103(14):1920–7.

58. Terrovitis J, Stuber M, Youssef A, et al. Magnetic resonance imaging overestimates ferumoxide-labeled stem cell survival after transplantation in the heart. Circulation 2008;117(12):1555–62.

59. Bergsmedh A, Ehnfors J, Spetz AL, et al. A Cre-loxP based system for studying horizontal gene transfer. FEBS Lett 2007;581(16):2943–6.

60. Bergsmedh A, Szeles A, Henriksson M, et al. Horizontal transfer of oncogenes by uptake of apoptotic bodies. Proc Natl Acad Sci U S A 2001;98(11): 6407–11.

61. Atsma DE, Fibbe WE, Rabelink TJ. Opportunities and challenges for mesenchymal stem cell-mediated heart repair. Curr Opin Lipidol 2007;18(6): 645–9.

62. Seeger FH, Tonn T, Krzossok N, et al. Cell isolation procedures matter: a comparison of different isolation protocols of bone marrow mononuclear cells used for cell therapy in patients with acute myocardial infarction. Eur Heart J 2007;28(6): 766–72.

63. Murry CE, Richard VJ, Reimer KA, et al. Ischemic preconditioning slows energy metabolism and delays ultra structural damage during a sustained ischemic episode. Circ Res 1990;66(4):913–31.

64. Schwarz ER, Reffelmann T, Kloner RA. Clinical effects of ischemic preconditioning. Curr Opin Cardiol 1999;14(4):340–8.

65. Diederich NJ, Goetz CG. The placebo treatments in neurosciences: new insights from clinical and neuroimaging studies. Neurology 2008;71(9): 677–84.

66. Mercado R, Constantoyannis C, Mandat T, et al. Expectation and the placebo effect in Parkinson 's disease patients with subthalamic nucleus deep brain stimulation. Mov Disord 2006;21(9):1457–61.

67. Tcheng JE, Madan M, O'Shea JC, et al. Ethics and equipoise: rationale for a placebo-controlled study design of platelet glycoprotein IIb/IIIa inhibition in coronary intervention. J Interv Cardiol 2003;16(2): 97–105.

68. Khurana R, Simons M. Insights from angiogenesis trials using fibroblast growth factor for advanced arteriosclerotic disease. Trends Cardiovasc Med 2003;13(3):116–22.

69. Packer M. The placebo effect in heart failure. Am Heart J 1990;120(6 Pt 2):1579–82.

70. Simons M, Annex BH, Laham RJ, et al. Pharmacological treatment of coronary artery disease with recombinant fibroblast growth factor-2: double-blind, randomized, controlled clinical trial. Circulation 2002;105(7):788–93.

71. Wagers AJ, Weissman IL. Plasticity of adult stem cells. Cell 2004;116(5):639–48.

72. Bu L, Jiang X, Martin-Puig S, et al. Human ISL1 heart progenitors generate diverse multipotent cardiovascular cell lineages. Nature 2009; 460(7251):113–7.

73. Cai CL, Liang X, Shi Y, et al. Isl1 identifies a cardiac progenitor population that proliferates prior to differentiation and contributes a majority of cells to the heart. Dev Cell 2003;5(6):877–89.

74. Moretti A, Caron L, Nakano A, et al. Multipotent embryonic isl1+ progenitor cells lead to cardiac, smooth muscle, and endothelial cell diversification. Cell 2006;127(6):1151–65.

75. Freed CR, Breeze RE, Schneck SA. Transplantation of fetal mesencephalic tissue in Parkinson's disease. N Engl J Med 1995;333(11):730–1.

76. Olanow CW, Freeman T, Kordower J. Transplantation of embryonic dopamine neurons for severe Parkinson's disease. N Engl J Med 2001;345(2): 146 [author reply 147].

Percutaneous Techniques for Mitral Valve Disease

Roberto J. Cubeddu, MD, Igor F. Palacios, MD*

KEYWORDS

- Mitral valve • Transcatheter • Valvular heart disease
- Mitral regurgitation

THE MITRAL VALVE

To appreciate the mechanistic role of current percutaneous therapies, it is important to understand the anatomic and functional properties of the mitral valve apparatus. The mitral valve is complex anatomic structure. Its proper function strictly depends on the structural and functional integrity of its individual components, which include the mitral valve annulus, leaflets, chordae tendineae, and subvalvular apparatus, including the papillary muscles and left ventricular wall (**Fig. 1**). Derangement of one or more these components characteristically typically results in flow-limiting (ie, stenosis) or regurgitant valvular dysfunction. In either case, a thorough appreciation of the disease mechanisms is essential for the conceptualization and development of alternative, less-invasive, percutaneous mitral valve therapies.

MITRAL STENOSIS—PERCUTANEOUS THERAPIES

Since its introduction in 1984 by Inoue and colleagues,[1] percutaneous mitral balloon valvuloplasty (PMV) has been used successfully as an alternative to open or closed surgical mitral commissurotomy in patients with symptomatic rheumatic mitral stenosis.[2–14] PMV is safe and effective and results in excellent immediate hemodynamic outcome, low complication rates, and improved clinical benefit. Sustained clinical and hemodynamic improvements have been previously reported and are similar to those of surgical

mitral commisssurotomy. Nevertheless, because of the less-invasive nature of PMV, currently it is considered the preferred therapy for relief of mitral stenosis in symptomatic patients with rheumatic heart disease.

Proper patient selection is a fundamental step when predicting the immediate results of PMV (**Fig. 2**). Candidates for PMV require precise assessment of mitral valve morphology.[1–5,15] The echocardiographic score (Echo-Sc) is currently the most widely used method for predicting PMV outcome.[7–11] Leaflet mobility, leaflet thickening, valvular calcification, and subvalvular disease are each scored from 1 to 4, yielding a maximum total Echo-Sc of 16.[14] An inverse relationship exists between the Echo-Sc and PMV success.

Both-Immediate, and intermediate follow-up studies have shown that patients with Echo-Sc less than or equal to 8 have superior results and significantly greater survival and combined event-free survival than patients with Echo-Sc greater than 8.[6,9,10] Long-term follow-up results, however, are scarce,[12,13,16] and although earlier studies have reported that PMV results in good immediate hemodynamic and clinical improvement in most patients with mitral rheumatic stenosis,[6–14,16] superior long-term follow-up results are seen in a selected group of patients with Echo-Sc less than or equal to 8. The authors have recently reported other clinical and morphologic predictors of long-term PMV success (**Fig. 3**) that include pre-(mitral valve area, history of previous surgical commissurotomy, age, and mitral

Interventional Cardiology and Structural Heart Disease, Massachusetts General Hospital, Harvard Medical School, Boston, MA 02114, USA
* Corresponding author.
E-mail address: ipalacios@partners.org (I.F. Palacios).

Cardiol Clin 28 (2010) 139–153
doi:10.1016/j.ccl.2009.09.006

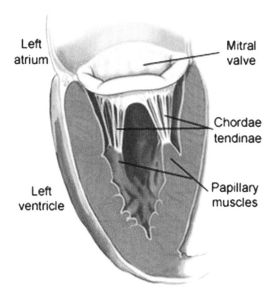

Fig. 1. The mitral valve apparatus.

left heart pressure measurements, cardiac output, and oxygen saturation determinations should be routinely performed before and after PMV. The mitral valve area (MVA) is calculated with the Gorlin formula. Left ventriculography is performed before and after PMV to assess the severity of MR using Sellers' classification. The effective balloon-dilating area by used is calculated using the standard geometric formulas normalized to body surface area.[19]

There has been some controversy as to whether or not the double-balloon or Inoue technique provides superior immediate and long-term results. The authors have reported that the double-balloon technique results in larger post-PMV mitral valve area and a lower incidence of severe post-PMV MR.[22] No significant differences in event-free survival at long-term follow-up between the two techniques were observed, however. Thus, the Inoue and the double-balloon techniques seem equally effective techniques of PMV. Failure rates of PMV are variable (1% to 15%) and highly dependent on operator experience. PMV-related morbidity and mortality are low and similar to surgical commissurotomy. It is estimated that the PMV procedural mortality rate ranges between 0% and 3%. Hemopericardium however may be seen in up to 12% of cases. Systemic embolization has been reported in 0.5% to 5% of cases. In spite of this, one of the most concerning complications of PMV is the development of severe MR after balloon inflation which occurs

regurgitation [MR]) and post-PMV variables (MR ≥3 and pulmonary artery pressure), that may be used in conjunction with the Echo-Sc to further optimally identify candidate patients for PMV.[17,18]

Percutaneous Mitral Balloon Valvuloplasty Technique

PMV is more frequently performed using the double-balloon (**Fig. 4**) or the Inoue single-balloon technique (**Fig. 5**).[1,19–22] In either case, right and

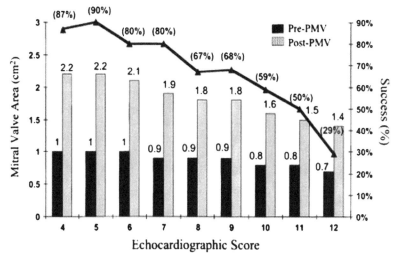

Fig. 2. Relationship between the Echo-Sc and changes in mitral valve area after PMV (*bar graph*) and relationship between the Echo-Sc and PMV success (*line with filled triangles*). Numbers at the top of rectangular bars represent mean mitral valve areas before (*black bars*) and after (*shaded bars*) PMV for each Echo-Sc. Percentages in parentheses represent PMV success rate at each Echo-Sc. (*From* Palacios IF, Sanchez PL, Harrell LC, et al. Which patients benefit from percutaneous mitral balloon valvuloplasty? Prevalvuloplasty and postvalvuloplasty variables that predict long-term outcome. Circulation 2002;105(12):1465–71; with permission.)

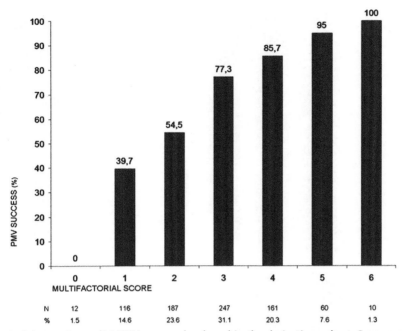

Fig. 3. Multifactorial score to predict PMV success developed in the derivation cohort. Score constructed by an arithmetic sum of the number of PMV success predictors (age <55 years, NYHA classes I and II, pre-PMV mitral valve area ≥ 1 cm^2, pre-PMV MR grade <2, Echo-Sc >8, and male gender) present for each patient. Rates of PMV success were calculated for various patient subgroups on the basis of the multifactorial score. Success increased incrementally as the PMV success predictor score increased (P<.001 by $\times2$ for trend). (*From* Cruz-Gonzalez I, et al. A multifactorial score. Am J Med 2009;122(6):581.e11–89; with permission.)

in 2% to 10% of patients and typically results from noncommissural leaflet tearing, particularly in patients less favorable anatomy. In these cases, urgent surgery is rarely required (<1% in experienced centers) but however, may be necessary when massive hemopericardium or severe MR results in hemodynamic collapse and refractory pulmonary edema.

Percutaneous Mitral Balloon Valvuloplasty Outcomes

The authors recently reported clinical results from 844 consecutive patients who underwent PMV at the Massachusetts General Hospital at a mean follow-up of 4.2 ($\pm$3.7) years.[17] For the entire population, there were 110 deaths (25 noncardiac), 234 mitral valve replacements (MVRs), and 54

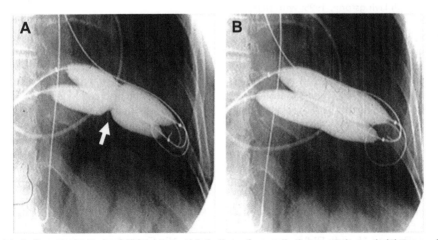

Fig. 4. Double-balloon technique of PMV. (*A*) Double balloon from mitral stenosis (*arrow*). (*B*) Successful balloon dilatation. *From* Palacios IF. Balloon dilation of the cardiac valves. In: Willerson JT, Kohn JN, editors. Cardiovascular Medicine, Second Edition. New York: Churchill Livingstone, 1995; with permission.

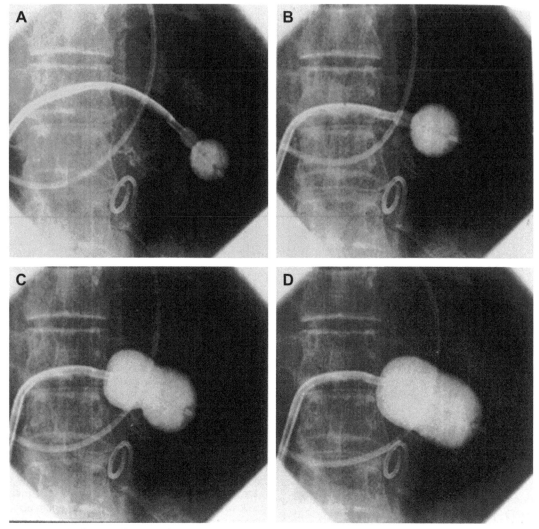

Fig. 5. Inoue balloon technique of PMV. Progressive balloon dilation across the mitral valve. *From* Palacios IF. Balloon dilation of the cardiac valves. In: Willerson JT, Kohn JN, editors. Cardiovascular Medicine, Second Edition. New York: Churchill Livingstone, 1995; with permission.

redo PMVs, accounting for a total of 398 patients with combined events (death, MVR, or redo PMV). Of the remaining 446 patients who were free of combined events, 418 (94%) were classified as New York Heart Association (NYHA) class I or II. Follow-up events occurred less frequently in patients with Echo-Sc less than or equal to 8 and included 51 deaths, 155 MVRs, and 39 redo PMVs, accounting for a total of 245 patients with combined events at follow-up. Of the remaining 330 patients who were free of combined events, 312 (95%) were in NYHA class I or II. Events in patients with Echo-Sc greater than 8 included 59 deaths, 79 MVRs, and 15 redo PMVs, accounting for a total of 153 patients with combined events at follow-up. Of the remaining 116 patients who

were free of any event, 105 (91%) were in NYHA class I or II.

Fig. 6 shows the estimated total survival curves for the overall population and for patients with Echo-Sc less than or equal to 8 and those greater than 8. As shown, survival rates were significantly better in patients with Echo-Sc less than or equal to 8 at a follow-up time of 12 years compared with patients with Echo-Sc greater than 8 (82% versus 57%, $P<.001$). **Fig. 7** shows the estimated event-free survival estimates (alive and free of MVR or redo PMV) for patients with Echo-Sc less than or equal to 8, 9 to 11, and Echo-Sc greater than 12. Event-free survival (38% versus 22%, $P<.0001$) at 12 years' follow-up were also significantly higher for patients with Echo-Sc less

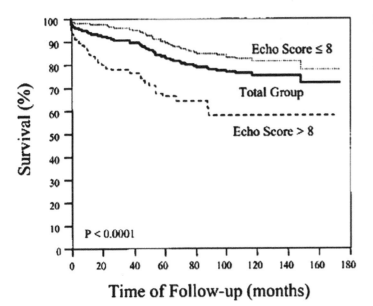

Fig. 6. Kaplan-Meier survival estimates for all patients and for patients with Echo-Sc ≤8 and >8. (*From* Palacios IF, et al. Circulation 2002;105(12):1465–71; with permission.)

than or equal to 8. Cox regression analysis identified post-PMV MR greater than or equal to 3+, Echo-Sc greater than 8, age, prior commissurotomy, NYHA class IV, pre-PMV MR greater than or equal to 2+, and post-PMV pulmonary artery pressure as independent predictors of combined events at long-term follow-up.

In summary, PMV results in excellent immediate and long-term results similar to those of surgical commissurotomy. Randomized trials have demonstrated no significant difference between strategies.[23–25] As previously discussed, patient selection is essential in predicting PMV results and requires proper preprocedural evaluation of mitral valve morphology. The determinants of

PMV success are multifactorial and include demographic, clinical, and hemodynamic variables in addition to the more important echocardiographic Wilkins score.[15] The recently reported multifactorial score may be used to further identify the subset patients who derive the greatest clinical benefit from PMV.[18]

MITRAL REGURGITATION—PERCUTANEOUS THERAPIES

MR remains one of the most common forms of valvular heart disease.[26] It is estimated that up to 20% of patients with heart failure and 12% of patients post–myocardial infarction have at least

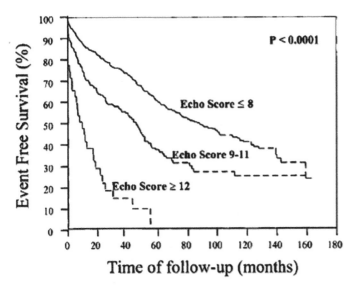

Fig. 7. Kalpan-Meier survival estimates (alive and free of MVR or redo PMV) for patients with Echo-Sc <8, 9 to 12, and >12. (*From* Palacios IF, et al. Circulation 2002;105(12):1465–71; with permission.)

moderate MR.[27,28] Mitral insufficiency typically results from primary valvular disease or as a consequence of a myopathic dilated left ventricle that results in downward papillary muscle displacement, leaflet tethering, annular dilatation, and progressive left ventricular remodeling. The latter is known as functional MR and has been associated with marked decrease in survival among heart failure, post–myocardial infarction, and perioperative surgical bypass patients. In either case, until recently, available treatment options were limited to open surgical repair or replacement, and, although this option exists, it is often challenging and associated with high operative morbidity, disease recurrence, and increased mortality.[29–31] Consequently, hundreds of thousands of patients are left untreated. In the European Heart Survey, up to one-third of patients with symptomatic severe valve disease were denied surgery, including one-half with severe symptomatic MR.[32] The pursuit of less-invasive, alternative, transcatheter therapies has been important. Currently, more than 10 percutaneous mitral regurgitant programs are being developed. Some are on the verge of mainstay therapy whereas others remain in preclinical stages. This article provides a comprehensive overview of the current status, applicability, and limitations of these novel emerging mitral regurgitant therapies. For practical purposes the may be divided into (1) percutaneous leaflet repair, (2) direct or indirect annuloplasty, and (3) transatrial or transventricular mitral valvular complex remodeling.

Percutaneous Leaflet Repair

In 2000, Alfieri and colleagues[33] introduced a simplistic and revolutionary surgical technique to treat degenerative and functional MR. Although initially poorly accepted, the Alfieri stitch, or edge-to-edge, technique gained increasing popularity among many surgeons.[34] By suturing the free edges of the middle anterior (A2) and posterior (P2) mitral leaflets and creating a double-orifice inlet valve, the edge-to-edge technique improves leaflet coaptation and thus decreases MR. Acceptable results have been reported for degenerative and functional MR, with 5-year freedom from recurrent MR greater than 2+ and reoperation rates of up to 90 (±5%).[35] The results have triggered the development of less-invasive transcatheter edge-to-edge techniques. To date, two major mitral valve programs have been developed to mimic the double-orifice strategy using a catheter-based approach: the MitraClip (Evalve, Menlo Park, California) and the MOBIUS (Edwards Lifesciences, Irvine, California) system.

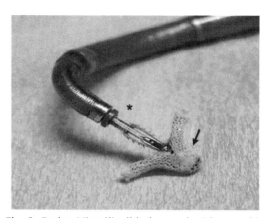

Fig. 8. Evalve MitraClip (*black arrow*) with steerable delivery system (*asterisk*) . (*From* Chiam PT, del Valle-Fernández R, Ruiz CE. [Percutaneous transcatheter valve therapy]. Rev Esp Cardiol 2008;61(Suppl 2): 10–24 [in Spanish].)

The MitraClip

The MitraClip is a unique device that is delivered using a triaxial catheter system to create a double-orifice mitral valve (**Fig. 8**). After the initial encouraging results in animal models, the revolutionary transcatheter technique was first implanted in humans in June 2003.[36] At 2-year follow-up, the 56-year-old woman with heart failure and severe 4+ MR remained symptom-free with less than 2+ MR.[37] Safety and feasibility results of the MitraClip system have now been tested in the Endovascular Valve Edge-to-Edge Repair Study (EVEREST) phase I and phase II study.[38] Preliminary results of the initial 107 patients (EVEREST I, 55, and EVEREST II, 52) with degenerative (79%) or functional MR (21%) are encouraging. Implant success occurred in 90% of patients, of which acute success (MR grade ≤2+) was reported in 84% of the cases. Among these patients, improvement in NYHA functional class was reported in 73% at 1-year follow-up. To date, approximately 400 patients have been treated with the MitraClip system. Importantly, reports of clip failure are well tolerated and do not preclude patients from surgical mitral valve repair or replacement.

Technically, the MitraClip system consists of three major subsystems: a guide catheter, a clip delivery system, and the MitraClip implant with two arms used to grasp and fasten together the valve leaflets. The guide catheter is 24F proximally and tapers to 22F distally. It is inserted from the femoral vein and advanced above the mitral valve following a transseptal puncture. The steering knob allows flexion and lateral movement of the distal tip so that the clip is positioned orthogonally over the three planes of the mitral valve and the origin of the regurgitant jet. The opened span of the clip is approximately 2 cm and the width is 4 mm. Leaflet tissue is secured between the closed arms and locked effectively to maintain coaptation of the two leaflets.

The degree of MR can be assessed during the procedure with the aid of a transesophageal echocardiography. If necessary, the clip can be reopened, the mitral leaflets released, and the clip repositioned. Once optimal reduction of MR is achieved, the clip is released from the clip delivery system, and the delivery system and guide catheter are withdrawn. Repeat hemodynamic, angiographic, and echocardiographic assessments are routinely performed. Heparin is routinely used during the procedure and administered to achieve an activated clotting time of 250 seconds or more. Aspirin (325 mg) and clopidogrel (75 mg) daily are ordinarily recommended after the procedure for 6 months and 30 days, respectively.

The final results of the EVEREST II trial are highly awaited. This prospective, randomized, multi-center study is expected to enroll 279 patients in the United States and Canada. Patients are randomized 2:1 to receive the MitraClip device. The study was initiated in 2005 and is intended to compare the Evalve MitraClip with current standard of care, including mitral valve surgery. The same sites are also enrolling patients in a high-risk registry. The favorable preliminary results on MR reduction, left ventricular reverse remodeling, and preservation of a subsequent surgical options strongly suggest that the MitraClip system may become a viable option for many patients.

The MOBIUS leaflet repair system

The MOBIUS Leaflet Repair system (Edwards Lifesciences), previously called the Milano Stitch, was introduced by Dr. Maurice Buchbinder as a similar catheter-based edge-to-edge technique. Contrary to the MitraClip, this strategy uses a small guiding catheter to stitch the free edges of the anterior and the posterior mitral leaflets, thus creating a double-orifice inlet valve. An innovative suction catheter is used to adhere the leaflets together and facilitate stitch placement under fluoroscopic and echocardiographic guidance.[39] After the successful animal model experience, the first human procedure was performed in Milan, Italy, in a 67-year-old woman with NYHC functional class III and severe MR secondary to a prolapsed posterior leaflet.[40] Subsequently, the percutaneous Alfieri-like stitch was tested in a feasibility trial of 15 patients with degenerative or functional MR. In this phase I study, acute procedure success occurred in 9 of 15 patients. Of these, three patients

required a single stitch, five required two stitches, and one patient required three stitches. At 30-day follow-up, only 66% of the patients (six of nine) had a successful stitch in place with at least one grade improvement in MR reduction. The acute failure patients (6 of 15) all underwent subsequent successful surgical repair. Unfortunately, the study's intermediate result has prompted the investigators to suspend further evaluation for this particular indication.

Percutaneous Annuloplasty

As previously discussed, mitral annular dilation is a common pathologic problem in patients with severe persistent MR. Accordingly, surgical annuloplasty results in septal-lateral annular shortening and decrease in MR severity.[41] Long-term safety and efficacy results after surgical annuloplasty report freedom from recurrent MR and need for reoperation in 82% and 95% of patients during 7-year follow-up, respectively.[42] Consequently, there has been a major drive to duplicate these results with catheter-based techniques.

Direct annuloplasty techniques

The Mitralign system The Mitralign system (Mitralign) is one of the first insightful direct endovascular percutaneous annuloplasty systems. It consists of a deflectable catheter that is manipulated and advanced retrogradely across the aortic valve through a 14F femoral sheath into the subvalvular mitral valve space. Once properly aligned, anchor pledgets are delivered from the left ventricle to the left atrium across the circumferential mitral valve annulus and pulled together with a guide wire to decrease the annulus septal-lateral dimension. The approach uses standard fluoroscopic imaging. The feasibility and durability of this technique were confirmed in early animal studies wherein significant reductions in MR were demonstrated.[42] Currently, the technique is being tested in a European-based safety and feasibility phase I clinical study; however, preliminary results have yet to be released.

The AccuCinch system The AccuCinch system (Guided Delivery Systems, California) is another promising strategy that is soon to commence its first clinical investigation with humans in Europe. It too uses a specific endovascular retrograde catheter that crosses the aortic valve and accommodates within the subannular mitral valve space. Once this first determinant step is accomplished, a series of interconnecting endomyocardial anchors are sequentially released across the subvalvular mitral annulus. An adjustable intercommunicating cinching wire permits effective septal-lateral annular reduction and MR improvement. To the authors' knowledge, the AccuCinch system has been successfully tested during open heart surgery in two patients with +2 MR and coronary disease undergoing routine coronary artery bypass grafting. The surgically implanted device resulted in sustained and successful reductions in MR severity (from +2 to 0) at 6- and 12-month follow-up. The first percutaneous implant in humans is expected to occur in Europe later this year.

The QuantumCor system The QuantumCor system (QuantumCor) is a unique and different concept that has yet to be tested in humans. It involves an end-loop catheter electrode system that delivers subablative radiofrequency energy to induce heating and shrinkage of the collagen tissue of the mitral annulus. The technique has been tested in acute and chronic sheep models where up to 20% reductions in septal-lateral annular dimensions have been reported.[43] Histopathologic examination has shown no evidence of undesirable injury among the vicinity of related structures.

Indirect annuloplasty—coronary sinus techniques

Considering the technical difficulties of percutaneous direct annuloplasty in the beating heart, other insightful, less-demanding technical approaches have been explored. Among them is the use of the coronary sinus, a distinct anatomic structure that lies in close relationship to the posterior-lateral circumference of the mitral valve annulus.[44] Any conformation change of the coronary sinus may be used advantageously to reduce the septal-lateral annular dimensions and improve MR severity. Interest in this approach is reflected by the many programs that have been developed based on this premise (discussed later).

The Monarc system The Monarc system (Edwards Lifesciences) is a percutaneously implanted coronary sinus device that is designed to improve MR severity over an estimated 3- to 6-week period. The rationale is to remodel the mitral annulus by implanting a bioabsorbable spring-like bridge that is connected between two self-expanding proximal and distal stents (**Fig. 9**). The procedure is performed through a 12-F catheter under local anesthesia via the right internal jugular vein. The stent anchors, once delivered, provide the force necessary to draw the proximal coronary sinus and distal great cardiac vein together while the interconnecting bridge tenses and foreshortens over time. The conformational changes invoked over the posterior annular segment presumably

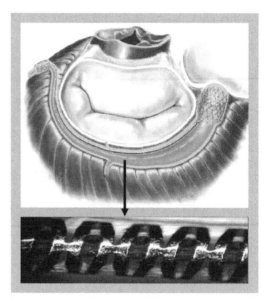

Fig. 9. Cartoon illustration of the Monarc system deployed within the coronary sinus (*top*). Bioabsorbable intercommunucating ridge (*bottom*).

shortens the septal-lateral dimensions to reduce MR severity.

The first human experience with the Monarc system was reported by Webb and colleagues[45] in 2006 and included five patients with chronic ischemic severe MR. Implantation was successful in four of the five patients and resulted in mean decrease in MR grade from +3.0 (±0.7) to +1.6 (±1.1). Nonetheless, loss of efficacy was later seen in three of the patients due to asymptomatic separation and fracture of the bridging segment. After device modification and reinforcement of the bridging segment, the EVOLUTION phase I study was conducted. In this study, successful implantation was achieved in 59 of the 72 patients (82%) with functional MR and heart failure. Freedom from death, MI, and cardiac tamponade at 30 days was 91%. Coronary artery compression was noted in 30% of patients. Major adverse events at 18 months included one death, three myocardial infarctions, two coronary sinus perforations, one anchor displacement, and four anchor separations. The study proved that the Monarc system is feasible to implant and, although efficacy data is encouraging, coronary compression and anchor separations remain concerns and limitations. The EVOLUTION phase II clinical trial is scheduled to commence this year and will hopefully serve to identify those that benefit most.

The Carillon Mitral Contour system The Carillon Mitral Contour System (Cardiac Dimensions) is another unique coronary sinus annuloplasty

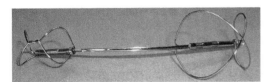

Fig. 10. Carillon Mitral Contour System. (*From* Chiam PT, del Valle-Fernández R, Ruiz CE. [Percutaneous transcatheter valve therapy]. Rev Esp Cardiol 2008;61(Suppl 2):10–24 [in Spanish].)

device. It consists of two helical anchors and an intercommunicating nitinol bridge. It is delivered percutaneously under fluoroscopic guidance from the right internal jugular vein (**Fig. 10**). Once access to the coronary sinus has been obtained and angiography performed, the distal smallest anchor is deployed and gradual tension applied so that the posterior annulus moves anteriorly and the septal-lateral dimensions shorten. The results are best appreciated by the immediate reduction in MR severity seen during transesophageal echocardiography. The Carillon system is simple and unique, as it is adjustable and recapturable in cases of malposition or inefficacy. Its delivery system measures 60 mm in length whereas the distal and proximal anchors vary in size from 7 to 14 mm and 12 to 20 mm, respectively. Initial experiments in dogs were encouraging and demonstrated acute and chronic reductions in mitral annular dimensions (from 2.7 [±0.2] cm to 2.3 [±0.1] cm, $P<.05$) and in the ratio of MR to left atrial area (from 16 [±4] to 4 [±1], $P = .052$).[46,47]

The device was first tested in humans by Joachim Schofer in Hamburg, Germany. Acute results from a European phase I safety and efficacy trial, Carillon Mitral Annuloplasty Device European Union Study (AMADEUS), were recently reported.[48] The study included patients with congestive heart failure, greater than or equal to 2+ functional MR, and depressed left ventricular systolic function (ejection fraction <40%). Successful implantation occurred in 70% of the patients (30 of 43) and resulted in improved functional class and MR severity of at least 1+ in 80% of the cases. Those who benefited most had evidence of congestive heart failure and greater than or equal to 2+ centric MR secondary to mitral annulus dilation. Major adverse events at 1 month follow-up included two myocardial infarctions, two coronary sinus perforations, one dissection, one anchor displacement, one contrast nephropathy, and one death. The device crossed the coronary arteries 84% of the time; however, left circum FLEX flow compromise was seen in only six patients (14%) in whom the device was immediately recaptured.

The Viacor Percutaneous Transvenous Mitral Annuloplasty device The Percutaneous Transvenous Mitral Annuloplasty (PTMA) device (Viacor) consists of a 7F polytetrafluoroethylene catheter through which different rigid elements are introduced into the coronary sinus from the right jugular or subclavian vein. Up to three rods of varying stiffness and length are inserted behind the P2 segment of the posterior mitral valve leaflet depending on the tension required to shorten the

A

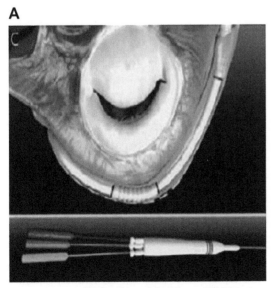

B

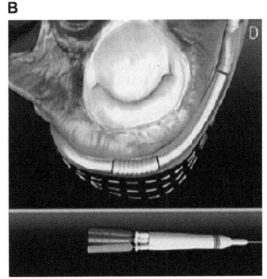

Fig. 11. Cartoon illustration of the Viacor PTMA system within the coronary sinus. Notice change in septal-lateral annular dimension between (*A*) and (*B*). (*Courtesy of* Viacor, Wilmington, MA.)

septal-lateral annular dimension (**Fig. 11**). The device may be retrieved in the absence of efficacy or in the presence of arterial compromise. Preliminary studies in sheep models were highly encouraging and resulted in decrease MR severity (from +3–4 to +0–1, P<.03) and associated with significant reductions in septal-lateral mitral annular dimensions (from 30 [±2.1] mm to 24 [±1.7] mm, P<.03).[49] The first feasibility and safety study in humans was reported by Dubreuil and colleagues[50] in 2007 and included four patients with ischemic MR and NYHA class II or III requiring surgical mitral annuloplasty. In this study, the device was temporally implanted, adjusted, and subsequently removed. The investigators report substantial reductions in regurgitant volumes (45.5 [±24.4] to 13.3 [±7.3] mL) due to the mechanically induced anterior-posterior diameter reduction (40.75 [±4.3] to 35.2 [±1.6] mm) in three patients. In one patient, the device could not be deployed due to extreme angulated anatomy. The study represents a small sample and did not include patients with mitral leaflet or mitral apparatus abnormality.

The recently reported Canadian and European phase I Percutaneous Transvenous Mitral Annuloplasty (PTOLEMY) trial included 27 patients with NYHA functional class II or III and moderate to severe functional MR Sack and colleagues.[51] Successful implantation was performed in 19 of the 27 patients. The remainder were excluded due to unsuitable coronary sinus anatomy. Of those who underwent successful implantation, 13 had a reduction in MR severity, and in six, the device was ineffective. Device removal was required in four patients due to fracture or device migration or diminished efficacy. Long-term success in MR reduction was seen in only 18.5% of the patients. The phase II PTOLEMY trial is currently under way in Europe, Canada, and the United States and is expected to enroll 60 patients with moderate to severe MR, class II to IV heart failure, and left ventricular dysfunction (ejection fraction 25% to 50%).

Remodeling of the Mitral Valvular Complex

An interesting group of transcatheter devices are those currently being developed to improve the paravalvular geometric distortion that is universally encountered in patients with nonorganic or functional MR. As discussed previously, functional MR is best defined a disease of the left ventricle that results in secondary mitral insufficiency and frequently seen in patients with dilated cardiomyopathies. Unfortunately, medical treatment options provide only minimal improvement in MR and the

remaining mechanical treatments fall only within the realm of open heart surgery, including annuloplasty repair or prosthetic MVR.[29,52]

The Percutaneous Septal Sinus Shortening system

The Percutaneous Septal Sinus Shortening system, also known as PS3 (Ample Medical) is a sophisticated transcatheter atrial/mitral annulus remodeling device that integrates several concepts and consists of three basic elements: (1) an atrial septal occluder, (2) an interconnecting cinching wire, and (3) permanent small coronary sinus T-bar element positioned behind P2 (**Fig. 12**). The interatrial occluder serves as a pivotal anchor and allows cinching to occur from the posterior annulus to the superior medial interatrial septum. The concept was developed based on the premise that previous animal studies showed unequivocal increase in posterior wall to interatrial septum dimensions in functional MR. The authors' initial experience with the PS3 device was first reported in 23 sheep with dilated cardiomyopathy and functional MR. Immediate and midterm results at 30 days revealed reductions in septal to lateral dimensions and MR severity.[53] Coronary arterial impingement was not observed, and the great cardiac vein was patent in all animals during follow-up histopathologic examination. Significant hemodynamic improvements and a drop in brain natriuretic peptide levels were observed. Finally, there was no evidence of device migration, erosion, or intra-atrial bridge thrombosis.

The feasibility and safety of this technique was first confirmed in two patients undergoing

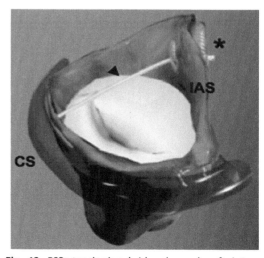

Fig. 12. PS3: tensioning bridge (*arrowhead*); interatrial septal anchor (*asterisk*). CS, coronary sinus; IAS, interatrial septum. (*Adapted from* Rogers JH, et al. Circulation 2006;113(19):2329–34.)

temporary implantation of the PS3 system before clinically indicated mitral valve repair surgery.[54] In the first patient, the PS3 resulted in a relative change of 29% in septal-lateral dimension and was associated with a 1+ decrease in MR severity. The MR severity in the second patient decreased from +3 to +1 after a 31% relative change in septal-lateral dimension. No procedural complications were reported. The CAFÉ trial is an ongoing phase I safety and feasibility study that will test the safety and efficacy of the chronic PS3 implant in humans with heart failure and severe functional MR. Promising preliminary results are expected and recently presented by Cubeddu at the transcatheter therapeutic meeting in San Francisco, CA in September 2009.

The iCoapsys

The iCoapsys (Myocor) left ventricular reshaping device was, until recently, a promising alternative percutaneous strategy developed to treat functional MR. Although no longer in use, the strategy represents a concept that is worthy of mention and may one day re-emerge through improved concepts. The iCoapsys transventricular system consists of an anterior and posterior epicardial pad tethered together by a subvalvular transventricular chord that travels through the left ventricle and between the papillary muscles (**Fig. 13**). After its implantation via subxyphoid pericardial approach, the chord length can be reduced and adjusted to establish optimal septal-lateral left ventricle and annular dimensions. Conformational changes are intended to reorient the papillary muscles and reduce left ventricle geometric distortion, resulting in decrease in regurgitant orifice and MR severity. Promising results were reported from the early animal experience.[55] Unfortunately, the Food and Drug Administration–approved Valvular and Ventricular Improvement Via iCoapsys Delivery (VIVID) feasibility study in humans was prematurely discontinued due to the inherent technical difficulties during device implantation, and suboptimal patient applicability.

PERIVALVULAR PROSTHETIC MITRAL REGURGITATION

Percutaneous repair of perivalvular prosthetic MR has evolved to become yet another attractive alternative strategy. Paravalvular MR is a well-recognized dreadful complication that may be seen in up to 7% of patients after prosthetic heart valve surgery.[56] Although the majority of affected patients are asymptomatic, heart failure, hemolytic anemia, or infective endocarditis may be seen.[57] In high-risk patients, redo operations are commonly challenging and associated with significantly increased procedural mortality.[58] Nevertheless, a series of percutaneous endovascular devices have been explored and used off-label with promising results.[59–61] Among them are the Amplatzer Vascular Plug, Amplatzer Septal Occluder, and Amplatzer Duct Occluder from AGA Medical (Golden Valley, Minnesota).

The percutaneous treatment of paravalvular mitral leaks is particularly challenging, one of the most difficult in interventional cardiology, mainly because of the increased need for catheter manipulation after transseptal puncture. Consequently,

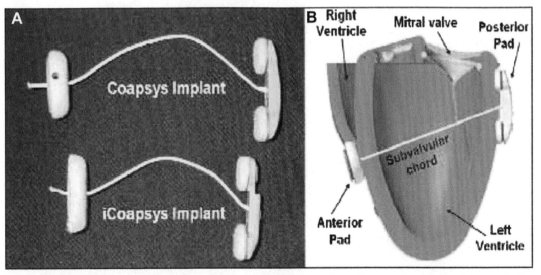

Fig. 13. Cartoon image of the iCoapsys system. (*A*) The epicardial pads and transventricular chord. (*B*) Illustration of the geometry relationship to the mitral valve apparatus. (*From* Pedersen WR, Feldman TE. Percutaneous treatment for FMR: a ventricular approach. Cardiac Interventions Today 2008;2(4):60; with permission.)

the use of steerable, bidirectional tip catheters often becomes necessary to identify and cross the regurgitant defect. In other instances, it is necessary to create an arteriovenous rail using a snaring catheter antegradely or retrogradely. In rare instances, a left ventricular apical puncture is required. The Amplatzer Duct Occluder is the most commonly used device. Oversizing of the device by 2 to 3 mm is typically recommended. Nevertheless, implantation of two or possibly three devices may be necessary. In the authors' experience, simultaneous 3-D transesophageal echocardiogram imaging should be encouraged in all cases, as it provides optimal information during device implantation (**Fig. 14**).[62] Although the feasibility and effectiveness of these techniques have been reported, it should be remembered that these devices were not specifically designed for this indication. Nevertheless, the authors are hopeful that the encouraging results will prompt the development of transcatheter-specific paravalvular closure techniques and are confident that these advances, and those related to intraoperative imaging (ie, 4-D TEE), will ultimately result in improved technical success and long-term clinical outcome.

SUMMARY

Over the past 10 years, novel nonsurgical strategies for the treatment of valvular heart disease have opened new options in patient care. Animal and early human studies indicate that many of these techniques are safe effective and feasible. Several clinical studies are currently under way and will likely determine the benefits of transcatheter mitral valve therapy. It is apparent, given the complexity of the mitral valve apparatus and its subvalvular structure, that a single device to treat all forms of MR is unlikely to be developed. The encouraging results of the MitraClip suggest, however, that this technique may eventually play a role in the treatment of organic MR. Furthermore, this technique has recently been applied successfully in several patients with functional MR. The role for isolated coronary sinus devices remains uncertain, however, and limited by the variable relationship between the coronary sinus and the

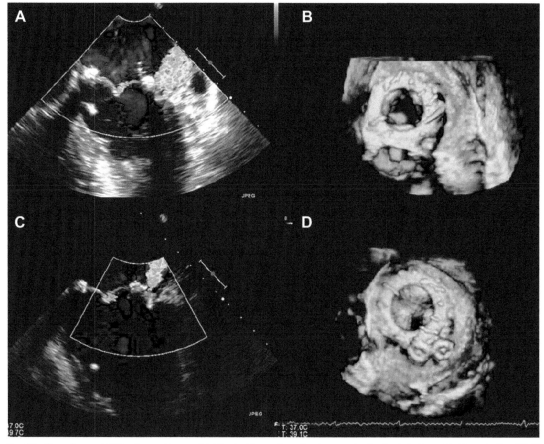

Fig. 14. Doppler and 3-D echocardiographic illustration of a mitral paravalvular leak before (*A, B*) and after (*C, D*) successful transcatheter closure using two side by side Amplatzer Duct Occluder devices.

mitral valve annulus. Ultimately, althrough the role of transcatheter left ventricular remodeling to treat functional MR is ideal, this strategy remains in the infancy of its development. Despite the substantial technical and financial efforts invested in transcatheter mitral valve therapy, most of the emerging devices remain early in their development and will ultimately need to be proven effective when compared to the gold standard open surgical repair. Finally, the applicability of many of these percutaneous interventions will require advanced training of highly qualified operators and interventional standards to prevent the widespread indiscriminant use of these techniques.

REFERENCES

1. Inoue K, Owaki T, Nakamura T, et al. Clinical application of transvenous mitral commissurotomy by a new balloon catheter. J Thorac Cardiovasc Surg 1984; 87(3):394–402.

2. Lock JE, Khalilullah M, Shrivastava S, et al. Percutaneous catheter commissurotomy in rheumatic mitral stenosis. N Engl J Med 1985;313(24):1515–8.

3. Palacios I, Block PC, Brandi S, et al. Percutaneous balloon valvotomy for patients with severe mitral stenosis. Circulation 1987;75(4):778–84.

4. Al Zaibag M, Ribeiro PA, Al Kasab S, et al. Percutaneous double-balloon mitral valvotomy for rheumatic mitral-valve stenosis. Lancet 1986;1(8484): 757–61.

5. Vahanian A, Michel PL, Cormier B, et al. Results of percutaneous mitral commissurotomy in 200 patients. Am J Cardiol 1989;63(12):847–52.

6. McKay RG, Lock JE, Safian RD, et al. Balloon dilation of mitral stenosis in adult patients: postmortem and percutaneous mitral valvuloplasty studies. J Am Coll Cardiol 1987;9(4):723–31.

7. McKay CR, Kawanishi DT, Rahimtoola SH. Catheter balloon valvuloplasty of the mitral valve in adults using a double-balloon technique. Early hemodynamic results. JAMA 1987;257(13):1753–61.

8. Abascal VM, Wilkins GT, O'Shea JP, et al. Prediction of successful outcome in 130 patients undergoing percutaneous balloon mitral valvotomy. Circulation 1990;82(2):448–56.

9. Herrmann HC, Wilkins GT, Abascal VM, et al. Percutaneous balloon mitral valvotomy for patients with mitral stenosis. Analysis of factors influencing early results. J Thorac Cardiovasc Surg 1988; 96(1):33–8.

10. Rediker DE, Block PC, Abascal VM, et al. Mitral balloon valvuloplasty for mitral restenosis after surgical commissurotomy. J Am Coll Cardiol 1988; 11(2):252–6.

11. Palacios IF, Block PC, Wilkins GT, et al. Follow-up of patients undergoing percutaneous mitral balloon valvotomy. Analysis of factors determining restenosis. Circulation 1989;79(3):573–9.

12. Abascal VM, Wilkins GT, Choong CY, et al. Echocardiographic evaluation of mitral valve structure and function in patients followed for at least 6 months after percutaneous balloon mitral valvuloplasty. J Am Coll Cardiol 1988;12(3):606–15.

13. Block PC, Palacios IF, Block EH, et al. Late (two-year) follow-up after percutaneous balloon mitral valvotomy. Am J Cardiol 1992;69(5):537–41.

14. Nobuyoshi M, Hamasaki N, Kimura T, et al. Indications, complications, and short-term clinical outcome of percutaneous transvenous mitral commissurotomy. Circulation 1989;80(4):782–92.

15. Wilkins GT, Weyman AE, Abascal VM, et al. Percutaneous balloon dilatation of the mitral valve: an analysis of echocardiographic variables related to outcome and the mechanism of dilatation. Br Heart J 1988;60(4):299–308.

16. Tuzcu EM, Block PC, Griffin BP, et al. Immediate and long-term outcome of percutaneous mitral valvotomy in patients 65 years and older. Circulation 1992;85(3): 963–71.

17. Palacios IF, Sanchez PL, Harrell LC, et al. Which patients benefit from percutaneous mitral balloon valvuloplasty? Prevalvuloplasty and postvalvuloplasty variables that predict long-term outcome. Circulation 2002;105(12):1465–71.

18. Cruz-Gonzalez I, Sanchez-Ledesma M, Sanchez PL, et al. Predicting success and long-term outcomes of percutaneous mitral valvuloplasty: a multifactorial score. Am J Med 2009;122(6):581. e11–89.

19. Chen CR, Cheng TO, Chen JY, et al. Long-term results of percutaneous mitral valvuloplasty with the Inoue balloon catheter. Am J Cardiol 1992; 70(18):1445–8.

20. Hung JS, Chern MS, Wu JJ, et al. Short- and long-term results of catheter balloon percutaneous transvenous mitral commissurotomy. Am J Cardiol 1991; 67(9):854–62.

21. Cribier A, Eltchaninoff H, Koning R, et al. Percutaneous mechanical mitral commissurotomy with a newly designed metallic valvulotome: immediate results of the initial experience in 153 patients. Circulation 1999;99(6):793–9.

22. Leon MN, Harrell LC, Simosa HF, et al. Comparison of immediate and long-term results of mitral balloon valvotomy with the double-balloon versus Inoue techniques. Am J Cardiol 1999;83(9):1356–63.

23. Turi ZG, Reyes VP, Raju BS, et al. Percutaneous balloon versus surgical closed commissurotomy for mitral stenosis. A prospective, randomized trial. Circulation 1991;83(4):1179–85.

24. Reyes VP, Raju BS, Wynne J, et al. Percutaneous balloon valvuloplasty compared with open surgical commissurotomy for mitral stenosis. N Engl J Med 1994;331(15):961–7.

25. Ben Farhat M, Ayari M, Maatouk F, et al. Percutaneous balloon versus surgical closed and open mitral commissurotomy: seven-year follow-up results of a randomized trial. Circulation 1998;97(3):245–50.

26. Nkomo VT, Gardin JM, Skelton TN, et al. Burden of valvular heart diseases: a population-based study. Lancet 2006;368(9540):1005–11.

27. Robbins JD, Maniar PB, Cotts W, et al. Prevalence and severity of mitral regurgitation in chronic systolic heart failure. Am J Cardiol 2003;91(3):360–2.

28. Bursi F, Enriquez-Sarano M, Nkomo VT, et al. Heart failure and death after myocardial infarction in the community: the emerging role of mitral regurgitation. Circulation 2005;111(3):295–301.

29. McGee EC, Gillinov AM, Blackstone EH, et al. Recurrent mitral regurgitation after annuloplasty for functional ischemic mitral regurgitation. J Thorac Cardiovasc Surg 2004;128(6):916–24.

30. Gillinov AM, Wierup PN, Blackstone EH, et al. Is repair preferable to replacement for ischemic mitral regurgitation? J Thorac Cardiovasc Surg 2001;122(6):1125–41.

31. Grossi EA, Goldberg JD, LaPietra A, et al. Ischemic mitral valve reconstruction and replacement: comparison of long-term survival and complications. J Thorac Cardiovasc Surg 2001;122(6):1107–24.

32. Iung B, Baron G, Butchart EG, et al. A prospective survey of patients with valvular heart disease in Europe: the Euro Heart Survey on Valvular Heart Disease. Eur Heart J 2003;24(13):1231–43.

33. Alfieri O, Maisano F, De Bonis M, et al. The double-orifice technique in mitral valve repair: a simple solution for complex problems. J Thorac Cardiovasc Surg 2001;122(4):674–81.

34. Maisano F, Caldarola A, Blasio A, et al. Midterm results of edge-to-edge mitral valve repair without annuloplasty. J Thorac Cardiovasc Surg 2003;126(6):1987–97.

35. Maisano F, Vigano G, Calabrese C, et al. Quality of life of elderly patients following valve surgery for chronic organic mitral regurgitation. Eur J Cardiothorac Surg 2009;36(2):261–6.

36. St Goar FG, Fann JI, Komtebedde J, et al. Endovascular edge-to-edge mitral valve repair: short-term results in a porcine model. Circulation 2003;108(16):1990–3.

37. Condado JA, Acquatella H, Rodriguez L, et al. Percutaneous edge-to-edge mitral valve repair: 2-year follow-up in the first human case. Catheter Cardiovasc Interv 2006;67(2):323–5.

38. Feldman T, Wasserman HS, Herrmann HC, et al. Percutaneous mitral valve repair using the edge-to-edge technique: six-month results of the EVEREST Phase I Clinical Trial. J Am Coll Cardiol 2005;46(11):2134–40.

39. Naqvi TZ, Zarbatany D, Molloy MD, et al. Intracardiac echocardiography for percutaneous mitral valve repair in a swine model. J Am Soc Echocardiogr 2006;19(2):147–53.

40. Naqvi TZ, Buchbinder M, Zarbatany D, et al. Beating-heart percutaneous mitral valve repair using a transcatheter endovascular suturing device in an animal model. Catheter Cardiovasc Interv 2007;69(4):525–31.

41. Tibayan FA, Rodriguez F, Liang D, et al. Paneth suture annuloplasty abolishes acute ischemic mitral regurgitation but preserves annular and leaflet dynamics. Circulation 2003;108(Suppl 1):II128–33.

42. Aybek T, Risteski P, Miskovic A, et al. Seven years' experience with suture annuloplasty for mitral valve repair. J Thorac Cardiovasc Surg 2006;131(1):99–106.

43. Heuser RR, Witzel T, Dickens D, et al. Percutaneous treatment for mitral regurgitation: the QuantumCor system. J Interv Cardiol 2008;21(2):178–82.

44. Maselli D, Guarracino F, Chiaramonti F, et al. Percutaneous mitral annuloplasty: an anatomic study of human coronary sinus and its relation with mitral valve annulus and coronary arteries. Circulation 2006;114(5):377–80.

45. Webb JG, Harnek J, Munt BI, et al. Percutaneous transvenous mitral annuloplasty: initial human experience with device implantation in the coronary sinus. Circulation 2006;113(6):851–5.

46. Maniu CV, Patel JB, Reuter DG, et al. Acute and chronic reduction of functional mitral regurgitation in experimental heart failure by percutaneous mitral annuloplasty. J Am Coll Cardiol 2004;44(8):1652–61.

47. Byrne MJ, Kaye DM, Mathis M, et al. Percutaneous mitral annular reduction provides continued benefit in an ovine model of dilated cardiomyopathy. Circulation 2004;110(19):3088–92.

48. Schofe J, Tuebler T, Treede H, et al. Eur Heart J 2008;29:780 [Abstract].

49. Liddicoat JR, Mac Neill BD, Gillinov AM, et al. Percutaneous mitral valve repair: a feasibility study in an ovine model of acute ischemic mitral regurgitation. Catheter Cardiovasc Interv 2003;60(3):410–6.

50. Dubreuil O, Basmadjian A, Ducharme A, et al. Percutaneous mitral valve annuloplasty for ischemic mitral regurgitation: first in man experience with a temporary implant. Catheter Cardiovasc Interv 2007;69(7):1053–61.

51. Sack S, Kahlert P, Biledeau L, et al. Circulation 2008;118:S808–9 [Abstract].

52. Hung J, Papakostas L, Tahta SA, et al. Mechanism of recurrent ischemic mitral regurgitation after annuloplasty: continued LV remodeling as a moving target. Circulation 2004;110(11 Suppl 1):II85–90.

53. Rogers JH, Macoviak JA, Rahdert DA, et al. Percutaneous septal sinus shortening: a novel procedure

for the treatment of functional mitral regurgitation. Circulation 2006;113(19):2329–34.

54. Palacios IF, Condado JA, Brandi S, et al. Safety and feasibility of acute percutaneous septal sinus shortening: first-in-human experience. Catheter Cardiovasc Interv 2007;69(4):513–8.

55. Pedersen WR, Block P, Leon M, et al. iCoapsys mitral valve repair system: percutaneous implantation in an animal model. Catheter Cardiovasc Interv 2008; 72(1):125–31.

56. Jindani A, Neville EM, Venn G, et al. Paraprosthetic leak: a complication of cardiac valve replacement. J Cardiovasc Surg 1991;32(4):503–8.

57. Safi AM, Kwan T, Afflu E, et al. Paravalvular regurgitation: a rare complication following valve replacement surgery. Angiology 2000;51(6):479–87.

58. Echevarria JR, Bernal JM, Rabasa JM, et al. Reoperation for bioprosthetic valve dysfunction. A decade of clinical experience. Eur J Cardiothorac Surg 1991;5(10):523–6 [discussion 527].

59. Pate GE, Al Zubaidi A, Chandavimol M, et al. Percutaneous closure of prosthetic paravalvular leaks: case series and review. Catheter Cardiovasc Interv 2006;68(4):528–33.

60. Kort HW, Sharkey AM, Balzer DT. Novel use of the Amplatzer duct occluder to close perivalvar leak involving a prosthetic mitral valve. Catheter Cardiovasc Interv 2004;61(4):548–51.

61. Webb JG, Pate GE, Munt BI. Percutaneous closure of an aortic prosthetic paravalvular leak with an Amplatzer duct occluder. Catheter Cardiovasc Interv 2005;65(1):69–72.

62. Johri AM, Yared K, Durst R, et al. Three-dimensional echocardiography-guided repair of severe paravalvular regurgitation in a bioprosthetic and mechanical mitral valve. Eur J Echocardiogr 2009;10(4):572–5.

Transcatheter Aortic Valve Implantation

Raquel del Valle-Fernández, MD,
Claudia A. Martinez, MD, Carlos E. Ruiz, MD, PhD*

KEYWORDS

- Aortic valve stenosis • Percutaneous treatment
- Heart valve prosthesis • Bioprosthesis

Surgical valve replacement has so far been the only effective treatment of symptomatic aortic stenosis (AS).[1,2] Charles Dotter[3] first suggested the possibility of transcatheter placement of prosthetic cardiac valves in 1981. Twenty years later, Cribier and colleagues[4] implanted the first transcatheter aortic valve. The introduction of transcatheter aortic valve implantation (TAVI) made it possible to offer a much less invasive alternative for those patients who are high-risk or nonsurgical candidates. Recent advances in percutaneous valve technology and the satisfactory early results of TAVI have led to a dramatic increase in the number of devices being developed[5,6] and the number of patients with severe AS undergoing percutaneous treatment.

Percutaneous aortic valve (PAV) interventions date back to the 1980s, when balloon aortic valvuloplasty (BAV) was first performed. However, this technique rapidly lost popularity because of the limited long-term benefits compared with medical therapy.[7–9] Thereafter, the concept of balloon-expandable and self-expandable transcatheter valve implantation was introduced. The first reported TAVI in humans, by Cribier and colleagues,[4] took place 7 years ago.

In 2009, there are at least 17 TAVI programs undergoing active research (**Table 1**),[5] and 2 of the transcatheter aortic valve prosthesis are currently approved for clinical use outside the United States: the balloon-expandable Edwards SAPIEN (Edwards Lifesciences Inc, Irving, CA) and the self-expandable CoreValve ReValving (Medtronic, Minneapolis, MN). The number of high-risk or nonsurgical candidate patients being treated with this technology has been growing quickly since these companies obtained CE mark approval in 2007, with more than 7000 implants worldwide to date. No valve has yet obtained US Food and Drug Administration (FDA) approval, and therefore all clinical experience in the United States comes from clinical trials. Furthermore, newer devices are being developed, and this article reviews the current status of these technologies.

PATIENT SELECTION

Selection criteria for TAVI are being developed. Currently, TAVI is available to high-risk surgical or nonsurgical candidates. There is no consensus on what constitutes high risk, but risk scoring systems are often used. The most common systems in use are the Logistic EuroSCORE (mostly in European studies) and the Society of Thoracic Surgeons (STS) score (in US studies), both of which have been validated for patients undergoing cardiac surgery, based on data from the 1990s.[10–13]

However, a recent validation of the EuroSCORE (additive and logistic) using contemporaneous surgical outcomes found substantial differences between the observed and expected mortality risks. The EuroSCORE tends to overestimate risk, whereas the STS risk model may underestimate the current risk of surgical aortic valve replacement (AVR).[14] Furthermore, an evaluation of outcomes of isolated surgical AVR in the STS database from 1997 to 2006 has shown a decrease in morbidity and mortality.[13] A third model,

Funding: Raquel del Valle-Fernández, MD, has a research grant from the Spanish Society of Cardiology.
Structural and Congenital Heart Disease, Lenox Hill Heart and Vascular Institute, 130 East 77th Street, 9th Floor Black Hall, New York, NY 10021-10075, USA
* Corresponding author.
E-mail address: cruiz@lenoxhill.net (C.E. Ruiz).

cardiology.theclinics.com

Table 1
Transcatheter aortic valve technologies

Balloon-expandable	Self-expandable	Other
Edwards SAPIEN	CoreValve ReValving	Direct Flow Medical
Paniagua ETR	Lotus (Sadra	
Entrata ATS 3f	AorTx (Hansen Medical)	
IHT Cordynamics	Sorin Perceval	
	Enable ATS 3f	
	Ventor-Embracer	
	Heart Leaflet Technology	
	JenaValve	
	PercValve (ABPS)	
	Paniagua (ETR)	
	Lutter Tissue	
	IHT Cordynamics	

validated and more specifically designed to predict in-hospital mortality after valve surgery with or without coronary artery bypass graft (CABG), is the Ambler model.[15] Comparisons of the logistic EuroSCORE, STS, and Ambler scores have demonstrated that the STS score is the most sensitive of these 3 models for assessing perioperative and long-term mortality for isolated AVR.[12]

Piazza and colleagues[16] described a patient selection algorithm based on 15 anatomic factors evaluated by noninvasive methods (echocardiography, cardiac tomography angiography [CTA], magnetic resonance imaging [MRI]) and angiography, to categorize patients as acceptable or not acceptable for the CoreValve ReValving system.

Assessment of the peripheral arteries is also crucial in selecting candidates for this procedure, and should be part of the inclusion criteria in any TAVI protocol. In addition to vessel caliber and tortuosity assessment with CTA or aortography, a noncontrast computerized tomography (CT) scan is useful to evaluate calcium in the peripheral vessels and the valve.

None of these scoring systems and imaging selection protocols take into consideration other important factors such as frailty index, and therefore it is expected that the results of the current TAVI studies will lead to the development of more specific risk algorithms to better select patients.

PROSTHESIS FOR TAVI
Clinically Approved (Outside United States) Devices

Edwards SAPIEN prosthesis
Technical background The commercially available Edwards SAPIEN prosthesis is the second generation of the Cribier-Edwards valve (**Fig. 1**B). This is a balloon-expandable valve consisting of a stainless steel frame covered by a Dacron skirt, in which 3 leaflets of pericardium are sutured. It is deployed in a subcoronary position during rapid ventricular pacing, via a retrograde transfemoral (TF) or transapical (TA) approach. The leaflets in the first generation were made of equine pericardium, and in the second generation they are made of bovine pericardium, with improvements in the suture to the frame and an increase in the skirt length to reduce aortic regurgitation. There are 2 commercialized sizes: 23 mm (diameter) × 14 mm (height), and 26 mm × 16 mm. The next-generation, lower-profile Edwards XT valve (not yet available commercially) has a new cobalt-chromium frame with a wider opening and modifications in the design of the leaflets. It is currently being tested in the ongoing PREVAIL EU CE Mark trial, which includes a premarket cohort to evaluate system performance and a post-market clinical follow-up phase up to 5 years.

The Edwards valve comes expanded and must be crimped carefully on the balloon with a dedicated device. The crimped profile of the valve will determine the size of the delivery sheath, which is a proprietary system (Retroflex) with torque capabilities. Four generations of this Retroflex system have been developed, with progressively lower profiles and increased flexibility to avoid aortic trauma. A 22F Retroflex-2 delivery sheath is needed for the 23-mm Edwards SAPIEN valve, and a 24F sheath for the 26-mm valve. The next-generation 26-mm Edwards XT valve navigates through a 22F Retroflex-2 sheath, and, in the ongoing PREVAIL EU trial, it is being tested with the 18F Retroflex-4 (Novaflex) delivery sheath.

The dedicated TA delivery system is called ASCENDRA. The initial 33F sheath has evolved to a shorter 26F sheath, which is easier to handle and better at confronting TA pitfalls.

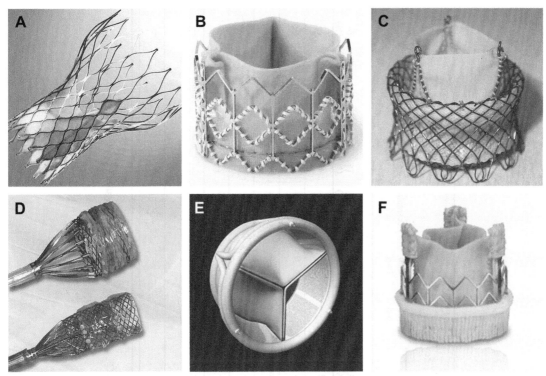

Fig. 1. Transcatheter aortic valve technologies. (*A*) CoreValve. (*Courtesy of* Medtronic, Minneapolis, MN.) (*B*) Edwards SAPIEN. (*Courtesy of* Edwards Life Science, Irvine, CA.) (*C*) HLT valve. (*Courtesy of* Heart Leaflet Technology, Inc., Maple Grove, MN.) (*D*) Lotus valve. (*Courtesy of* Sadra Medical, Inc, Campbell, CA.) (*E*) Direct Flow. (*Courtesy of* Direct Flow Medical, Inc, Santa Rosa, CA.) (*F*) ATS 3f Entrata. (*Courtesy of* ATS Medical, Inc, Minneapolis, MN.)

Clinical status

Antegrade TF (transseptal) approach Initial first-in-man (FIM) and feasibility trials with the 23-mm Cribier-Edwards valve (I-REVIVE and RECAST trials) were developed on a compassionate-use basis for patients who had been rejected for surgery (**Table 2**).[17,18] The procedural success rate in these feasibility trials was 75%, with consistent improvements achieved in the aortic valve area (from 0.60 ± 0.09 cm^2 to 1.70 ± 0.11 cm^2) and in the transvalvular mean gradient (37 ± 13 mm Hg to 9 ± 2 mm Hg). Nevertheless, 30-day event rates were high due to the severe comorbidities of the patients, with a 26% rate of major adverse cardiovascular clinical events (MACCE).[18] Deployment of the prosthesis in these series was mainly transseptal, and the initial experience showed that this approach carried high risk for serious mitral valve injury.[18] Consequently, the transseptal approach was abandoned in favor of the retrograde TF or the TA approach.

Retrograde TF approach A dedicated deflectable sheath (Retroflex) was developed to ease the advancement of the prosthesis and delivery catheter through the aorta and to facilitate crossing the stenotic valve. This delivery catheter was used

initially in the feasibility trials, the Canadian special access trial, and in the multicenter REVIVE II and REVIVAL II. Experience with this approach showed significant improvement on procedural success and 30-day outcomes.[19,20] A learning curve was evident, as procedure success rates increased from 76% in the initial 25 patients to 97% in the following 25 patients. The 30-day mortality figures decreased significantly, from 16% to 8%, in a group of patients with an expected 30-day mortality of 28%.[19,20] Retrograde TAVI produced significant hemodynamic improvement, with a decrease in the mean transaortic valve gradient (from 46 ± 17 mm Hg to 11 ± 5 mm Hg) and an increase in valve area (from 0.6 ± 0.2 cm^2 to 1.7 ± 0.4 cm^2). No valve deterioration occurred at the maximum follow-up of 359 days, and significant improvement in left ventricular ejection fraction and reduction in the grade of mitral regurgitation were also evident at follow-up.[20]

Improvements in the delivery systems may be related to improvements in procedural outcomes. In a recently published article on acute outcomes using the Retroflex-2 system (in 22 patients with the Edwards SAPIEN valve and in 3 patients with the Edwards XT valve), procedural success rate was 100% and no deaths were reported at

Table 2
Summary of Edwards SAPIEN clinical studies

Study	Type	No. of Patients	Access TF	Access TA	Device success (AR<2) TF (%)	Device success (AR<2) TA (%)	Euro SCORE TF	Euro SCORE TA	Survival 30-d TF (%)	Survival 30-d TA (%)	Survival 1 y TF (%)	Survival 1 y TA (%)	Survival 2 y TF (%)	Survival 2 y TA (%)	Stroke 30-d TF (%)	Stroke 30-d TA (%)	AMI 30-d TF (%)	AMI 30-d TA (%)	Pacemaker 30-d TF (%)	Pacemaker 30-d TA (%)	Surgery 30-d TF (%)	Surgery 30-d TA (%)	Valve embolization TF (%)	Valve embolization TA (%)	NYHA I-II 1 year TF (%)	NYHA I-II 1 year TA (%)	MACCE 30-d (%)
RECAST-REVIVE	R	36	26AG 7 RG	—	85 AG 57 RG	—	12	—	75	—	—	—	22	—	2.70	—	0	—	1	—	—	—	?5.5	—	19	—	26
REVIVE II	R	106	106	0	70	NA	28.9 ± 13.4	NA	87	NA	73	NA	—	NA	3	NA	10.5	NA	3.8	NA	1	NA	—	0.60	28–59	NA	—
TRAVERCE	R	172	0	172	NA	90	NA	26.7 ± 12.7	NA	85	NA	65	NA	59	NA	3	NA	1	NA	5.8	NA	6	—	1.70	—	5–16	—
REVIVALII	R	95	55	40	88.9	83.8	34.1 ± 18.0	36.2 ± 15.7	92.7	82.4	—	54.7	—	—	9.2	5.5	16.4	15.2	7.3	2.5	1.90	1.90	—	12.50	—	QOL	—
PARTNER-EU	R	130	61	69	91	91	25.7 ± 11.5	33.8 ± 14.7	92	81	78	50	—	—	3	2	2	5	1.6	4.4	2	3	3.2	1.4	—	—	—
SOURCE	R	1038	463	575	92.4	90.8	25.70	29.20	93.7	89.7	—	—	—	—	2.4	2.6	0.20	0.70	6.7	7.3	1.70	3.50	0	0.50	—	—	—
PARTNER-IDE	RCT	1040	—	—	—	—	—	—	—	—	—	—	—	—	—	—	—	—	—	—	—	—	—	—	—	—	—
PREVAIL-EU 2008	NRC	150	—	—	—	—	—	—	—	—	—	—	—	—	—	—	—	—	—	—	—	—	—	—	—	—	—

Device success is composite including AR less than 2.

Abbreviations: AG, antegrade; AMI, acute myocardial infarction; AR, aortic regurgitation; MACCE, major adverse cardiac/cerebrovascular events; NRC, nonrandomized confirmatory; R, registry; RG, retrograde; RCT, randomized controlled trial; TA, transapical; TF, transfemoral.

30 days.[21] However, the reporting investigators are among the most experienced in TAVI procedures.

The results of 2 prospective European postmarket registries, the SOURCE and the PARTNER EU trial, were presented at EuroPCR 2009 (see **Table 2**). Despite encouraging results, randomized trials are essential to determine whether transcatheter techniques for AVR are a sound alternative to conventional surgical AVR. Determining this is the aim of the ongoing, randomized, PARTNER-US Investigational Device Exemption (IDE) trial. This trial plans to randomize 1040 patients with severe AS, stratified by estimated surgical risk and the severity of the peripheral arterial disease. Patients in whom surgery is considered a reasonable option are randomized to surgery or transcatheter implant (TA in those cases with poor vascular access and TF in the rest), patients with suitable femoral access and prohibitive surgical risk will be randomized to TF aortic valve implantation or conservative management. Patients who do not qualify for surgical AVR, and who have poor vascular access, will not be randomized. More than 700 patients have been recruited to date, and, according to the company, recruitment of the nonsurgical cohort (350 patients) has been completed.

Antegrade TA approach Specifically designed for those patients with peripheral arteriopathy, access to the left ventricle is achieved through a minimally invasive left anterior thoracotomy. This approach is not recommended in patients with previous left ventricle surgery (such as a Dor procedure), calcified pericardium, or severe respiratory insufficiency. Procedural success in the initial studies of this approach was high[22,23]; the FDA feasibility study reported a 10% rate of implant failure. In the European experience, actuarial survival rates at 30 days, 6 months, and 12 months were 92% ($\pm$3.8%), 73.9% ($\pm$6.2%) and 71.4% ($\pm$6.5%) respectively.[24] John Webb at CRT 2009 reported the procedural results from the TRAVERCE trial, to assess the feasibility of the TA approach.

Currently, 36 ongoing studies involving the Edward-SAPIEN and the ASCENDRA valve have been identified, of which 21 have completed enrolment (source: cvPipeline).

Therefore, this TAVI approach is certainly not only a viable alternative for patients with severe AS who also have advanced peripheral vascular disease, but, as technology evolves, a truly percutaneous TA approach may become an attractive alternative, especially if the incidence of cerebrovascular accidents (CVAs) is significantly smaller than with the retrograde transarterial approach.

CoreValve ReValving PAV

Technical background The CoreValve ReValving system consists of 3 leaflets of porcine pericardium mounted on a self-expandable nitinol frame (**Fig. 1**A), which expands from the left ventricular outflow tract to the ascending aorta. The initial device had a 25F profile, but rapidly evolved through a 21F to the current 18F device. This model has facilitated the conversion of this method into a strictly percutaneous technique. The currently available third generation device measures 50 mm in height, and has 3 clearly differentiated sections: (1) an inflow portion that is designed to fix the valve to the annulus that has the highest radial strength, (2) an outflow portion (40 mm in diameter in the third generation valve) that has the lowest radial force and is designed to attach the frame to the ascending aorta to stabilize it, and (3) a central portion that is constrained to avoid obstructing the coronaries and allow coronary perfusion through the struts of the frame. Despite this valve being implanted intra-annularly, its function (coaptation point) is supra-annular. Available sizes are 26 and 29 mm in diameter, designed for annuli between 20 and 27 mm.

Clinical status

TF approach Because technical improvements in the delivery system have occurred quickly, only 14 patients were treated with the 25F system and 52 patients with the 21F system (**Table 3**). More than 3500 implantations have been performed to date with the 18F device. Reports on the first 25 enrolled patients showed a procedural success rate with the first- and second-generation devices of 84%, with a marked improvement in the aortic valve gradient. In-hospital mortality and MACCE occurred in 20% and 32% of the patients, respectively.[25]

A subsequent report on the second-generation (50 patients) and third-generation (36 patients) devices showed a combined acute device success of 88% with an increase in the aortic valve area from 0.60 $\pm$ 0.16 to 1.67 $\pm$ 0.41 cm^2, and overall mortality at 30 days of 12%.[25,26]

A recently published single-center study compared the 3 generations of the CoreValve in 136 patients.[27] Procedural success improved significantly from the first and second generations to the third (70% and 70.8% vs 91.2%, $P = .003$), although it is not possible to isolate the influence of increased operator experience from that of the lower profile of the third generation device. Procedural MACCE also improved with the third generation (20.0% and 16.7% vs 3.9%, $P = .008$). Twelve-month outcome data revealed a rate of death of 40% for the first-generation device,

Table 3
Summary of CoreValve studies

Study	Type	No. of Patients	Access	Device Success (%)	Euro SCORE	Survival 30 d (%)	2 y	1 y	CVA 0-d (%)	AMI 0-d (%)	PPM 30-d (%)	Emergency Surgery (%)	Valve Embolization (%)	NYHC I-II 1 y (%)
S&E Study (CE marking)	R	112	TF	86.50	23.4 ± 13	84.80	—	—	6.30	3.60	26.90	—	—	>30–40
European Registry (post-CE mark)	R	1500	TF	97.30	23 ± 14	89.60	—	—	—	—	—	—	—	—
Australian New Zealand Trial	R	150	TF	98.30	17.6	91.90	—	—	—	—	—	—	—	—
Lange	R	137	TF	98.50	—	87.60	—	—	—	—	—	—	—	—
Grube	R	102	TF	91.20	—	89.20	—	—	1.7/2.5	—	19/28	1.1/0	—	—
U. Pisa Subclavian Revalving	R	393	355TF-38SC	93.5–100	23/26	—	—	—	—	—	—	—	—	—
CoreValve Extended Registry - SC	R	79	79SC	100	28.2 ± 17	90.60	—	—	3.80	0.00	37.50	0	—	—
Laborde	R	584	529TF-55SC	99–100	—	—	—	—	—	—	—	—	—	—

Device success is composite including AR less than 2.
Abbreviations: AMI, acute myocardial infarction; PPM, permanent pacemaker; R, registry; SC, subclavian; TF, transfemoral.

20.8% for the second-generation device, 16% for the third-generation device, and a rate of stroke of 10%, 8.3%, and 3%, respectively.[27]

The most recent results of the postmarket-surveillance CoreValve Multicenter Expanded Evaluation Registry (with the third generation device), including more than 1500 patients, were reported at EuroPCR09 by Patrick Serruys (**Table 3**).

TA approach According to the company, the FIM TA ReValving system implantation was performed in 5 patients in 2007. However, this approach was not pursued further, and the alternative subclavian approach for patients with extensive peripheral vascular disease was explored.

Subclavian approach Left and right subclavian artery access has been reported in several small series, with a 100% procedural success rate and a mortality rate of 6.9%.[28] Jean Claude Laborde presented his experience with the CoreValve Re-Valving system using the subclavian approach at EuroPCR09, and reported a 100% success rate on 79 consecutive patients. These results suggest that this approach may emerge as an alternative for patients with ileofemoral arteries unsuitable for TAVI.

Valve-in-valve The ReValving system has also been implanted successfully in degenerated surgical tissue prostheses (the "valve-in-valve" concept).[29] This is an exciting alternative for patients with significant degenerative changes of previously implanted bioprosthesis with high surgical risk. Positioning may be easier in these cases, as the previous prosthetic ring serves as a marker; however, the current experience is limited. The ReValving system has also been deployed within a previously placed transcatheter valve prosthesis that was positioned incorrectly.[30]

Forty-five other ongoing studies have been identified outside the United States, including single and multicenter registries, of which 17 have completed enrolment (source: cvPipeline).

Complications related to these valve implantations

The rapid increase in the number of patients treated and the longer follow-up available have provided important insights into the complications of these techniques. Previously uncommon complications in the catheter laboratory have gained notoriety since the introduction of TAVI, because of the greater complexity of the procedure and the size of the devices in a high-risk group of patients. Increased operator experience, improved patient selection, and refinements in technology are expected to lower complication rates in the future (**Table 4**).

Vascular injury Initial reports suggested that vascular injury was a serious limitation with retrograde approaches.[6] The rate of vascular complications in a pooled analysis of the retrograde TF REVIVE II and REVIVAL trial was 15.5%, as reported by Susheel Kodali at TCT 2008. These included a series of 50 patients in which 1 aortic rupture, 1 iliac perforation, 2 other iliac injuries requiring surgical repair, and 2 access site infections were reported.[20]

Vascular complications increase mortality. At TCT 2008, William Gray reported an in-hospital mortality of 36% in those patients in the REVIVE II/REVIVAL trial with vascular complications, compared with 10.3% in those without vascular complications. Therefore, a detailed evaluation of the vascular access is mandatory before any potential implant. Vessel diameter, calcification, tortuosity, and existing lesions in the ileofemoral vessels and in the abdominal and thoracic aorta must be evaluated carefully. According to Martin Leon during the 2009 SCAI Scientific Sessions, the percentage of patients with vascular complications in the REVIVE trial decreased from 30% before the introduction of the vascular core-laboratory to 6% afterwards. In cases with unsuitable femoral access, a TA approach should be considered.

Valve malpositioning Valve malpositioning has been described with the balloon-expandable[20,31] and the CoreValve[32] prostheses. Malpositioning can lead to significant regurgitation,[32] or to impingement of the anterior leaflet of the mitral valve, if the valves are deployed too low in the left ventricular outflow tract. If deployed too high in the aorta, coronary obstruction, with the possibility of clinically relevant ischemia and prosthesis migration,[18,20] have been described.[20,33] A better understanding of the aortic root anatomy, and a detailed knowledge of the anatomic characteristics of each patient, will help in device selection and optimal valve positioning. Recent reports have described the anatomic characteristics defined with CT imaging of the aortic root in patients with severe AS,[34] as a first step in defining those anatomic variables that might be related to procedural outcomes. The optimal preprocedural imaging strategy has yet to be determined.

Cardiac perforation and tamponade Cardiac perforation and tamponade have been described.[18,25] In most cases tamponade is due to perforation of cardiac structures with a rigid guide wire; care in manipulation of devices and wires reduces this risk.

Conduction abnormalities Infranodal conduction disturbances are well-known complications of

Table 4
Complications of TAVI

| | Edwards TF | Edwards TA | | CoreValve TF | | | Piazza et al. EuroInterv 2008;4:242–49 |
| | Webb et al. Circulation. 2007;116:755–63 | Walther et al. Eur J Cardiothor Surgery 2008;33:983–8 | Svensson et al. Ann Thorac Surg 2008;86:46–55 | Grube et al. Circ Cardiovasc Intervent 2008;1:167–75 | | | |
				First Generation	Second Generation	Third Generation	
Mean EuroSCORE	28	27		18.3	21.1	24.5	23.1
Procedural success	97 (first cohort) 76 (second cohort)	89.8	90	70.0	70.4	91.2	97
Migration/embolization	4	0	10	NR			NR
Procedural mortality	2	NR	NR	10	8.3	0	1.5
In-hospital mortality	NR	13.6	22.5	40	8.3	9.8	NR
30-d mortality	12	13.6	17.5	40	8.3	10.8	8
30-d MACCE	16	NR	35	40.0	20.8	14.7	9.3
Procedural CVA	4	3.4	0	10	4.2	2.9	0.6
30-d stroke	NR	NR	5	10	8.3	2.9	1.9
Procedural MI	2	NR	NR	0	4.2	1	0.5
30-d MI	NR	NR	15	0	4.2	2	0.6
Tamponade	2	NR	NR	0	0	2	1.4
Heart block	4	NR	NR	NR			NR
Open surgery	0	6.8	2.5	10	16.7	0	0.5
Valve-in-valve	NR	NR	NR	2.9			2.6
Pacemaker	NR	NR	NR	10	13.6	33.3	9.3

Abbreviation: NR, not reported.

surgical AVR. Initial experience indicates that they are also frequent after TAVI, with a reported 5.7% incidence of new left bundle branch block with the Edwards SAPIEN valve[35] and 40% with the Core-Valve.[36,37] The need for permanent pacemaker implantation after TAVI is still unclear, but it has ranged from 5.7% to 18%,[35–37] although many of the implants in the second cohort have been prophylactic. With the CoreValve ReValving System, the risk of conduction disturbances is higher than with the Edwards SAPIEN valve, and seems to be related to a deeper implantation in the left ventricle outflow tract.[36]

Aortic regurgitation Although postprocedural mild to moderate aortic regurgitation has been described in more than 50% of the patients,[18,20,37] regurgitation of grade 3 or higher is uncommon. In the preliminary results of the PARTNER EU trial presented by John Webb at EuroPCR09, postprocedural paravalvular regurgitation decreased over time (41% of the patients with grade 2 postprocedure vs 32% at 12 months, and the rate of grade 1 regurgitation increased from 28% to 42%). These data suggest that, even though the severity of leaks decreased over time, the rate of leaks did not. The long-term consequences of new aortic regurgitation in ventricles that have decreased compliance secondary to hypertrophy remain to be evaluated.

Stroke Stroke rates have ranged between 2% and 9%,[6] but this outcome variable has not been reported consistently. The Bonn-Cerebral Embolism Study will compare the incidence of silent and clinically apparent cerebral embolism among conventional, TF, and TA aortic valve repair, and will provide greater detail regarding neurologic outcomes of the procedure.

Myocardial infarction The risk of myocardial infarction with TAVI needs better definition. Reported rates have varied greatly, ranging from 1%[37] to 16%,[6] and correlates of periprocedural myocardial infarction are not well understood. Standardization of the diagnostic criteria and careful review of each case are essential.

Others The long-term durability of a percutaneous prosthesis is unknown and must be compared with surgical valve prostheses.

Non-Clinically Approved Devices

Direct Flow Medical Valve
The Direct Flow Medical Valve (Direct Flow Medical, Santa Rosa, CA) is a stentless, nonmetallic, expandable device that consists of bovine pericardial leaflets sewed to a Dacron fabric cuff, with an inflatable ring on the aortic side and another on the ventricular side (**Fig. 1E**), designed for TF delivery. Once the valve is positioned, the rings are inflated with saline and contrast until the position and function has been confirmed. The diluted contrast is then exchanged for an active polymeric medium that, when polymerized, hardens and forms the final support structure. This valve is therefore repositionable and retrievable before complete deployment. This prosthesis is currently available in sizes 23 mm (diameter) × 16 mm (height), 25 mm (diameter) × 17 mm (height) (outer ring 4mm larger), and 27 mm (diameter). It was deployed initially through a 22F sheath but, more recently, an 18F delivery system has been developed.[38,39]

Clinical results FIM was performed in 2006 by Adrian Ebner and colleagues[39] in Paraguay. Currently, a prospective multicenter European study is ongoing (n = 50 in 4 centers), in which at least 31 patients had been enrolled by May 2009.[40] At the 2009 SCAI Scientific Sessions, Khun Keong Yeo reported on the successful implantation in 22 of the 31 patients enrolled, and indicated that 18 of them had been discharged alive. Procedural success rate was 80% and the mean residual pressure gradient was 14 mm Hg. During AATS-2009, Hendrik Treede reported no paravalvular leaks (PVLs) in 58% of the patients, and 1 or more PVL in 42% at 6 months. The latest follow-up results on 18 implanted patients reported by Joachim Schoefer MD at EuroPCR09 indicated that 1 patient suffered stroke (4.5%), 2 required permanent pacemaker implantation (9%), all patients survived 30 days, and 89% were alive at 6 months (1 patient died of causes not related to the procedure, and another of an indeterminate cause). The longest available follow-up is 19 months.

Lotus Valve
The Lotus Valve (Sadra Medical Inc, Saratoga, CA) is a bioprosthesis consisting of 3 bovine pericardial leaflets suspended in a self-expanding and self-centering braided nitinol stent frame (**Fig. 1D**). It has an active shortening-locking mechanism and an external polyurethane sealing membrane to prevent PVL. The valve is delivered retrograde via a TF approach. The stent has a dual-state design: although in the delivery catheter it is in its longitudinal form, with low radial force and small profile, once the valve has been positioned and the outer catheter is retracted, the prosthesis expands radially, gaining radial force and losing height, effectively locking the valve in place. Unlocking the prosthesis, repositioning it,

and again relocking it can be done for fine adjustments of the position. Currently available in 23-mm size, it was initially delivered through a 21F system,[41] and Eberhard Grube reported a second-generation 18 to 19F delivery system at CRT 2009. There is no need for rapid pacing during the delivery because flow through the valve orifice is preserved during the entire deployment.

Clinical results Grube and colleagues[41] performed FIM implantation of the 21F system in 2007, and the results of this cohort of 10 patients were presented during CRT 2009. Of the 10 patients, 6 were implanted successfully with a mean postprocedure gradient of 4 mm Hg and no PVL. There was 1 postprocedure mortality that was not device related. The longest follow-up in 1 patient was 18 months.

AorTx Device
The AorTx Device (Hansen Medical Inc, Mountain View, CA) is a sutureless prosthesis that consists of a pericardial-tissue valve attached to a self-expanding, solid nitinol frame. This frame is folded before deployment. It is repositionable and retrievable. This valve has been designed for a TA and transarterial approach through an 18F delivery system, and is currently undergoing technical refinement for precise robotic placement.

Clinical results The FIM temporary implants were performed by Adrian Ebner in Paraguay, and presented at CRT 2006 by Peter Fitzgerald. The first 8 patients who underwent temporary surgical implants, and were taken off pump for 20 minutes before undergoing surgical AVR, had a 100% procedural success with no embolization and excellent hemodynamic results.

Paniagua Heart Valve
The Paniagua Heart Valve (Endoluminal Technology Research, Miami, FL) is a biologic valve with a collapsed profile of 2 mm that must be manually crimped on to a delivery balloon, but that also exists as a self-expanding model. It can be inserted through a 10F to 18F sheath, depending on the mounting frame and the final valve diameter. This valve was designed to be used in any heart valve position.

Clinical results In 2005, Paniagua and colleagues[42] reported the retrograde implant of a prosthetic aortic valve as compassionate use in a severely ill patient with severe AS and left ventricular dysfunction. Acute hemodynamic results were satisfactory, although the patient died on day 5 after the procedure, with normal valve function on echocardiography. There is no recent clinical activity on this valve, although it is still under development.

The Ventor-Embracer Technology
The Ventor-Embracer Technology (Medtronic, Minneapolis, MN) is a self-expandable pericardial-tissue prosthesis with a composite nitinol proprietary frame. The outer frame has a crown-shape, with troughs that flare out to anchor the valve in the sinuses. An inner frame has an hourglass shape and is designed to minimize pressure loss at inlet and maximize pressure recovery at outlet, and thereby optimizing fluid dynamics (based on the Venturi effect). This valve was originally designed for TA delivery in sizes of 12 to 29 mm, but, more recently, a TF version with a 16F delivery system has been developed.

Clinical results Falk and colleagues[43] reported the FIM implantation of this valve, and implantation in 11 patients was reported during TCT 2008 by Ehud Schwammenthal with a 100% procedural success rate. However, 2 patients died at postoperative days 4 and 7 (1 from ischemic colitis, the other from cardiac arrest). The latest report by Frederic Mohr[43] at the STS 2009 meeting mentioned that the University of Leipzig experience with the TA approach was 14 patients. The FIM-Embracer TF study is underway and results are pending.

Heart Leaflet Technology
The Heart Leaflet Technology (HLT; Maole Grove, MN) is a porcine pericardial trileaflet valve mounted in a self-inverting nitinol cuff, with 3 nitinol support hoops and with an antireflux collar (**Fig. 1**C). Available in 4 sizes (19, 21, 23, and 25 mm), it is delivered through a 16F to 17F delivery system with repositioning capability.

Clinical results FIM experience with acute human implants was performed at Monzino Hospital, Milan, Italy by Robert Wilson, and reported at TCT 2008. He presented results on the 8 patients who underwent temporary implant on cardiopulmonary bypass before undergoing surgical AVR, demonstrating adequate radial force without interference with mitral valve opening or coronary blood flow. The hemodynamic results in an ovine model showed a low transvalvular gradient on implantation without significant clinical changes at 5 months.

ATS 3f Series
The ATS 3f Series (ATS Medical, Minneapolis, MN) is a self-expandable bioprosthesis mounted in a tubular nitinol frame designed for surgical (ATS 3f Enable) and percutaneous (ATS 3f Entrata) deployments (**Fig. 1**F). Six sizes are available, from 19 to 29 mm.

Clinical results There are several ongoing pivotal clinical studies in Europe using the surgical ATS 3f Enable,[44] the largest of which has included more than 100 patients. Although a transcatheter delivery technology has been developed for this valve, to date there are no known implants.

Perceval-Percutaneous
The Perceval-Percutaneous (Sorin Group, Milan, Italy) is a self-expandable bovine pericardial valve with a nitinol panel frame matching the anatomy of the aortic root and sinuses of Valsalva. It has a double sheath that provides enhanced sealing and nonexpandable support rods.

Clinical results The available clinical experience is from ongoing studies with the surgical versions of this device, the Freedom SOLO valve (currently undergoing a pivotal trial in Europe) and the Perceval S aortic valve.[45] At EACTS 2008, Thierry Folliguet reported the results in 30 patients who underwent Perceval S implantation: 30-day mortality was 3.3%, postprocedure mean aortic gradient was 11 mm Hg, and the paravalvular leak rate was 3.3%. There have been no implants with the transcatheter device to date.

Jena Clip
The Jena Clip (JenaValve Technology GmbH, Munich, Germany) is a bioprosthetic pericardial-tissue valve mounted in a self-expanding nitinol stent (the JenaClip) that is built up of 2 layers of "paper clip–like" structures (3 in each layer) that are compressed in a dedicated delivery catheter. It has been designed anatomically to fit in the sinuses of Valsalva with a clip-based anchoring system. The initial concept was developed in 1995,[46] and the first stent prototype was completed in 1999.[47] Once the delivery catheter is in the ascending aorta, it is retracted to allow the outer layer of the stent to open and be positioned in the native aortic cusps. Once in an adequate position, the catheter is pushed forward to open the inner layer of clips and unfold the valve. The native leaflets are held between the 2 clip layers and pressed against the aortic wall. The valve can be repositioned and retrieved before its final deployment. Systems for TF and TA implants are being developed simultaneously.

Preclinical studies The Jena valve human proof of concept is underway. The initial animal studies were reported by Ferrari and colleagues[48] in 6 pigs that underwent implantation via the subclavian artery with a 67% success rate of implantation. The results demonstrated the feasibility of this approach in the beating animal heart and after pharmacologic stress. Lauten and colleagues[49] reported the results of the Jena clip using the TA approach in 15 sheep, with a primary deployment success rate of 80% and no significant hemodynamic changes after implantation, but ventricular fibrillation occurred in 13% of the sheep, and mitral regurgitation in 13%. The study demonstrated the feasibility of a leaflet-fixation device in nondiseased aortic valves.

Bailey-Palmaz PercValve
The Bailey-Palmaz PercValve (Advanced Bio Prosthesis Surfaces, Ltd. San Antonio, TX) is a completely mechanical valve consisting of a monolithic structure of nanosythesized nitinol in a self-expanding cage and nitinol leaflets that also has a nitinol membrane at the base of the valve to reduce paravalvular regurgitation. This new nanosynthetic material has improved stress and fracture resistance and has allowed for a device with a smaller profile, which can be delivered through a 10F sheath. It is designed to be repositionable and retrievable, and to be delivered by retrograde, antegrade, or TA approach.

Preclinical studies Julio Palmaz and Steven Bailey developed the technology at the University of Texas Health Science (San Antonio, TX). Early animal studies have shown the valve to be competent and 100% endothelized within 10 days after implantation. At CRT 2009, Bailey reported the implantation of the valve in a porcine iliac vein model, demonstrating complete endothelization at 28 days.

HOCOR PAV
HOCOR PAV (HOCOR Cardiovascular Technologies, LLC, Honolulu, HI) is a novel design that involves ablation of the native valve with a unique delivery and deployment system. First, a stent is place across the aortic valve to ablate the native leaflets, and subsequently the PAV is deployed in the native aortic valve inside the ablation stent. Ho[50,51] recently described a miniaturizing strategy to assemble the PAV in a piecemeal fashion from smaller components to be delivered through smaller-diameter catheters. No animal study has been reported.

FUTURE OF TAVI AND SUMMARY

Surgical AVR, the gold standard treatment of severe AS, is now firmly challenged by the growing enthusiasm and encouraging results of percutaneous techniques, with the emphasis on high-risk groups. However, TAVI requires much additional study to define patient selection criteria, which should be based on the results of ongoing trials and nonrandomized experiences.

In addition to data from randomized clinical trials, mandatory longitudinal registries are needed to evaluate long-term prosthesis behavior (durability and function), procedure-related events, and outcomes. Multiple single site studies and many individual country registries are currently being conducted outside the United States for clinically approved valves, and it is difficult to obtain the results of the overall clinical experience. Large centralized registries to collect and maintain all available clinical data in an unbiased manner would be extremely useful. Such registries can only be possible with the joint efforts of device manufacturers and the large medical societies. Registries should be mandatory for all implanting sites, and they must be independent of industry.

The ideal TAVI device must be low profile, repositionable and retrievable, and with proven durability. Several devices that might satisfy these requirements are being studied, and might become alternatives to the current surgical standard of care for patients with severe AS.

REFERENCES

1. Culliford AT, Galloway AC, Colvin SB, et al. Aortic valve replacement for aortic stenosis in persons aged 80 years and over. Am J Cardiol 1991;67: 1256–60.
2. Rosengart TK, Feldman T, Borger MA, et al. Percutaneous and minimally invasive valve procedures: a scientific statement from the American Heart Association Council on Cardiovascular Surgery and Anesthesia, Council on Clinical Cardiology, Functional Genomics and Translational Biology Interdisciplinary Working Group, and Quality of Care and Outcomes Research Interdisciplinary Working Group. Circulation 2008;117:1750–67.
3. Doter CT. Interventional radiology – review of an emerging field. Semin Roentgenol 1981;16:7–12.
4. Cribier A, Eltchaninoff H, Bash A, et al. Percutaneous transcatheter implantation of an aortic valve prosthesis for calcific aortic stenosis: first human case description. Circulation 2002;106:3006–8.
5. Chiam PT, Ruiz CE. Percutaneous transcatheter aortic valve implantation: evolution of the technology. Am Heart J 2009;157:229–42.
6. Serruys PW. Keynote address–EuroPCR 2008, Barcelona, May 14th, 2008. Transcatheter aortic valve implantation: state of the art. EuroIntervention 2009;4(5):558–65.
7. Lieberman EB, Bashore TM, Hermiller JB, et al. Balloon aortic valvuloplasty in adults: failure of procedure to improve long-term survival. J Am Coll Cardiol 1995;26:1522–8.
8. Otto CM, Mickel MC, Kennedy JW, et al. Three-year outcome after balloon aortic valvuloplasty. Insights into prognosis of valvular aortic stenosis. Circulation 1994;89:642–50.
9. Cribier A, Savin T, Berland J, et al. Percutaneous transluminal balloon valvuloplasty of adult aortic stenosis: report of 92 cases. J Am Coll Cardiol 1987;9:381–6.
10. Roques F, Michel P, Goldstone AR, et al. The logistic EuroSCORE. Eur Heart J 2003;24:881–2.
11. Edwards FH, Grover FL, Shroyer AL, et al. The Society of Thoracic Surgeons National Cardiac Surgery Database: current risk assessment. Ann Thorac Surg 1997;63:903–8.
12. Dewey TM, Brown D, Ryan WH, et al. Reliability of risk algorithms in predicting early and late operative outcomes in high-risk patients undergoing aortic valve replacement. J Thorac Cardiovasc Surg 2008;135(1):180–7.
13. Brown JM, O'Brien SM, Sikora JA, et al. Isolated aortic valve replacement in North America comprising 108,687 patients in 10 years: changes in risks, valve types, and outcomes in the Society of Thoracic Surgeons National Database. J Thorac Cardiovasc Surg 2009;137(1):82–90.
14. Osswald BR, Gegouskov V, Badowski-Zyla D, et al. Overestimation of aortic valve replacement risk by EuroSCORE: implications for percutaneous valve replacement. Eur Heart J 2009;30:74–80.
15. Ambler G, Omar RZ, Royston P, et al. Generic, simple risk stratification model for heart valve surgery. Circulation 2005;112:224–31.
16. Piazza N, Grube E, Gerckens U, et al. Procedural and 30-day outcomes following transcatheter aortic valve implantation using the third generation (18 Fr) corevalve revalving system: results from the multicentre, expanded evaluation registry 1-year following CE mark approval. EuroIntervention 2008;4(2):242–9.
17. Cribier A, Eltchaninoff H, Tron C, et al. Early experience with percutaneous transcatheter implantation of heart valve prosthesis for the treatment of end stage inoperable patients with calcific aortic stenosis. J Am Coll Cardiol 2004;43:698–703.
18. Cribier A, Eltchaninoff H, Tron C, et al. Treatment of calcific aortic stenosis with the percutaneous heart valve. Mid-term follow-up from the initial feasibility studies: the French experience. J Am Coll Cardiol 2006;47:1214–23.
19. Webb JG, Chandavimol M, Thompson CR, et al. Percutaneous aortic valve implantation retrograde from the femoral artery. Circulation 2006;113:842–50.
20. Webb JG, Pasupati S, Humphries K, et al. Percutaneous transarterial aortic valve replacement in selected high-risk patients with aortic stenosis. Circulation 2007;116:755–63.
21. Webb JG, Altwegg L, Masson JB, et al. A new transcatheter aortic valve delivery system. J Am Coll Cardiol 2009;53(20):1855–8.

22. Svensson LG, Dewey T, Kapadia S, et al. United States feasibility study of transcatheter insertion of a stented aortic valve by the left ventricular apex. Ann Thorac Surg 2008;86:46–55.

23. Walther T, Falk V, Kempfert J, et al. Transapical minimally invasive aortic valve implantation; the initial 50 patients. Eur J Cardiothorac Surg 2008;33:983–8.

24. Walther T, Simon P, Dewey T, et al. Transapical minimally invasive aortic valve implantation. Multicenter experience. Circulation 2007;116(Suppl I):I240–5.

25. Grube E, Schuler G, Buellesfeld L, et al. Percutaneous aortic valve replacement for severe aortic stenosis in high-risk patients using the second- and current third-generation self-expanding CoreValve prosthesis: device success and 30-day clinical outcome. J Am Coll Cardiol 2007;50:69–76.

26. Grube E, Gerckens U, Wenaweser P, et al. Percutaneous aortic valve replacement with CoreValve prosthesis (reply). J Am Coll Cardiol 2008;51:170–1.

27. Grube E, Buellesfeld L, Mueller R, et al. Progress and current status of percutaneous aortic valve replacement: results of three device generations of the CoreValve ReValving System. Catheter Cardiovasc Interv 2008;1:167–75.

28. Bauernschmitt R, Schreiber C, Bleiziffer S, et al. Transcatheter aortic valve implantation through the ascending aorta: an alternative option for no-access patients. Heart Surg Forum 2009;12(1):E63–4.

29. Wenaweser P, Buellesfeld L, Gerckens U, et al. Percutaneous aortic valve replacement for severe aortic regurgitation in degenerated bioprosthesis: the first valve in valve procedure using the CoreValve Revalving system. Catheter Cardiovasc Interv 2007;70:760–4.

30. Ruiz CE, Laborde JC, Condado JF, et al. First percutaneous transcatheter aortic valve-in-valve implant with three year follow-up. Catheter Cardiovasc Interv 2008;72:143–8.

31. Al Ali AM, Altwegg L, Horlick EM, et al. Prevention and management of transcatheter balloon-expandable aortic valve malposition. Catheter Cardiovasc Interv 2008;72(4):573–8.

32. Grube E, Laborde JC, Gerckens U, et al. Percutaneous implantation of the CoreValve self-expanding valve prosthesis in high-risk patients with aortic valve disease: the Siegburg first-in-man study. Circulation 2006;114(15):1616–24.

33. Schofer J, Schluter M, Treede H, et al. Retrograde transarterial implantation of a nonmetallic aortic valve prosthesis in high–surgical-risk patients with severe aortic stenosis a first-in-man feasibility and safety study. Circ Cardiovasc Intervent 2008;1:126–33.

34. Tops LF, Wood DA, Delgado V, et al. Noninvasive evaluation of the aortic root with multislice computed tomography: implications for transcatheter aortic valve replacement. JACC Cardiovasc Imaging 2008;1(3):321–30.

35. Sinhal A, Altwegg L, Pasupati S, et al. Atrioventricular block after transcatheter balloon expandable aortic valve implantation. JACC Cardiovasc Interv 2008;1:305–9.

36. Piazza N, Onuma Y, Jesserun E, et al. Early and persistent intraventricular conduction abnormalities and requirements for pacemaking after percutaneous replacement of the aortic valve. JACC Cardiovasc Interv 2008;1:310–6.

37. Piazza N, Grube E, Gerckens E, et al. - on Behalf of the Clinical Centers that Participated in the Study. Procedural and 30-days outcomes following transcatheter aortic valve implantation using the third generation (18F) Corevalve revalving system. Results from the Multicenter, expanded evaluation registry 1-year following CE mark approval. EuroIntervention 2008;4:242–9.

38. Bolling SF, Rogers JH, Babaliaros V, et al. Percutaneous aortic valve implantation utilising a novel tissue valve: preclinical experience. EuroIntervention 2008;4(1):148–53.

39. Low RI, Bolling SF, Ebner A. Direct Flow medical percutaneous aortic valve: proof of concept. EuroIntervention 2008;4(2):256–61.

40. Treede H, Schofer J, Tuebler T, et al. The direct flow valve: first in man experience with a repositionable and retrievable pericardial valve for percutaneous aortic valve replacement. ATTS 89th meeting abstract book 2009. p. 197–8. Available at: http://www.aats.org/annualmeeting/Abstracts/2009/T1.html. Accessed October 13, 2009.

41. Buellesfeld L, Gerckens U, Grube E. Percutaneous implantation of the first repositionable aortic valve prosthesis in a patient with severe aortic stenosis. Catheter Cardiovasc Interv 2008; 71:579–84.

42. Paniagua D, Condado JA, Besso J, et al. First human case of retrograde transcatheter implantation of an aortic valve prosthesis. Tex Heart Inst J 2005;32:393–8.

43. Falk V, Schwammenthal EE, Kempfert J, et al. New anatomically oriented transapical aortic valve implantation. Ann Thorac Surg 2009;87(3):925–6.

44. Martens S, Ploss A, Sirat S, et al. Sutureless aortic valve replacement with the 3f Enable aortic bioprosthesis. Ann Thorac Surg 2009;87(6):1914–7.

45. Shrestha M, Khaladj N, Bara, et al. A staged approach towards interventional aortic valve implantation with sutureless valve: initial human implants. Thorac Cardiovasc Surg 2008;56(7):398–400.

46. Figulla HR, Ferrari M. Perkutan. Implantierbare aortenklappe: de JenaValve-konzept-evolution [Percutaneously implantable aortic valve: the JenaValve concept evolution]. Herz 2006;31:685–7 [in German].

47. JenaValve Technologies official webpage. Available at: http://www.jenavalve.de/index.php?id=Company. Accessed July 16, 2008.

48. Ferrari M, Figulla HR, Schlosser M, et al. Transarterial aortic valve replacement with a self expanding stent in pigs. Heart 2004;90:1326–31.

49. Lauten A, Ferrari M, Ensminger SM, et al. Experimental evaluation of the JenaClip transcatheter aortic valve. Catheter Cardiovasc Interv 2009;74(3):514–9.

50. Ho PC. Percutaneous aortic valve replacement: a novel design of the delivery and deployment system. Minim Invasive Ther Allied Technol 2008;17(3):190–4.

51. Ho PC. Percutaneous aortic valve replacement: a novel design of the delivery and deployment system (part 2): miniaturization of the delivery system based on the novel temporary valve technology. Minim Invasive Allied Technol 2009;1:172–7.

Percutaneous Left Ventricular Support Devices

Kunal Sarkar, MBBS, Annapoorna S. Kini, MD, MRCP, FACC*

KEYWORDS

- Left ventricular • IMELLA • TandemHeart • IABP

Patients presenting with cardiogenic shock, severely compromised left ventricular (LV) dysfunction, and complex coronary lesions (such as unprotected left main disease, complex multivessel disease, last remaining conduit vessel, and bypass graft disease) are at increased risk of early and long-term major adverse cardiac events (MACEs) because of significant ischemia from balloon inflations, dissections, abrupt vessel closure, malignant arrhythmias, or no-reflow phenomenon.[1,2] This is reflected in the high in-hospital mortality rates of 10% to 15% in these patients.[3] Prophylactic insertion of circulatory support devices in the catheterization laboratory can prevent acute hemodynamic collapse, protect and preserve LV function by unloading the left ventricle, and maintain perfusion to vital organs.[4,5] The advent of drug-eluting stents, enhanced deliverability of devices, operator experience, and periprocedural pharmacotherapy[6,7] have facilitated the successful use of percutaneous coronary intervention (PCI) in high-risk patients and complex lesion subsets that were hitherto considered unamenable to percutaneous revascularization.

Cardiogenic shock complicates 7% to 10% of cases of ST segment elevation myocardial infarction (STEMI) presenting to the hospital and remains the most important cause of in-hospital mortality in patients with STEMI.[8] Mechanical unloading of the myocardium during ischemia and reperfusion can limit infarct size, sustain end-organ perfusion, and decrease LV filling pressures thereby reducing LV pressure work and myocardial oxygen consumption.[9,10] Surgically implanted LV assist devices (LVADs) have been used to provide mechanical circulatory support in these patients.[11] However, implantation of these devices is a cumbersome procedure requiring a midline sternotomy with its associated significant morbidity. In addition, patients with STEMI who required temporary circulatory support with an LVAD had a very high mortality rate.[12] Further, these devices are not readily available in many institutions, which limits their use in routine clinical practice. Percutaneous circulatory support devices have long been of major interest to operators to provide partial or total hemodynamic support to patients with cardiogenic shock and during high-risk PCI, without the need for surgical implantation. It is estimated that there are approximately 100 to 150,000 cases of cardiogenic shock and an additional 100,000 cases of complex intervention every year that could benefit from the use of circulatory support devices.

In this article, the authors discuss (1) the percutaneous circulatory support devices presently available and routinely used in the catheterization laboratory, (2) the technical aspects involved with insertion and removal, and (3) relevant data from randomized trials, meta-analyses, and registries about the benefits emanating from their use in patients with cardiogenic shock complicating STEMI and in those with significant LV systolic dysfunction undergoing complex PCI. Currently available percutaneous LVADs are given in **Table 1**.

There is no conflict of interest either real or perceived of any author in the publication of this manuscript.
Cardiac Catheterization Laboratory of the Cardiovascular Institute, Mount Sinai Hospital, One Gustave Levy Place, New York, NY, 10029 USA
* Corresponding author.
E-mail address: annapoorna.kini@mountsinai.org (A.S. Kini).

cardiology.theclinics.com

Table 1
Percutaneous ventricular assist devices

Device	Pump	Speed (rpm)	Duration	Cardiac Support (L/min)	Anticoagulation	Motor
TandemHeart	Centrifugal	3000–7500	Up to 14 d	Up to 4	Required ACT (250–300 s)	Rotor powered by electromagnetic coupling
Impella Recover LP2.5	Axial	Up to 50,000	Up to 5 d	Up to 2.5	Required ACT (250–300 s) ACT>300 s if using Bivalirudin	Integrated electric motor
Reitan catheter pump	Axial	Up to 13,000	Up to 5.5 h	Up to 20 (in vitro)	Required ACT (250–300 s)	Drive unit connected to propeller by wire

Abbreviation: ACT, activated clotting time.

Desirable features of a percutaneous circulatory support device (**Box 1**).

- Accessibility: The device should be readily accessible and be placed within a short time in the catheterization laboratory.
- Hemodynamic efficacy: The device should provide an output of 2 to 4 L/min to ensure adequate hemodynamic support, reduce LV filling pressures, decrease myocardial oxygen consumption, and improve supply/demand ratio.
- Safety: The device-insertion procedure should ideally be simple, without an external blood circuit, and avoid ischemia at the arterial insertion site.
- Dwelling time: It should be possible to leave the device in place for a period of several hours to 2 to 3 days without the risk of thrombosis, hemolysis, or infection.
- Weaning and removal: The device removal at the time of transition to the next intermediate or long-term support device, definitive therapy, or at the end of PCI should be relatively benign without significant bleeding or vascular complications.

HISTORICAL PERSPECTIVE

The femorofemoral cardiopulmonary support system was one of the earlier devices used to provide circulatory support during elective PCI. Although the device provided adequate hemodynamic support, it required a perfusionist to direct the circulation and was associated with complications at the insertion site, including bleeding, femoral neuropathy, skin infection, and necrosis. These complications occurred in equal frequency in percutaneous and cutdown cannulation.[13] Thirty percent of patients required blood transfusion, because the activated clotting time (ACT) required to maintain the system was more than 400 seconds.[14] Another LVAD, the Hemopump Cardiac Assist System (Medtronic, Inc,

Minneapolis, MN, USA), also fell out of favor because of increased morbidity and mortality associated with the use of large-size arterial cannulas, thromboembolic complications, and the need for anesthetists and perfusionists.[15,16] Currently available percutaneous LVADs include the TandemHeart (Cardiac Assist Inc, Pittsburg, PA, USA), the Impella LP2.5 system (Abiomed Europe GmbH, Aachen, Germany), and the Reitan catheter pump (RCP) (CardioBridge GmbH, Hechingen, Germany).

THE INTRA-AORTIC BALLOON PUMP

The intra-aortic balloon pump (IABP) was first used clinically by Kantrowitz and colleagues[17] in a series of patients with cardiogenic shock in the setting of acute myocardial infarction (MI). Since then, its use has progressively increased to provide circulatory support to patients with decompensated heart failure and postoperative LV dysfunction and prophylactically to provide hemodynamic support in patients undergoing complex PCI. In the United States, the IABP is used in more than 30% of patients undergoing complex procedures.[18] The present-day iteration of the IABP is an over-the-wire balloon catheter that can be inserted readily through a 7.5F introducer sheath (**Fig. 1**). This allows for a smaller arteriotomy and occupies decreased cross-sectional area in the iliofemoral vessels, thus allowing better distal flow in cases of significant peripheral arterial disease. The catheter is equipped with a fiberoptic sensor that allows timing accuracy and beat-to-beat adjustment, depending on the hemodynamic status of the patient.

Hemodynamic Effects

In animal models, use of the IABP was associated with the restoration of epicardial blood flow, improved myocardial tension time index, and peripheral blood flow.[19] The effects of the IABP include decreases in heart rate, LV end-diastolic pressure, mean left atrial pressure, afterload, and myocardial oxygen consumption by at least 20% to 30%. The IABP also increases coronary perfusion pressure and decreases the right atrial pressure, pulmonary artery pressure, and pulmonary vascular resistance.[20] It had little effect on microvascular flow in the setting of acute MI. No significant changes in the mean aortic pressure have been observed, and IABP provides only modest enhancement in cardiac output and reduction in pulmonary capillary wedge pressure. The IABP requires a certain residual level of LV function to be effective. A meta-analysis of randomized trials of the use of IABP in STEMI

Box 1
Desirable features of a percutaneous circulatory support device

Hemodynamic efficacy

Rapid access and placement

Safety

Adequate dwelling time

Benign weaning and removal

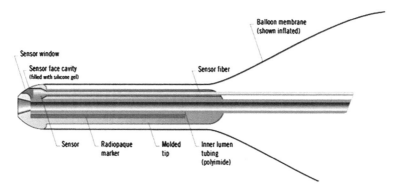

Fig. 1. Schematic diagram of a present-day IABP catheter. The fiberoptic sensor facilitates faster calibration and reduces signal delay in comparison with older fluid-filled systems.

showed neither a 30-day survival benefit nor an improved LV ejection fraction while being associated with significantly higher stroke and bleeding rates (**Fig. 2**A).[21] The use of IABP was apparently beneficial when used as an adjunct to thrombolysis. However, the data were limited by significant confounding and bias (see **Fig. 2**B). The use of IABP is a representative example of a treatment based on a concept that becomes clinical practice. The IABP has evolved into an amateur technology 4 decades after its introduction. Owing to the ease of percutaneous implantation, the low cost, and the beneficial hemodynamics at a low complication rate, it continues to be the most common mechanical cardiac assistance method in the catheterization laboratory.

TANDEM HEART

The TandemHeart percutaneous LVAD (**Fig. 3**A) is a left atrial-to-femoral bypass system that can provide rapid short-term circulatory support, with resolution of pulmonary edema and deranged metabolism in patients with cardiogenic shock.[22] In an animal model of acute MI and cardiogenic shock, the left atrial-to-femoral artery bypass assist device restored endocardial (microvascular) and epicardial blood flow to baseline and resulted in a substantial reduction in the infarct size.[23]

The TandemHeart can be implanted percutaneously and provides rapid hemodynamic support regardless of the native heart rhythm. It has been used in various situations, including (1) high-risk patients with PCI,[24] (2) acute MI complicated by cardiogenic shock, and (3) decompensated heart failure with myocarditis. It has also been used to preoperatively unload the left ventricle and to provide mechanical circulatory support during the peri- and postoperative period until cardiac function sufficiently recovers or an LVAD can be

surgically implanted for long-term hemodynamic support.

There are 3 subsystems that make up the TandemHeart system (see **Fig. 3**B–D). The first subsystem is a 21F venous transseptal inflow cannula that is made of polyurethane. This cannula has a curved design at its end to facilitate ideal tip placement in the left atrium and contains a large end hole at its distal tip and 14 side holes to aspirate oxygenated blood from the left atrium. The obturator is tapered at its tip to allow for easy insertion into the left atrium. The cannula is attached to a continuous flow centrifugal blood pump, which in turn is driven by a 3-phase, brushless, direct current servomotor that is capable of delivering up to 5.0 L/min of blood flow. The design features a hydrodynamic fluid bearing that supports the spinning rotor. The fluid bearing is supplied by a unique lubrication system, which feeds a nominal 10 mL/h of saline to which an anticoagulant (typically heparin) has been added. The fluid acts as a coolant and lubricant for the seal that separates the rotor chamber from the blood chamber, and the anticoagulant is delivered to the blood chamber precisely at the seal interface to minimize the risk of thrombus formation. Power is supplied by a direct current, brushless electromagnetic motor that operates at a range of 3000 to 7500 rpm. Blood is delivered from the pump to the femoral artery with an arterial perfusion catheter. This catheter ranges from 15F to17F and pumps blood from the left atrium to the right femoral artery. Alternatively, two 12F arterial perfusion catheters pump blood into the right and left femoral arteries.

The pump is driven by an external microprocessor-based controller. A pressure transducer monitors the infusion pressure and identifies any disruption in the infusion line. An in-line air bubble detector monitors for the presence of air in the infusion line.

Contraindications

Patients who have a ventricular septal defect are not good candidates for the TandemHeart because of the risk of hypoxemia due to right-to-left shunting. Because the left ventricle can become distended in the setting of severe LV dysfunction and impede subendocardial perfusion, aortic insufficiency is another contraindication to the TandemHeart. The TandemHeart can induce critical limb ischemia in patients who have severe peripheral vascular disease.

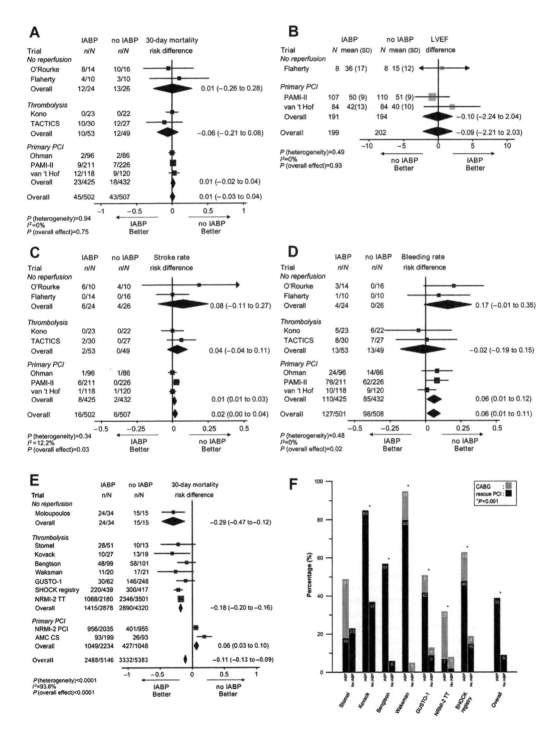

Implantation

The TandemHeart is implanted in the cardiac catheterization laboratory. With a few minor variations, the typical implantation procedure involves the following steps:

Femoral artery preclosure with the Perclose device (Abbott Laboratories, Abbott Park, IL, USA) using the preclosure technique

- An ipsilateral oblique projection femoral artery angiogram using a 4F arterial sheath dilator is obtained before upsizing to a larger French arterial sheath. The purpose of this angiogram is to delineate the angiographic anatomy of the iliofemoral system and to rule out peripheral vascular disease.
- If the vessel anatomy is found conducive (stick in the common femoral artery, artery size>5 mm), the 4F sheath dilator is exchanged for a 6F sheath. If the stick is found to be in the superficial femoral artery or profunda femoris artery, the 4F sheath dilator is removed, manual compression is applied, and hemostasis is achieved. Using the angiographic anatomy obtained previously, a higher stick is then attempted under fluoroscopy and a 6F sheath is introduced into the common femoral artery.
- The 6F introducer sheath is then removed, leaving the J-tip wire in the artery. The 2 Perclose devices are then sequentially deployed at 90° angles to each other (2-o'clock and 11-o'clock positions), yielding 2 sets of suture limbs spaced at 90° intervals. These were then harvested and secured using artery forceps.
- At this stage, care should be taken not to advance the suture knots down to the arterial wall. The 6F sheath is then reinserted over the J wire.

- This access site is used for subsequent placement of the arterial cannula of the TandemHeart.

Transseptal puncture and cannula placement

- The femoral vein is accessed for transseptal puncture, which is performed under fluoroscopic guidance using the Brockenbrough needle and a Mullins sheath, as is done during balloon mitral valvuloplasty.
- After confirming the position of the Mullins sheath in the left atrium, unfractionated heparin is given to achieve a target ACT of more than 300 seconds.
- The Mullins sheath is exchanged for the 14F/21F 2-stage dilator over a 0.038-in J-tip 260-cm Amplatz Super Stiff Guidewire (Boston Scientific Corp, Natick, MA, USA).
- Next, the 21F TandemHeart transseptal cannula is advanced along with the 14F obturator over the Amplatz Super Stiff Guidewire and placed in the left atrium.
- The position of the cannula in the left atrium is confirmed by injecting dye and drawing blood and assessing the saturation level.
- The obturator and the wire are then removed and clamps applied for temporary homeostasis. Care should be taken to place all the side holes of the TandemHeart cannula into the left atrium to avoid possible right-to-left shunting during device operation.
- The peripheral end of the cannula is sutured to the skin of the patient's thigh and clamped. The left femoral artery 6F sheath is then exchanged for the 15F arterial perfusion cannula of the TandemHeart device,

---

Fig. 2. (*A*) Meta-analysis of randomized clinical trials of IABP therapy in STEMI. All meta-analyses show effect estimates for the individual trials, for each type of reperfusion therapy, and for the overall analysis. The size of each square is proportional to the weight of the individual trial. (*Top left*) The risk differences in 30-day mortality. (*Top right*) The mean differences in left ventricular ejection fraction (LVEF). (*Bottom left and right*) The risk differences in stroke and major bleeding rate. (*B*) Meta-analysis of cohort studies of IABP therapy in STEMI complicated by cardiogenic shock. (*Top*) The risk differences in 30-day mortality for the individual studies, for each type of reperfusion therapy, and for the overall analysis. The size of each square is proportional to the weight of the individual study. (*Bottom*) The revascularization procedures, that is, rescue PCI (*dark blue*) and coronary artery bypass grafting (CABG) (*light blue*) in the thrombolysis studies by IABP group and no IABP group, and the weighted overall revascularization rate. Single-colored bars are used if separate figures for PCI and coronary artery bypass grafting could not be given. IABP denotes IABP, NRMI (National Registry of Myocardial Infarction)-2TT denotes cohort from NRMI-2 study of patients treated with thrombolysis, and NRMI-2 PCI denotes cohort from NRMI-2 study of patients treated with primary PCI. (*From* Sjauw KD, Engström AE, Vis MM, et al A systematic review and meta-analysis of intra-aortic balloon pump therapy in ST-elevation myocardial infarction: should we change the guidelines? Eur Heart J 2009;30(4):459–68; with permission.)

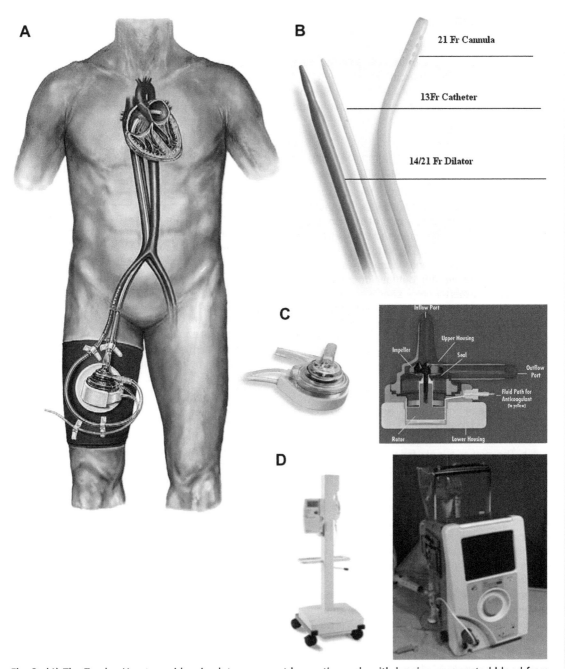

A

B

21 Fr Cannula

13Fr Catheter

14/21 Fr Dilator

C

Inflow Port

Upper Housing

Impeller

Seal

Outflow Port

Fluid Path for Anticoagulant (in yellow)

Rotor

Lower Housing

D

Fig. 3. (*A*) The TandemHeart provides circulatory support by continuously withdrawing oxygenated blood from the left atrium by way of a transseptal cannula placed in the femoral vein. The pump then returns blood by way of the femoral artery. The hemodynamic effects of the TandemHeart include an increase in cardiac output and blood pressure and a decrease in afterload and preload, thus decreasing myocardial oxygen demand. (*B*) A 21F venous transseptal inflow cannula made of polyurethane contains a large end hole and 14 side holes to allow for aspiration of the oxygenated blood from the left atrium. A 2-stage (14F/21F) dilator is used to dilate the transseptal puncture after a 0.035-in pigtail guidewire is inserted into the left atrium. The obturator is tapered at its tip to allow for easy insertion into the left atrium. (*C*) (*Left*) The continuous flow centrifugal blood pump contains a hydrodynamic fluid bearing to support a 6-bladed rotating impeller that provides up to 4 L/min of pump flow. (*Right*) Cutaway section of TandemHeart. The TandemHeart has a dual-chamber pump. The upper housing provides a conduit for inflow and outflow of blood. The lower housing provides communication with the controller, the ability to rotate the impeller, and a fluid path for a constant 10 mL/h flow of saline with unfractionated heparin, which is infused into the pump to provide (1) fluid bearing for the rotor, (2) local anticoagulation for the pump chamber to prevent the formation of thrombus, (3) systemic lubrication, and (4) cooling of the unit. (*D*) TandemHeart controller is a custom-designed system for driving the pump and supplying the lubrication fluid. It includes 2 controllers, a primary and a back up, which are constantly monitoring each other and are ready for use. (*Courtesy of* CardiacAssist, Pittsburgh, PA.)

with the distal end of the cannula lying above the aortic bifurcation.

- The peripheral end of the cannula is similarly sutured to the patient's thigh and clamped.

Connecting cannulas with the pump, de-airing, and initiation of mechanical support

- After the air is purged from the extracorporeal system, the transseptal cannula is attached to the inflow port of the centrifugal blood pump in the standard wet-to-wet fashion with 3/8-in Tygon tubing.
- The femoral arterial cannula is similarly connected to the outflow conduit of the TandemHeart pump after performing de-airing according to the specified protocol.
- A heparinized saline infusion is started according to the product specification, which provides hydrodynamic bearing, anticoagulation, and local cooling for the motor of the pump.
- The pump is then connected to the TandemHeart controller, and its speed is adjusted to provide a support of 2.5 to 3.0 L/min.
- The power supply for the TandemHeart is subsequently connected to the microprocessor-based controller.

In experienced centers, the entire insertion, assembly, and mechanical circulatory support can be accomplished in 30 minutes or less. At the authors' institution, the average time for the entire procedure has varied between 14 and 25 minutes.[24]

Because of the risk of thromboembolic complications, systemic anticoagulation with unfractionated heparin is mandatory to maintain an ACT of 400 seconds during insertion and 250 to 300 seconds during support. The TandemHeart has been used for up to 14 days. On removal, a small iatrogenic atrial septal defect is left after the explantation of the transseptal cannula, which resolves after 4 to 6 weeks or has no clinically significant left-to-right shunt. Explantation of the device is easily achieved by percutaneous removal of cannulas after discontinuing the heparin infusion and switching off the pump motor.

Hemodynamic Effects

The TandemHeart provides circulatory support by diverting oxygenated blood from the left atrium into systemic circulation, which increases cardiac output and blood pressure and decreases afterload and preload, thus decreasing myocardial

oxygen demand. The increase in mean arterial pressure may optimize the supply and demand of oxygen in the myocardium at risk and increase tissue perfusion at the coronary and peripheral level.[22] This increase in tissue perfusion leads to the reversal of metabolic acidosis and a decrease in serum lactate levels in patients with cardiogenic shock.

Potential Complications

The transseptal puncture required for the TandemHeart is a potential source of complications. Inadvertent puncture of the aortic root, coronary sinus, or posterior free wall of the right atrium can lead to disastrous complications, including death. Thromboembolism can be another potential source of complication. Cerebral thromboembolism has been reported secondary to thrombus formation at the edge of a large ventricular septal defect and at the site of the left atrial puncture despite anticoagulation with unfractionated heparin. Because unfractionated heparin is needed to achieve a high ACT, bleeding (especially from the groin) can occur with the TandemHeart. Systemic hypothermia can occur when contact of the system circuit with room temperature leads to the cooling of the blood flowing through the pump. Accidental dislodgement of the arterial cannula has led to acute decompensation and death from cardiogenic shock.[22] Local infections, bacteremia, and sepsis are potential complications with any implantable device.

Potential Applications

In addition to providing hemodynamic support in patients with cardiogenic shock and in high-risk PCI patients, potential applications for the TandemHeart include high-risk aortic valvuloplasty, percutaneous aortic valve replacement, and function as a percutaneous right ventricular assist device for right heart failure.[25]

IMPELLA LP2.5 SYSTEM

The Impella LP2.5 LVAD is a catheter-based, impeller-driven, axial flow pump, which pumps blood directly from the left ventricle into the ascending aorta. The device provides circulatory assistance in acute MI, cardiogenic shock or low-output states, or during high-risk PCI for up to 5 days (**Fig. 4**A).

The intracardiac axial flow pump contains an Archimedes screw–like rotor that is driven by an electrical motor and has an inflow cannula. The LV pump can provide up to 2.5 L/min of cardiac

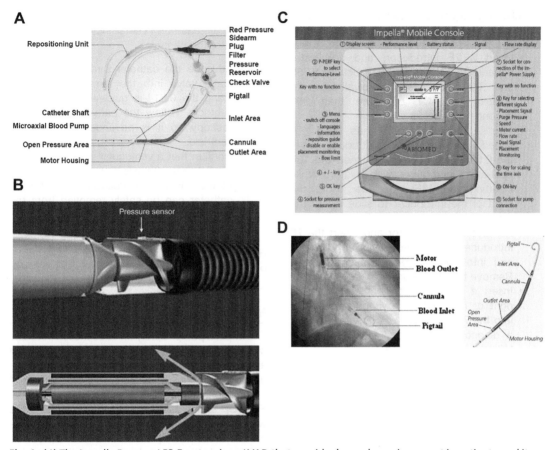

Fig. 4. (A) The Impella Recover LP2.5 system is an LVAD that provides hemodynamic support in patients, and it can be inserted percutaneously. The pigtail tip is inserted into the left ventricle to withdraw blood into the aorta. (B) (*Top*) The intracardiac axial flow pump contains a rotor that is driven by an electrical motor and has an inflow cannula. Blood is drawn in at the tip of the cannula and is expelled at the sides upstream from the motor into the aorta. A differential pressure sensor measures the difference in pressure between the inflow and outflow of the pump. (*Bottom*) The Impella motor is continuously purged with a glucose solution (10%) that is drawn into a 50-mL syringe with heparin (2500 IU). The purge flow rates normally range from 2 to 6 mL/h to continuously rinse and prevent thrombus formation in the pump. (C) The mobile console permits the management of the rotational speed of the pump and displays the differences of pressure between the inflow and outflow. It provides 60 minutes of battery time and 9 flow settings. (D) Confirmation of Impella catheter placement in left ventricle. (*Courtesy of* CardiacAssist, Pittsburgh, PA.)

output, depending on the speed of the rotor (which can operate at a maximum of 50,000 rpm) and the difference between aortic blood pressure and LV pressure, which is constantly monitored by a differential pressure sensor located in front of the rotor (see **Fig. 4**B). The appropriate position of the flow pump can be confirmed by the pressure difference between the aorta and the left ventricle. The catheter is connected to a mobile console that manages the rotational speed of the pump and displays the pressure differential between the left ventricle and the aorta (see **Fig. 4**C). The pump is continuously purged with a glucose solution (10%) that is drawn into a 50-mL syringe with

heparin (2500 IU). The purge flow rates normally range from 2 to 6 mL/h to continuously rinse and prevent thrombus formation in the pump.

Implantation

Similar to the TandemHeart, the Impella system is placed in the catheterization laboratory.

The initial part of the implantation involves iliofemoral angiography to rule out severe peripheral vascular disease and tortuosity. Once suitability of the femoral artery for Impella insertion has been determined, 2 Perclose sutures are deployed with the preclose technique as described earlier.

The following sequence of steps ensures correct device placement and functioning:

- Insert a 7F introducer, and administer heparin (to achieve an ACT between 250 and 300 seconds) or bivalirudin (to achieve an ACT of more than 300 seconds).
- After a therapeutic ACT has been obtained, remove the 7F introducer over the 0.035-in guidewire and insert the 13F peel-away introducer with dilator. While inserting the 13F introducer, hold the shaft of the introducer to slide it into the artery.
- Remove the 13F dilator and insert the 7F introducer with dilator over a guidewire and into the 13F peel-away introducer. Remove the 7F dilator.
- Insert a 6F diagnostic catheter (Judkins right or multipurpose) without side holes into the 7F introducer and advance it over a diagnostic 0.035-in guidewire into the left ventricle.
- Remove the diagnostic guidewire and insert the supplied 0.014-in Platinum PLUS guidewire.
- Advance the 0.014-in guidewire into the left ventricle until the floppy end and 3 to 4 cm of the stiffer part of the guidewire are visible in the left ventricle.
- Remove the 6F diagnostic catheter and 7F introducer.

Wet the cannula and backload the pigtail section of the catheter onto the 0.014-in guidewire. Straighten the cannula to ensure that the guidewire exits on the inner radius of the cannula. The pigtail is a very short monorail. It is important to keep the wire parallel to the cannula and advance the catheter in small increments to avoid bending of the cannula.

- Advance the catheter through the hemostatic valve into the femoral artery and along the 0.014-in guidewire into the left ventricle. Follow the catheter under fluoroscopy as it is advanced into the left ventricle.
- Confirm that a ventricular waveform is displayed on the Impella console (see **Fig. 4**D).
- At the end of the procedure, the Impella catheter can be safely removed from the left ventricle.

An advantage of the Impella over the TandemHeart is that there is no need for a transseptal puncture and no extracorporeal blood.

Hemodynamic Effects

The Impella pump rapidly unloads the left ventricle by delivering blood into the ascending aorta. In an animal model, the Impella pump reduced myocardial oxygen consumption during ischemia and reperfusion, leading to a reduced infarct size (see **Fig. 4**C).[26] Patients with cardiogenic shock treated with the Impella pump system showed improvements in cardiac output and mean blood pressure and a reduction in pulmonary capillary wedge pressure.[27] Compared with the IABP, the Impella pump improved cardiac and systemic hemodynamics during acute mitral regurgitation in an animal model (**Table 2**).[28]

The average pressure-volume loops demonstrate a reduction in the LV end-diastolic pressure (18–11 mm Hg), end-diastolic volume (345–321 mL), and stroke volume (94–76 mL).[29]

Table 2
Effect of IABP and Impella 2.5 device on important hemodynamic parameters[a]

Hemodynamic Parameter	%change	
	IABP (1:1)	Impella (Full)
Cardiac output	+4	+25
Aortic pressure	+11	+17
Carotid flow	+8	+48
Diastolic coronary flow	+96	+69
LV work	−4	−46

[a] Although the diastolic coronary flow augmentation is more with IABP, the Impella device provides better overall reduction in LV work.

(*Data from* Reesink KD, et al. Miniature intracardiac assist device provides more effective cardiac unloading and circulatory support during severe left heart failure than intraaortic balloon pumping. Chest 2004;126(3):896–902.)

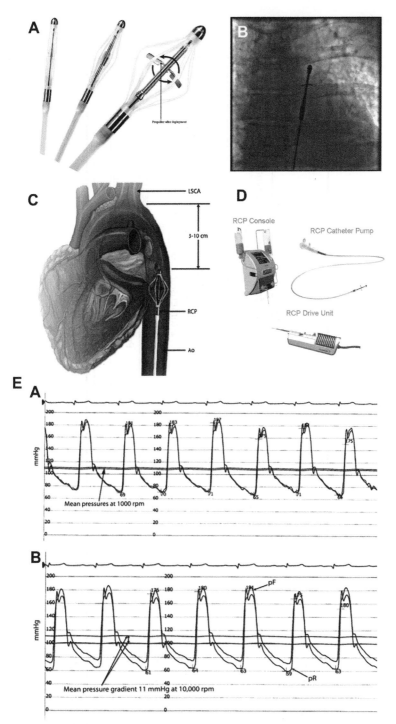

Fig. 5. (*A*) The RCP head deployed. The propeller is deployed ex vivo surrounded by longitudinal polymer filaments forming a cage protecting the aortic wall from the rotating propeller. (*B*) Fluoroscopic image of the deployed pump head in vivo. The pump head has been deployed fluoroscopically in the descending aorta. The polymer filaments are not visible. (*C*) The correct positioning of the RCP in the descending aorta. The deployed pump head (RCP) sits in the descending aorta (Ao) 3 to 10 cm distal to the origin of the left subclavian artery (LSCA). (*D*) The RCP system. (*E*) Simultaneous radial and femoral pressure traces pre- and post-RCP activation. (*Top*) Simultaneous radial and femoral pressure traces are demonstrated pre- and postpump activation. After pump insertion, the pump is routinely started at 1000 rpm to ensure appropriate pump function and reduce thrombotic risk. Radial and femoral pressure traces are superimposed, with no significant pressure gradient generated. (*Bottom*) The pump is activated when propeller rotation exceeds 8000 rpm. In this case, propeller rotation at 10,000 rpm results in an increase in femoral pressure (pF) and a decrease in radial pressure (pR), resulting in a mean transaortic pressure gradient of 11 mm Hg. (*Courtesy of* Impella CardioSystems, Aachen, Germany.)

Table 3
Recent trials comparing IABP with Impella 2.5 device

Trial	Device	Comparator	Patient Characteristics	End Point	Conclusions
PROTECT I	Impella 2.5	None	N = 20. High-risk PCI	Efficacy: freedom from hemodynamic compromise during PCI Safety: 30-d MACE	+
ISAR-SHOCK	Impella 2.5	IABP	N = 26. CS	Primary = CPO ↑from baseline Secondary = 30-d MACE	+
AMC-MACH2	Impella 2.5	IABP	N = 20. Anterior STEMI (Pre-CS)	Reduction in infarct size/↑in LVEF by 2-dimensional echo at 3 d and 120 d	+
PROTECT II	Impella 2.5	IABP	N = 654. High-risk PCI	Primary = 30-day MACE Secondary = CPO ↑from baseline	+
RECOVER II	Impella 2.5	IABP	N = 346	Primary = MACE Secondary = CPO ↑from baseline	Ongoing
EUROPELLA (multicenter registry)	Impella 2.5	None	N = 144. High-risk PCI	In-hospital and 30-d MACE	+

Abbreviations: CPO, cardiac power output; CS, cardiogenic shock; LVEF, left ventricular ejection fraction; N, number of patients; ↑, increase.

Contraindications

In addition to severe peripheral vascular disease, the Impella 2.5 system is contraindicated in the following situations:

1. Mural thrombus in the left ventricle
2. The presence of a mechanical aortic valve or heart constrictive device
3. Moderate aortic stenosis (aortic stenosis graded as $\geq$ +2 equivalent to an orifice area of 1.5 cm^2 or less) or moderate to severe aortic insufficiency (echocardiographic assessment of aortic insufficiency graded as $\geq$ +2)
4. Abnormalities of the aorta that would preclude surgery, including aneurysms and extreme tortuosity or calcifications
5. Renal failure (creatinine $\geq$ 4 mg/dL)
6. Liver dysfunction or markedly abnormal coagulation parameters (defined as platelet count $\leq$ 75,000/μL or international normalized ratio $\geq$ 2.0 or fibrinogen $\leq$ 1.50 g/L)
7. Recent (within 3 months) stroke or transient ischemic attack

Potential Complications

Meyns and colleagues[27] reported the loss of the sensor signal in 3 patients, which did not affect pump function. Displacement of the pump back into the aorta can also occur, but the addition of the pigtail catheter tip minimizes displacement potential. Similar to the TandemHeart, the percutaneous blood cannulas pose the inherent risk of infectious complications in the form of local infections, bacteremia, and sepsis. In a meta-analysis, hemolysis as measured by measurements of free hemoglobin was significantly higher and a trend toward higher rates of packed red blood cells and plasma transfusion was noted with use of Impella in comparison with IABP.[30]

THE REITAN CATHETER PUMP

The RCP is a novel, fully percutaneous circulatory support system (**Fig. 5A–E**) consisting of a catheter-mounted distal pump head with a foldable propeller and surrounding cage (an interface unit and an external drive unit with user console). The closed pump head is delivered through a 14F sheath via the femoral artery and positioned in the proximal descending aorta, distal to the left subclavian artery. In situ the cage is deployed and the propeller arms are extended and rotated. The pump creates a pressure gradient within the aorta, which has been demonstrated to reduce afterload and increase organ perfusion in animal studies.[31,32] The RCP does not require electrocardiography (ECG) synchronization and can be used in the presence of aortic regurgitation. In contrast to Impella, the RCP is not deployed within the LV cavity, and therefore, it is not contraindicated in the presence of LV thrombus.

Implantation

- Femoral arterial access is obtained initially using a 6F sheath, and angiography of the proximal descending aorta is performed to confirm a diameter of 22 mm or more to ensure safe deployment of the pump head.

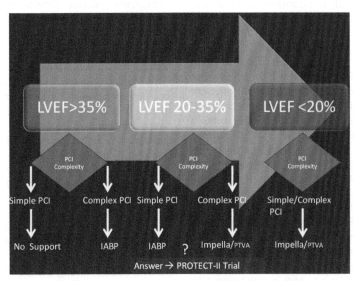

Fig. 6. Algorithm for device selection.

- Peripheral angiography is performed to exclude obstructive femoroiliac disease or severe tortuosity.
- As decribed for TandemHeart and Impella devices, 2 Perclose device sutures are inserted with the preclose technique before the introduction of a 30-cm 14F introducer sheath (Ultimum EV, St. Jude Medical, MN, USA; external diameter 5.5 mm).
- The sheath is advanced with a tapered dilator over a 0.38-in guidewire into the distal descending aorta.
- The dilator and wire are removed, and the collapsed pump head is delivered directly into the aorta. The device is positioned fluoroscopically 3 to 10 cm distal to the origin of the left subclavian artery, and the pump head is deployed.
- The propeller is rotated at 8000 to 13,000 rpm to maintain a target radial to femoral transaortic pressure gradient of 10 mm Hg. ACT is maintained at 250 to 300 seconds
- After pump removal, femoral hemostasis is achieved by deploying the 2 Perclose sutures inserted at the start of the procedure.

The RCP may offer more effective cardiac support than the IABP while being less invasive in comparison with Impella VR LP2.5, which requires positioning within the left ventricle, and the TandemHeart. The RCP and the IABP work in series with the heart, which means that the left ventricle ejects the total cardiac output through the aortic valve. The IABP modifies intra-aortic pressure to reduce afterload but requires ECG synchronization and has limited pump function itself. Because the RCP is a continuous nonphasic pump, it may be more effective than the IABP in the setting of atrial fibrillation or recurrent tachyarrhythmias. As a consequence of its folding propeller design, the pump can generate high flow rates up to 20 L/min at 12,000 rpm in vitro. In vivo, this high flow creates a pressure gradient inside the aorta thereby increasing the femoral pressure and reducing the radial pressure. In its present form, the pump itself has limitations related to the PCI procedure. First, the design of the pump head cage does not yet permit simultaneous cardiac catheterization from the femoral route, necessitating a radial PCI approach in all cases. Second, the pump head size currently necessitates a 14F sheath, which cannot be inserted in small, diseased, or tortuous femoral or iliac vessels. Incorporation of several design improvements has led to the development of a 10F compatible device, and a mechanism to provide transverse protection of the propeller to allow simultaneous femoral catheterization is being considered. In addition, conversion of the RCP to an over-the-wire technology is being developed, which may further reduce the risk of vascular complications. Prolonged cardiac support using the RCP is currently being investigated in the ongoing hemodynamic efficacy study of the device in patients with decompensated chronic left heart failure.

RECENT STUDIES AND RANDOMIZED TRIALS

Recent trials are summarized in **Table 3**.

PROTECT I

PROTECT I was a prospective multicenter feasibility study for Impella 2.5. Twenty patients underwent high-risk PCI circulatory support using the Impella 2.5 system.[33] All patients had poor LV function (ejection fraction ≤35%) and underwent PCI on an unprotected left main coronary artery or last patent coronary conduit. The primary safety end point was the incidence of MACE at 30 days. The primary efficacy end point was freedom from hemodynamic compromise during PCI (defined as a decrease in mean arterial pressure below 60 mm Hg for>10 minutes). The results showed that the Impella 2.5 device was implanted successfully in all patients. The mean duration of circulatory support was 1.7 ± 0.6 hours (range, 0.4–2.5 hours). Mean pump flow during PCI was 2.2 ± 0.3 L/min. At 30 days, the incidence of MACEs was 20%. There was no evidence of aortic valve injury, cardiac perforation, or limb ischemia. Two patients (10%) developed mild, transient hemolysis without clinical sequelae. This trial successfully demonstrated the safety and feasibility of Impella 2.5 during high-risk PCI.

ISAR-SHOCK

This study tested the feasibility and safety of using the Impella device in patients with cardiogenic shock caused by acute MI.[34] Twenty-six patients were randomized to Impella or an IABP. The primary end point was the change of the cardiac index (CI) from baseline to 30 minutes after implantation. Secondary end points were lactic acidosis, hemolysis, and mortality at 30 days. The results showed that the CI after 30 minutes of support was significantly increased in patients with the Impella compared with patients with an IABP (increase in CI of 0.49 vs 0.11 L/min/m²). There was no difference in 30-day mortality (46% in both groups). Among the survivors, there was no difference in the LV ejection fraction at discharge

(35% ± 17% in the Impella group vs 45% ± 17% in the IABP group, P = .34). The results suggested that Impella can be used safely in patients with cardiogenic shock and that it is associated with an improved cardiac output compared with an IABP, without any evident difference in clinical outcome.

IMPRESS in STEMI

IMPRESS is a multicenter, randomized trial of the Impella Recover LP2.5 (LV assist) device versus IABP therapy for patients with large anterior acute STEMI who are treated with primary PCI. The primary objective of this study is to determine whether treatment with Impella compared with IABP therapy after primary PCI reduces infarct size and results in a higher residual LV ejection fraction in acute anterior wall MI treated by PCI.

PROTECT II

PROTECT II is a prospective, randomized multicenter trial comparing IABP with Impella 2.5 in the setting of nonemergent high-risk PCI. The primary end point is 30-day MACE, composite rate of intraprocedural and postprocedural major events. Secondary end point is maximum cardiac power output decrease from baseline.

RECOVER II

RECOVER II is a prospective, randomized multicenter trial comparing IABP with Impella 2.5 in the setting of acute MI and hemodynamic instability. The primary end point is 30-day MACE, composite rate of intraprocedural and postprocedural major events. Secondary end point is maximum cardiac power output decrease from baseline.

Fig. 6 depicts the institutional algorithm to help in the selection of appropriate circulatory support device. The results of several important ongoing trials are expected to delineate a simplified approach toward percutaneous circulatory support.

SUMMARY

Several new-generation percutaneous support devices are available or are in different stages of development for use in high-risk PCI, cardiogenic shock, and for other indications. Preliminary studies have demonstrated the feasibility and safety of these devices and their beneficial effect on hemodynamic parameters. However, no effect on the 30-day mortality and other MACEs has been observed in the limited studies till now. Ongoing studies are expected to provide answers to these important questions. The use may grow substantially, if ongoing trials, such as PROTECT II, show survival benefit over IABP. Technologic advances in design and device profile are expected to embellish the armamentarium of an interventionalist and allow complex and high-risk PCI cases to be performed with greater success with the use of these LVADs.

REFERENCES

1. Ellis SG, Tamai H, Nobuyoshi M, et al. Contemporary percutaneous treatment of unprotected left main coronary stenoses: initial results from a multicenter registry analysis 1994–1996. Circulation 1997; 96(11):3867–72.
2. Kosuga K, Tamai H, Ueda K, et al. Initial and long-term results of angioplasty in unprotected left main coronary artery. Am J Cardiol 1999;83(1):32–7.
3. Valgimigli M, Malagutti P, Aoki J, et al. Sirolimus-eluting versus paclitaxel-eluting stent implantation for the percutaneous treatment of left main coronary artery disease: a combined RESEARCH and T-SEARCH long-term analysis. J Am Coll Cardiol 2006;47(3):507–14.
4. Kar B, Adkins LE, Civitello AB, et al. Clinical experience with the TandemHeart percutaneous ventricular assist device. Tex Heart Inst J 2006;33(2): 111–5.
5. Kar B, Butkevich A, Civitello AB, et al. Hemodynamic support with a percutaneous left ventricular assist device during stenting of an unprotected left main coronary artery. Tex Heart Inst J 2004;31(1):84–6.
6. Hamon M, Rasmussen LH, Manoukian SV, et al. Choice of arterial access site and outcomes in patients with acute coronary syndromes managed with an early invasive strategy: the ACUITY trial. EuroIntervention 2009;5(1):115–20.
7. Mehran R, Lansky AJ, Witzenbichler B, et al. Bivalirudin in patients undergoing primary angioplasty for acute myocardial infarction (HORIZONS-AMI): 1-year results of a randomised controlled trial. Lancet 2009 [Epub ahead of print].
8. Babaev A, Frederick PD, Pasta DJ, et al. Trends in management and outcomes of patients with acute myocardial infarction complicated by cardiogenic shock. JAMA 2005;294(4):448–54.
9. Laschinger JC, Cunningham JN Jr, Catinella FP, et al. 'Pulsatile' left atrial-femoral artery bypass. A new method of preventing extension of myocardial infarction. Arch Surg 1983;118(8):965–9.
10. Laschinger JC, Grossi EA, Cunningham JN Jr, et al. Adjunctive left ventricular unloading during myocardial reperfusion plays a major role in minimizing myocardial infarct size. J Thorac Cardiovasc Surg 1985;90(1):80–5.
11. Catinella FP, Cunningham JN Jr, Glassman E, et al. Left atrium-to-femoral artery bypass: effectiveness

in reduction of acute experimental myocardial infarction. J Thorac Cardiovasc Surg 1983;86(6):887–96.

12. Chen JM, DeRose JJ, Slater JP, et al. Improved survival rates support left ventricular assist device implantation early after myocardial infarction. J Am Coll Cardiol 1999;33(7):1903–8.

13. Vogel RA, Shawl F, Tommaso C, et al. Initial report of the National Registry of Elective Cardiopulmonary Bypass Supported Coronary Angioplasty. J Am Coll Cardiol 1990;15(1):23–9.

14. Shawl FA, Domanski MJ, Wish MH, et al. Percutaneous cardiopulmonary bypass support in the catheterization laboratory: technique and complications. Am Heart J 1990;120(1):195–203.

15. Scholz KH, Dubois-Rande JL, Urban P, et al. Clinical experience with the percutaneous hemopump during high-risk coronary angioplasty. Am J Cardiol 1998;82(9):1107–10, A6.

16. Scholz KH, Tebbe U, Chemnitius M, et al. Transfemoral placement of the left ventricular assist device "Hemopump" during mechanical resuscitation. Thorac Cardiovasc Surg 1990;38(2):69–72.

17. Kantrowitz A, Tjonneland S, Freed PS, et al. Initial clinical experience with intraaortic balloon pumping in cardiogenic shock. JAMA 1968;203(2):113–8.

18. Cohen M, Urban P, Christenson JT, et al. Intra-aortic balloon counterpulsation in US and non-US centres: results of the Benchmark Registry. Eur Heart J 2003; 24(19):1763–70.

19. Moulopoulos SD, Kwan-Gett CS, Collan R, et al. Intra-aortic balloon pumping. Effect in sheep with a ligated coronary artery. Minn Med 1970;53(3):261–5.

20. Nanas JN, Nanas SN, Charitos CE, et al. Hemodynamic effects of a counterpulsation device implanted on the ascending aorta in severe cardiogenic shock. ASAIO Trans 1988;34(3): 229–34.

21. Sjauw KD, Engström AE, Vis MM, et al. A systematic review and meta-analysis of intra-aortic balloon pump therapy in ST-elevation myocardial infarction: should we change the guidelines? Eur Heart J 2009;30(4):459–68.

22. Thiele H, Lauer B, Hambrecht R, et al. Reversal of cardiogenic shock by percutaneous left atrial-to-femoral arterial bypass assistance. Circulation 2001;104(24):2917–22.

23. Fonger JD, Zhou Y, Matsuura H, et al. Enhanced preservation of acutely ischemic myocardium with transseptal left ventricular assist. Ann Thorac Surg 1994;57(3):570–5.

24. Rajdev S, Krishnan P, Irani A, et al. Clinical application of prophylactic percutaneous left ventricular assist device (TandemHeart) in high-risk percutaneous coronary intervention using an arterial preclosure technique: single-center experience. J Invasive Cardiol 2008;20(2):67–72.

25. Rajdev S, Benza R, Misra V, et al. Use of TandemHeart as a temporary hemodynamic support option for severe pulmonary artery hypertension complicated by cardiogenic shock. J Invasive Cardiol 2007; 19(8):E226–9.

26. Meyns B, Stolinski J, Leunens V, et al. Left ventricular support by catheter-mounted axial flow pump reduces infarct size. J Am Coll Cardiol 2003;41(7): 1087–95.

27. Meyns B, Dens J, Sergeant P, et al. Initial experiences with the Impella device in patients with cardiogenic shock—Impella support for cardiogenic shock. Thorac Cardiovasc Surg 2003;51(6):312–7.

28. Reesink KD, Dekker AL, Van Ommen V, et al. Miniature intracardiac assist device provides more effective cardiac unloading and circulatory support during severe left heart failure than intraaortic balloon pumping. Chest 2004;126(3):896–902.

29. Valgimigli M, Steendijk P, Sianos G, et al. Left ventricular unloading and concomitant total cardiac output increase by the use of percutaneous Impella Recover LP 2.5 assist device during high-risk coronary intervention. Catheter Cardiovasc Interv 2005; 65(2):263–7.

30. Cheng JM, den Uil CA, Hoeks SE, et al. Percutaneous left ventricular assist devices vs. intra-aortic balloon pump counterpulsation for treatment of cardiogenic shock: a meta-analysis of controlled trials. Eur Heart J 2009;30(17):2102–8.

31. Reitan O, Ohlin H, Peterzén B, et al. Initial tests with a new cardiac assist device. ASAIO J 1999;45(4): 317–21.

32. Reitan O, Steen S, Ohlin H. Hemodynamic effects of a new percutaneous circulatory support device in a left ventricular failure model. ASAIO J 2003; 49(6):731–6.

33. Dixon SR, Henriques JP, Mauri L, et al. A prospective feasibility trial investigating the use of the Impella 2.5 system in patients undergoing high-risk percutaneous coronary intervention (The PROTECT I Trial): initial U.S. experience. JACC Cardiovasc Interv 2009;2(2):91–6.

34. Seyfarth M, Sibbing D, Bauer I, et al. A randomized clinical trial to evaluate the safety and efficacy of a percutaneous left ventricular assist device versus intra-aortic balloon pumping for treatment of cardiogenic shock caused by myocardial infarction. J Am Coll Cardiol 2008;52(19):1584–8.

Index

Note: Page numbers of article titles are in **boldface** type.

Cardiol Clin 28 (2010) 185–189
doi:10.1016/S0733-8651(09)00124-6

cardiology.theclinics.com

Moving?

Make sure your subscription moves with you!

To notify us of your new address, find your **Clinics Account Number** (located on your mailing label above your name), and contact customer service at:

Email: journalscustomerservice-usa@elsevier.com

800-654-2452 (subscribers in the U.S. & Canada)
314-447-8871 (subscribers outside of the U.S. & Canada)

Fax number: 314-447-8029

Elsevier Health Sciences Division
Subscription Customer Service
3251 Riverport Lane
Maryland Heights, MO 63043

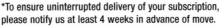
*To ensure uninterrupted delivery of your subscription, please notify us at least 4 weeks in advance of move.

ELSEVIER